W9-DFC-866

UNDERSTANDING HEALTH POLICY
A Clinical Approach

EIGHTH EDITION

Thomas Bodenheimer, MD
Professor Emeritus
Department of Family & Community Medicine
University of California, San Francisco

Kevin Grumbach, MD
Professor and Chair
Department of Family & Community Medicine
University of California, San Francisco

Mc Graw Hill

New York   Chicago   San Francisco   Athens   London   Madrid   Mexico City
New Delhi   Milan   Singapore   Sydney   Toronto

Understanding Health Policy: A Clinical Approach, Eighth Edition

1 2 3 4 5 6 7 8 9 LCR 25 24 23 22 21 20

ISBN 978-1-260-45426-0
MHID 1-260-45426-6
ISSN 1080-9465

Notice

Medicine is an ever-changing science. As new research and clinical experience broaden our knowledge, changes in treatment and drug therapy are required. The authors and the publisher of this work have checked with sources believed to be reliable in their efforts to provide information that is complete and generally in accord with the standards accepted at the time of publication. However, in view of the possibility of human error or changes in medical sciences, neither the authors nor the publisher nor any other party who has been involved in the preparation or publication of this work warrants that the information contained herein is in every respect accurate or complete, and they disclaim all responsibility for any errors or omissions or for the results obtained from use of the information contained in this work. Readers are encouraged to confirm the information contained herein with other sources. For example, and in particular, readers are advised to check the product information sheet included in the package of each drug they plan to administer to be certain that the information contained in this work is accurate and that changes have not been made in the recommended dose or in the contraindications for administration. This recommendation is of particular importance in connection with new or infrequently used drugs.

This book was set in Minion Pro by MPS Limited.
The editors were Kay Conerly and Kim J. Davis.
The production supervisor was Catherine Saggese.
Project management was provided by Poonam Bisht, MPS Limited.

This book is printed on acid-free paper.

Contents

Preface

Understanding Health Policy: A Clinical Approach is a book about health policy as well as individual patients and caregivers and how they interact with each other and with the overall health system. We, the authors, are practicing primary care physicians—one in a public hospital and clinic and the other, for many years, in a private practice. We are also analysts of our nation's health care system. In one sense, these two sides of our lives seem quite separate. When treating a patient's illness, health expenditures as a percentage of gross domestic product or variations in surgical rates between one city and another seem remote if not irrelevant—but they are neither remote nor irrelevant. Health policy affects the patients we see on a daily basis. Managed care referral patterns determine to which specialist we can send a patient; the coverage gaps for outpatient medications in the Medicare benefit package affects how we prescribe medications for our elderly patients; and differences in access to care between families on Medicaid and those with private coverage influences which patients end up seeing one of us in the private sector over the other in a public hospital. In *Understanding Health Policy*, we hope to bridge the gap separating the microworld of individual patient visits and the macrouniverse of health policy.

THE AUDIENCE

The book is primarily written for health science students—medical, nursing, nurse practitioner, physician assistant, pharmacy, social work, public health, and others—who will benefit from understanding the complex environment in which they will work. Physicians feature prominently in the text, but in the actual world of clinical medicine, patients' encounters with other health care givers are an essential part of their health care experience. Physicians would be unable to function without the many other members of the health care team. Patients seldom appreciate the contributions made to their well-being by public health personnel, research scientists, educators, and many other health-related professionals. We hope that the many nonphysician members of the clinical care, public health, and health science education teams as well as students aspiring to join these teams will find the book useful. Nothing can be accomplished without the combined efforts of everyone working in the health care field.

THE GOAL OF THE BOOK

Understanding Health Policy attempts to explain how the health care system works. We focus on basic principles of health policy in hopes that the reader will come away with a clearer, more systematic way of thinking about health care in the United States, its problems, and the alternatives for managing these problems. Most of the principles also apply to understanding health care systems in other nations.

Given the public's intense concerns about health care in the United States, we call out the failings as well as the successes of the US approach to financing and organizing care. Only by recognizing the difficulties of the system can we begin to fix its problems. The goal of this book, then, is to help all of us understand the health care system so that we can better work in the system and change what needs to be changed.

CLINICAL VIGNETTES

In our attempt to unify the overlapping spheres of health policy and health care encounters by individuals, we use clinical vignettes as a central feature of the book. These short descriptions of patients, physicians, and other caregivers interacting with the health care system are based on our own experiences as physicians, the experiences of colleagues, or cases reported in the medical literature or popular press. Most of the people and institutions presented in the vignettes have been given fictitious names to protect privacy. Some names used are emblematic of the occupations, health problems, or attitudes portrayed in the vignettes; most do not have special significance.

OUR OPINIONS

In exploring the many controversial issues of health policy, our own opinions as authors inevitably color and shade the words we use and the conclusions we reach. We present several of our most fundamental values and perspectives here.

THE RIGHT TO HEALTH CARE

We believe that health care should be a right enjoyed equally by everyone. Certain things in life are considered essential. No one gets excited if someone is turned away from a movie or concert because he or she cannot afford a ticket. But sick people who are turned away from a medical practice can make headlines, and rightly so. A simple statement of the right to health care reads something like this: All people should have equal access to a reasonable level of appropriate health services, regardless of ability to pay.

In 2009, the United States entered into a fierce debate over whether health care should be a right. The debate focused on President Barack Obama's campaign to enact universal health insurance. Following a year of public ferment, Congress passed the Affordable Care Act, which moves in the direction of guaranteeing health care as a right. Yet, at the time of writing this edition of *Understanding Health Policy*, the controversy continues.

THE IMPERATIVE TO CONTAIN COSTS

We believe that limits must be placed on the costs of health care. Cost controls can be imposed in a manner that does relatively little harm to the health of the public. The rapidly rising costs of health care are in part created by scientific advances that spawn new, expensive technologies. Some of these technologies truly improve health, some are of little value or harmful, and others are of benefit to some patients but are inappropriately used for patients whom they do not benefit. Eliminating medical services that produce no benefit is one path to "painless" cost control (see Chapter 8).

Reduction in the rapidly rising cost of administering the health care system is another route to painless cost containment. Administrative excess wastes money that could be spent for useful purposes, either within or outside the health care sector. While large bureaucracies do have the advantage of creating jobs, the nation and the health care system have a great need for more socially rewarding and productive jobs (e.g., home health aides, drug rehabilitation counselors, childcare workers, and many more) that could be financed from funds currently used for needless administrative tasks.

There is a growing consensus that health care cost increases are bad for the economy. Employers complain that the high cost of health insurance for employees reduces international competitiveness. If government health expenditures continue their rapid rise, other publicly financed programs essential to the nation's economy (e.g., education and transportation) will be curtailed and the unsustainable government budget deficits will strain the future of the nation's well-being.

Rising costs are harmful to everyone because they make health services and health insurance unaffordable. Many companies are shifting more health care costs onto their employees. As government health budgets balloon, cutbacks are inevitable, generally hurting the elderly and the poor. Individuals with no health insurance or inadequate coverage have a far harder time paying for care as costs go up. As a general rule, when costs go up, access goes down.

For these reasons, we believe that health care costs should be contained, using strategies that do the least harm to the health of the population.

THE NEED FOR POPULATION-BASED MEDICINE

Most physicians, nurses, and other health professionals are trained to provide clinical care to individuals. Yet clinical care is not the only determinant of health status; standard of living and public health measures have an even greater influence on the health of a population (see Chapter 3). Health care, then, should have another dimension: concern for the population as a whole. Individual physicians may be first-rate in caring for their patients' heart attacks, but may not worry enough about the prevalence of hypertension, smoking, elevated cholesterol levels, uncontrolled diabetes, and lack of exercise in their city, in their neighborhood, or among the group of patients enrolled in their practices. For years, clinical medicine has divorced itself from the public health community, which does concern itself with the health of the population. We believe that health caregivers should be trained to add a population orientation to their current role of caring for individuals.

ACKNOWLEDGMENTS

We could not have written this book by ourselves. The circumstances encountered by hundreds of our patients and dozens of our colleagues provided the insights we needed to understand and describe the health care system. Any inaccuracies in the book are entirely our responsibility. Our warmest thanks go to our families, who have provided both encouragement and patience.

Earlier versions of Chapters 2, 4, 5, 8, 9, and 16 were published serially as articles in the *Journal of the American Medical Association* (1994;272:634–639, 1994;272:971–977, 1994;272:1458–1464, 1995;273:160–167, 1995;274:85–90, and 1996;276:1025–1031) and are published here with permission (copyright, 1994, 1995, and 1996, American Medical Association).

CONCLUSION

This is a book about health policy. As such, we will cite technical studies and will make cross-national generalizations. We will take matters of profound personal meaning—sickness, health, caring for individuals in need—and discuss them using the detached language of "inputs and outcomes," "providers and consumers," and "cost-effectiveness analysis." As practicing physicians, however, we are daily reminded of the human realities of health policy. *Understanding Health Policy: A Clinical Approach* is fundamentally about the people we care for: the under-insured janitor with high-deductible insurance enduring the pain of a gallbladder attack because surgery might be unaffordable, or the retired university professor who sustains a stroke and whose life savings are disappearing in nursing home bills uncovered by her Medicare or private insurance plans.

Almost every person, whether a mother on public assistance, a working father, a well-to-do physician, or a millionaire insurance executive, will someday become ill, and all of us will die. Everyone stands to benefit from a system in which health care for all people is accessible, affordable, appropriate in its use of resources, and of high quality.

Thomas Bodenheimer
Kevin Grumbach
San Francisco, California

Introduction: The Paradox of Excess and Deprivation

Louise Brown was an accountant with a 25-year history of diabetes. Her physician taught her to monitor her glucose at home, and her health coach helped her follow a diabetic diet. Her diabetes was brought under good control. Diabetic retinopathy was discovered at yearly eye examinations, and periodic laser treatments of her retina prevented loss of vision. Ms. Brown lived to the age of 92, a success story of the US health care system.

Angela Martini grew up in an inner-city housing project, never had a chance for a good education, became pregnant as a teenager, and has been on public assistance while caring for her four children. Her Medicaid coverage allows her to see her family physician for yearly preventive care visits. A mammogram ordered by her family physician detected a suspicious lesion, which was found to be cancer on biopsy. She was referred to a surgical breast specialist, underwent a mastectomy, was treated with a hormonal medication, and has been healthy for the past 15 years.

For people with private or public insurance who have access to health care services, the melding of high-quality primary and preventive care with appropriate specialty treatment can produce the best medical care in the world. The United States is blessed with thousands of well-trained physicians, nurses, pharmacists, and other health caregivers who compassionately provide up-to-date medical attention to patients who seek their assistance. This is the face of the health care system in which we can take pride. Success stories,

however, are only part of the reality of health care in the United States.

EXCESS AND DEPRIVATION

The health care system in the United States has been called "a paradox of excess and deprivation" (Enthoven & Kronick, 1989). Some persons receive too little care because they are uninsured, inadequately insured, or have Medicaid coverage that many physicians will not accept.

James Jackson was unemployed for more than a year but unable to qualify for Medicaid because his state did not expand Medicaid under the 2010 Patient Protection and Affordable Care Act. At age 34, he developed abdominal pain but did not seek care for 10 days because he had no insurance and feared the cost of treatment. He began to vomit, became weak, and was finally taken to an emergency room by his cousin. The physician diagnosed a perforated ulcer with peritonitis and septic shock. The illness had gone on too long; Mr. Jackson died on the operating table. Had he received prompt medical attention, his illness would likely have been cured.

Betty Yee was a 68-year-old woman with angina, high blood pressure, and diabetes. Her total bill for medications, which were only partly covered under her Medicare plan, came to $200 per month. She was unable to afford the medications, her blood pressure went out of control, and she suffered a stroke. Ms. Yee's final lonely years were spent in a nursing home; she was paralyzed on her right side and unable to speak.

Mary McCarthy became pregnant but could not find an obstetrician who would accept her Medicaid card. After 7 months, she began to experience severe headaches, went to the emergency room, and was found to have hypertension and preeclampsia. She delivered a stillborn baby.

While some people cannot access the care they need, others receive too much care that is costly and may be harmful.

At age 66, Daniel Taylor noticed that he was getting up to urinate twice each night. It did not bother him much. His family physician sent him to a urologist, who found that his prostate was enlarged (though with no signs of cancer) and recommended surgery. Mr. Taylor did not want surgery. He had a friend with the same symptoms whose urologist had said that surgery was not needed. Since Mr. Taylor never questioned doctors, he went ahead with the procedure anyway. After the surgery, he became incontinent of urine.

Consuelo Gonzalez had a moderate pain in her back which was relieved by over-the-counter acetaminophen. She went to an orthopedist who ordered an MRI, which showed a small disc protrusion. The doctor recommended surgery, after which Ms. Gonzalez' pain became much worse. She consulted a general internist who told her that the MRI abnormality was not serious, that the surgery had been unnecessary, and that physical therapy might help. After a year of physical therapy, the pain subsided back to its original level.

▶ Too Little Care

In 2018, 4 years after the Affordable Care Act was fully implemented, 27.5 million people in the United States remained without health insurance (US Census Bureau, 2019). In addition, many people with health insurance have inadequate coverage. In 2016, 33% of American adults reported having trouble affording health care (Osborn et al., 2016).

▶ Too Much Care

According to health services expert Robert Brook:

. . . almost every study that has seriously looked for overuse has discovered it, and virtually every time at least double-digit overuse has been found. If one could extrapolate from the available literature, then perhaps one-fourth of hospital days, one-fourth of procedures, and two-fifths of medications could be done without. (Brook, 1989)

A 2003 study found that elderly patients in some areas of the country receive 60% more services—hospital days, specialty consultations, and medical procedures—than similar patients in other areas; the patients receiving fewer services had the same mortality rates, quality of care, access to care, and patient satisfaction as those receiving more services (Fisher et al., 2003a, 2003b). In 2012, waste in health care was estimated at between $558 and $910 billion per year—from 21% to 34% of total health care expenditures (Berwick & Hackbarth, 2012).

THE PUBLIC'S VIEW OF THE HEALTH CARE SYSTEM

Health care in the United States encompasses a wide spectrum, ranging from the highest-quality, most compassionate treatment of those with complex illnesses, to the turning away of the very ill because of lack of ability to pay; from well-designed protocols for prevention of illness to inappropriate high-risk surgical procedures performed on uninformed patients. While the past decades have been witness to major upheavals in health care, one fundamental truth remains: the United States has the least universal, most costly health care system in the industrialized world (Osborn et al., 2016).

Many people view the high costs of care and the lack of universal access as indicators of serious failings in the health care system. In 2017, 73% of people in the United States believed that the system is working poorly (Pearl, 2018).

UNDERSTANDING THE CRISIS

In order to correct the weaknesses of the health care system while maintaining its strengths, it is necessary to understand how the system works. How is health care financed? What are the causes and consequences of incomplete access to care? How are physicians paid, and what is the effect of their mode of reimbursement on health care costs? How are health care services organized and quality of care enhanced? Is sufficient attention paid to the prevention of illness, and what are different strategies for preventing illness?

How can the problems of health care be solved? Did the Affordable Care Act enacted in 2010 provide the answer? Can costs be controlled in a manner that does not reduce access? Can access be expanded in a manner that does not increase costs? How have other nations done it—or attempted to do it? How might the health care system in the United States change in the future?

REFERENCES

Berwick DM, Hackbarth AD. Eliminating waste in US health care. *JAMA*. 2012;307:1513–1516.

Brook RH. Practice guidelines and practicing medicine. *JAMA*. 1989;262:3027–3030.

Enthoven A, Kronick R. A consumer-choice health plan for the 1990s. *N Engl J Med*. 1989;320:29–37.

Fisher ES, et al. The implications of regional variations in Medicare spending. Part 1: the content, quality, and accessibility of care. *Ann Intern Med*. 2003a;138:273–287.

Fisher ES, et al. The implications of regional variations in Medicare spending. Part 2: health outcomes and satisfaction with care. *Ann Intern Med*. 2003b;138:288–298.

Osborn R, et al. In new survey of 11 countries, US adults still struggle with access to and affordability of health care. *Health Affairs*. 2016;35:2327–2336.

Pearl R. 7 surveys that say a lot about US healthcare. *Forbes*. June 5, 2018.

US Census Bureau. Health insurance coverage in the United States: 2018. Report number P60-267. September 2019. www.census.gov/library/publications/2019/demo/p60-267.html.

Paying for Health Care

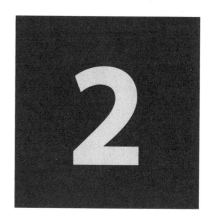

Health care is not free. Someone must pay. But how? Does each person pay when receiving care? Do people contribute regular amounts in advance so that their care will be paid for when they need it? When a person contributes in advance, might the contribution be used for care given to someone else? If so, who should pay how much?

Health care financing in the United States evolved to its current state through a series of social interventions. Each intervention solved a problem but in turn created its own problems requiring further intervention. This chapter will discuss the historical process of the evolution of health care financing. The enactment in 2010 of the Patient Protection and Affordable Care Act, commonly referred to as the Affordable Care Act, ACA, or "Obamacare," created major changes in the financing of health care in the United States.

MODES OF PAYING FOR HEALTH CARE

The four basic modes of paying for health care are out-of-pocket payment, individual private insurance, employment-based group private insurance, and government financing (Table 2–1). These four modes can be viewed both as a historical progression and as a categorization of current health care financing.

▶ Out-of-Pocket Payments

Fred Farmer broke his leg in 1913. His son ran 4 miles to get the doctor, who came to the farm to splint the leg. Fred gave the doctor a couple of chickens to pay for the visit. His great-grandson, Ted, *who was uninsured, broke his leg in 2013. He was driven to the emergency room, where the physician ordered an x-ray and called in an orthopedist who placed a cast on the leg. The cost was $8,800.*

One hundred years ago, people like Fred Farmer paid physicians and other health care practitioners in cash or through barter. In the first half of the twentieth century, out-of-pocket cash payment was the most common method of payment. This is the simplest mode of financing—direct purchase by the consumer of goods and services (Fig. 2–1).

People in the United States purchase most consumer items and services, from gourmet restaurant dinners to haircuts, through direct out-of-pocket payments. This is not the case with health care (Arrow, 1963; Evans, 1984), and one may ask why health care is not considered a typical consumer item.

Need Versus Luxury

Whereas a gourmet dinner is a luxury, health care is regarded as a basic human need by most people.

For 2 weeks, Marina Perez has had vaginal bleeding and has felt dizzy. She has no insurance and is terrified that medical care might eat up her $500 in savings. She scrapes together $100 to see her doctor, who finds that her blood pressure falls to 90/50 mm Hg upon standing and that her hematocrit is 26%. The doctor calls Marina's sister Juanita to drive her to the hospital. Marina gets into the car and tells Juanita to take her home.

Table 2–1. Health care financing in 2017[a]

Type of Payment	Percentage of National Health Expenditures, 2017
Out-of-pocket payment	11%
Individual private insurance	6%
Employment-based private insurance	30%[b]
Government financing	43%
Other	10%
Total	100%
Principal Source of Coverage	**Percentage of Population, 2017**
Uninsured	9%
Individual private insurance	9%
Employment-based private insurance	46%
Government financing	36%
Total	100%

Sources: Data extracted from U.S. Census Bureau: *Health Insurance Coverage* in the United States, 2017, September 2018. https://www.census.gov/library/publications/2018/demo/p60-264.html; Claxton G et al. Health benefits in 2018: modest growth in premiums, higher worker contributions at firms with more low-wage workers. *Health Aff (Millwood)*. 2018;37:1892–1900; Martin AB et al. National health spending in 2017. *Health Affairs*. 2019;38:96–106.
[a]Because private insurance tends to cover healthier people, the percentage of expenditures is less than the percentage of population covered. Public expenditures are higher per population because the elderly and disabled are concentrated in the public Medicare and Medicaid programs.
[b]This includes private insurance obtained by federal, state, and local employees which is in part purchased by tax funds.

If health care is a basic human right, then people who are unable to afford health care must have a payment mechanism available that is not reliant on out-of-pocket payments.

Unpredictability of Need and Cost

Whereas the purchase of a gourmet meal is a matter of choice and the price is shown to the buyer, the need for and cost of health care services are unpredictable. Most people do not know if or when they may become severely ill or injured or what the cost of care will be.

> Jake has a headache and visits the doctor, but he does not know whether the headache will cost $100 for a physician visit plus the price of a bottle of ibuprofen, $1,200 for an MRI, or $500,000 for surgery and irradiation for brain cancer.

The unpredictability of many health care needs makes it difficult to plan for these expenses. The medical costs associated with serious illness or injury usually exceed a middle-class family's savings.

Patients Need to Rely on Physician Recommendations

Unlike the purchaser of a gourmet meal, a person in need of health care may have little knowledge of what he or she is buying at the time when care is needed.

> Jenny develops acute abdominal pain and goes to the hospital to purchase a remedy for her pain. The physician tells her that she has acute cholecystitis or a perforated ulcer and recommends hospitalization, an abdominal CT scan, and

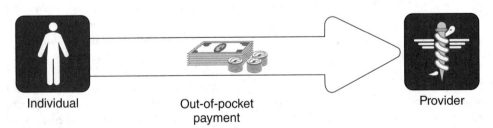

Individual   Out-of-pocket payment   Provider

▲ **Figure 2–1.** Out-of-pocket payment is made directly from patient to provider.

upper endoscopic studies. Will Jenny, lying on a gurney in the emergency room and clutching her abdomen with one hand, use her other hand to leaf through a textbook of internal medicine to determine whether she really needs these services, and should she have brought along a copy of Consumer Reports to learn where to purchase them at the cheapest price?

Health care is the foremost example of asymmetry of information between providers and consumers (Evans, 1984). A patient with abdominal pain is in a poor position to question a physician who is ordering laboratory tests, x-rays, or surgery. When health care is elective, patients can weigh the pros and cons of different treatment options, but even so, recommendations may be filtered through the biases of the physician providing the information. Compared with the voluntary demand for gourmet meals, the demand for health services is partially involuntary and is often physician rather than consumer-driven.

For these reasons among others, out-of-pocket payments are flawed as a dominant method of paying for health care services. Because the direct purchase of health services became increasingly difficult for consumers and was not meeting the needs of hospitals and physicians to be reliably paid, health insurance came into being.

▶ Individual Private Insurance

In 2012, Bud Carpenter was self-employed. To pay the $800 monthly premium for his individual health insurance policy, he had to work extra jobs on weekends, and the $5,000 deductible

meant he would still have to pay quite a bit of his family's medical costs out of pocket. Mr. Carpenter preferred to pay these costs rather than take the risk of spending the money saved for his children's college education on a major illness. When he became ill with leukemia and the hospital bill reached $80,000, Mr. Carpenter appreciated the value of health insurance. Nonetheless he had to feel disgruntled when he read a newspaper story listing his insurance company among those that paid out on average less than 60 cents for health services for every dollar collected in premiums.

With private health insurance, a third party, the insurer, is added to the patient and health care provider, who are the two basic parties of the health care transaction. While the out-of-pocket mode of payment is limited to a single financial transaction, private insurance requires two transactions—a premium payment from the individual to an insurance plan (also called a health plan), and a payment from the insurance plan to the provider (Fig. 2–2). Most insurance plans require patients to pay the first portion of their health expenses each year before the insurance coverage kicks in; these deductibles may be on the order of $2,000 or more per year. In addition, insurance plans often require patients to pay part of the cost of each service as coinsurance (e.g., patients pay 20% of the cost of a physician visit), or copayment (e.g., patients pay $20 for each prescription filled).

In nineteenth-century Europe, voluntary benefit funds were set up by guilds, industries, and mutual societies. In return for paying a monthly sum, people received assistance in case of illness. This early form

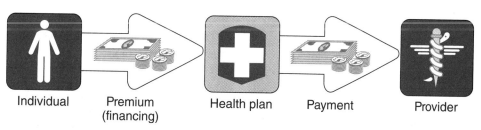

▲ Figure 2–2. Individual private insurance. A third party, the insurance plan (health plan), is added, dividing payment into a financing component and a payment component. The ACA added an individual coverage mandate for those not otherwise insured and federal subsidy to help individuals pay the insurance premium.

of private health insurance was slow to develop in the United States. In the early twentieth century, European immigrants set up some small benevolent societies in US cities to provide sickness benefits for their members. During the same period, two commercial insurance companies, Metropolitan Life and Prudential, collected 10 to 25 cents per week from workers for life insurance policies that also paid for funerals and the expenses of a final illness. The policies were paid for by individuals on a weekly basis, so large numbers of insurance agents had to visit their clients to collect the premiums as soon after payday as possible. Because of the huge administrative costs, individual health insurance never became a dominant method of paying for health care (Starr, 1982).

In 2014, Bud Carpenter signed up for individual insurance for his family of four through Covered California, the state exchange set up under the Affordable Care Act. Because his family income was 200% of the federal poverty level, he received a subsidy of $1,373 per month, meaning that his premium would be only $252 per month for a silver plan with Kaiser Permanente. His deductible was $2,000. Insurance companies were no longer allowed to deny coverage for his preexisting leukemia.

The Affordable Care Act (ACA) provides federal subsidies, like the one Bud Carpenter enjoyed, for individuals and families to obtain individual private health insurance through federal or state health insurance exchanges. Subsidies are available for individuals and families with incomes between 100% and 400% of the federal poverty level ($25,750 to $103,000 for a family of four) (see Table 2–2). The ACA initially required US citizens and legal residents to have insurance coverage meeting a federally determined "essential benefits" standard. Those who failed to purchase insurance and did not have employer-sponsored insurance, or did not qualify for Medicaid, Medicare, or veteran's health care benefits, had to pay a tax penalty. In 2017, the tax penalty was repealed. The ACA established federal and state-based insurance exchanges to assist people seeking individual coverage to shop for insurance plans meeting the federal standards. Insurance companies are no longer able to deny coverage for medical conditions that

Table 2–2. Summary of the individual health insurance provisions of the Affordable Care Act (ACA), 2019

As enacted in 2010, US citizens and legal residents were required to have health coverage with exemptions available for such issues as financial hardship. Those who chose to go without coverage paid a tax penalty. In 2017, the tax penalty was reduced to $0, essentially eliminating the original individual mandate (the requirement that people without health insurance purchase an individual insurance plan). As of 2019, other provisions of the ACA regarding purchase of individual insurance had not changed.

Tax credits to help pay health insurance premiums increase in size as family incomes rise from 100% to 400% of the Federal Poverty Level. In addition cost-sharing subsidies reduce the amount of out-of-pocket costs individuals and families must pay; the amount of the subsidy varies by income.

Uninsured individuals and families purchase individual insurance though insurance marketplaces called health insurance exchanges. Fifteen states have elected to set up their own exchanges; other states have state-federal partnership exchanges, and the remainder of states are covered by the federal exchange, Healthcare.gov.

Insurance companies marketing their plans through the exchanges offer four benefit categories:

- Bronze plans represent minimum coverage, with the insurer paying for 60% of a person's health care costs, with high out-of-pocket costs but low premiums
- Silver plans cover 70% of health care costs, with fewer out-of-pocket costs and higher premiums
- Gold plans cover 80% of costs, with low out-of-pocket costs and high premiums
- Platinum plans cover 90% of costs, with very low out-of-pocket costs and very high premiums

Most people who have obtained insurance through the exchanges have picked Bronze or Silver plans, and 87% have received a subsidy. A family of four with income of $40,000 receives an average 2019 subsidy of $16,000 that pays for most of a Silver plan premium of $18,000.

Source: Kaiser Family Foundation. Explaining health care reform: questions about health insurance subsidies. Issue brief. November 2018. https://www.kff.org/health-reform/issue-brief/explaining-health-care-reform-questions. Accessed September 19, 2019.

existed prior to the purchase of the insurance. The benefit packages offered by plans in the exchanges vary depending on whether individuals purchase a low-premium bronze plan with high out-of-pocket costs, a high-premium platinum plan with lower out-of-pocket costs, or intermediate silver or gold plans (Kaiser Family Foundation, 2013) (Table 2–2). The contentious politics of the ACA are discussed in Chapter 15.

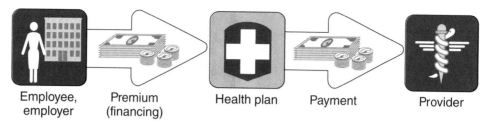

▲ **Figure 2–3.** Employment-based private insurance. In addition to the direct employer subsidy, indirect government subsidies occur through the tax-free status of employer contributions for health insurance benefits.

Employment-Based Private Insurance

Betty Lerner and her schoolteacher colleagues each paid $6 per year to Prepaid Hospital in 1929. Ms. Lerner suffered a heart attack and was hospitalized at no cost. The following year Prepaid Hospital built a new wing and raised the teachers' prepayment to $12.

Rose Riveter retired in 1961. Her health insurance premium for hospital and physician care, formerly paid by her employer, had been $25 per month. When she called the insurance company to obtain individual coverage, she was told that premiums at age 65 cost $70 per month. She could not afford the insurance and wondered what would happen if she became ill.

The development of private health insurance in the United States was impelled by the increasing effectiveness and rising costs of hospital care. Hospitals became places not only in which to die, but also in which to get well. However, many patients were unable to pay for hospital care, and this meant that hospitals were unable to attract "customers."

In 1929, Baylor University Hospital agreed to provide up to 21 days of hospital care to 1,500 Dallas schoolteachers such as Betty Lerner if they paid the hospital $6 per person per year. As the Great Depression deepened and private hospital occupancy in 1931 fell to 62%, similar hospital-centered private insurance plans spread. These plans (anticipating health maintenance organization [HMO] plans), restricted care to a particular hospital. The American Hospital Association built on this prepayment movement and established statewide Blue Cross hospital insurance plans allowing free choice of hospital. By 1940, 39 Blue Cross plans controlled by the private hospital industry had enrolled over 6 million people. The Great Depression reduced the amount patients could pay physicians out of pocket, and in 1939, the California Medical Association set up the first Blue Shield plan to cover physician services. These plans, controlled by state medical societies, followed Blue Cross in spreading across the nation (Starr, 1982; Fein, 1986).

In contrast to the consumer-driven development of health insurance in European nations, coverage in the United States was initiated by health care providers seeking a steady source of income. Hospital and physician control over the "Blues," a major sector of the health insurance industry, guaranteed that payment would be generous and that cost control would remain on the back burner (Law, 1974; Starr, 1982).

The rapid growth of employment-based private insurance was spurred by an accident of history. During World War II, wage and price controls prevented companies from granting wage increases, but allowed the growth of fringe benefits. With a labor shortage, companies competing for workers began to offer health insurance to employees such as Rose Riveter as a fringe benefit. After the war, unions picked up on this trend and negotiated for health benefits. The results were dramatic: Enrollment in group hospital insurance plans grew from 12 million in 1940 to 142 million in 1988.

With employment-based health insurance, employers pay a portion of the premium that purchases health insurance for their employees (Fig. 2–3). However, this flow of money is not as simple as it looks. The federal government views employer premium payments as a tax-deductible business expense. The government does not treat the health insurance fringe benefit as taxable income to the employee, even though the payment of premiums could be interpreted as a form of employee income. Because each premium dollar of employer-sponsored health insurance results in a reduction in taxes collected, the government is in essence subsidizing employer-sponsored health insurance. This subsidy is enormous, estimated at $280 billion in 2018.

The ACA made a change in employer-based health insurance, requiring employers with 50 or more full-time employees to offer coverage or pay a fee to the government; the fee is meant to discourage employers from dropping employee health insurance, which they might be tempted to do since their employees could buy individual insurance through the health insurance exchanges (Kaiser Family Foundation, 2018a). The ACA also imposed new rules on individual and employer-based insurance. Private health insurance plans are required to include young adults up to age 26 under their parents' policies. The ACA also prohibits denial of coverage based on preexisting conditions and limits variation in premium costs to a maximum ratio of three-to-one between a plan's highest and lowest premium charge for the same benefit package.

The growth of employment-based health insurance attracted commercial insurance companies to the health care field to compete with the Blues for customers. The commercial insurers changed the entire dynamic of health insurance. The new dynamic was called **experience rating**. (The following discussion of experience rating can be applied to individual as well as employment-based private insurance.)

Healthy Insurance Company insures three groups of people—a young healthy group of bank managers, an older healthy group of truck drivers, and an older group of coal miners with a high rate of chronic illness. Under experience rating, Healthy sets its premiums according to the experience of each group in using health services. Because the bank managers rarely use health care, each pays a premium of $600 per month. Because the truck drivers are older, their risk of illness is higher, and their premium is $700 per month. The miners, who have high rates of black lung disease, are charged a premium of $800 per month. The average premium income to Healthy is $700 per member per month.

Blue Cross insures the same three groups and needs the same $700 per member per month to cover health care plus administrative costs for these groups. Blue Cross sets its premiums by the principle of community rating. For a given health insurance policy, all subscribers in a community pay the same premium. The bank managers, truck drivers, and mine workers all pay $700 per month.

Health insurance provides a mechanism to distribute health care more in accordance with human need rather than exclusively on the basis of ability to pay. To achieve this goal, funds are redistributed from the healthy to the sick, a subsidy that helps pay the costs of those unable to purchase services on their own.

Community rating achieves this redistribution in two ways:

1. Within each group (bank managers, truck drivers, and mine workers), people who become ill receive benefits in excess of the premiums they pay, while people who remain healthy pay premiums while receiving few or no health benefits.
2. Among the three groups, the bank managers, who use less health care than their premiums are worth, help pay for the miners, who use more health care than their premiums could buy.

Experience rating is less redistributive than community rating. Within each group, those who become ill are subsidized by those who remain well, but among the different groups, healthier groups (bank managers) do not subsidize high-risk groups (mine workers). Thus the principle of health insurance, which is to distribute health care more in accordance with human need rather than exclusively on the ability to pay, is weakened by experience rating (Light, 1992).

In the early years, Blue Cross plans set insurance premiums by the principle of community rating, whereas commercial insurers used experience rating as a "weapon" to compete with the Blues (Fein, 1986). Commercial insurers such as Healthy Insurance Company could offer cheaper premiums to low-risk groups such as bank managers, who would naturally choose a Healthy commercial plan at $600 over a Blue Cross plan at $700. Experience rating helped commercial insurers overtake the Blues in the private health insurance market. While in 1945 commercial insurers had only 10 million enrollees, compared with 19 million for the Blues, by 1955 the score was commercials 54 million and the Blues 51 million.

Many commercial insurers would not market policies to such high-risk groups as mine workers, leaving Blue Cross with high-risk patients who were paying relatively low premiums. To survive the competition from the commercial insurers, Blue Cross had no choice but to seek younger, healthier groups by abandoning community rating and reducing the premiums for those groups. In this way, many Blue Cross and Blue Shield plans switched to experience rating. Without community rating, older and sicker groups became less and less able to afford health insurance.

From the perspective of the elderly and those with chronic illness, experience rating is discriminatory. Healthy persons, however, might have another viewpoint and might ask why they should voluntarily transfer their wealth to sicker people through the insurance subsidy. The answer lies in the unpredictability of health care needs. When purchasing health insurance, an individual does not know if he or she will suddenly change from a state of good health to one of illness. Thus, *within a group*, people are willing to risk paying for health insurance, even though they may not use it. *Among different groups*, however, healthy people have no economic incentive to voluntarily pay for community rating and subsidize another group of sicker people. This is why community rating cannot survive in a market-driven competitive private insurance system (Aaron, 1991).

In a major reform contained within the ACA, insurers are severely limited in using experience rating to set premiums; they can only vary premiums based on family size, geographic location, age, and smoking status. The ACA also limits how much premiums can differ between older and younger individuals (HealthCare.gov).

The most positive aspect of health insurance—that it assists people with serious illness to pay for their care—has also become one of its main drawbacks—the difficulty in controlling costs in an insurance environment. With direct purchase, the "invisible hand" of each individual's ability to pay holds down the price and quantity of health care. However, if a patient is well insured and the cost of care causes no immediate fiscal pain, the patient will use more services than someone who must pay for care out of pocket. In addition, particularly before the advent of fee schedules, health care providers could increase fees more easily if a third party was available to foot the bill.

Thus health insurance was originally an attempt by society to solve the problem of unaffordable health care under an out-of-pocket payment system, but its very capacity to make health care more affordable created a new problem. If people no longer had to pay out of their own pockets for health care, they would use more health care; and if health care providers could charge insurers rather than patients, they could more easily raise prices, especially during the era when the major insurers (the Blues) were controlled by hospitals and physicians. The solution of insurance fueled the problem of rising costs. As private insurance became largely experience rated and employment based, persons who had low incomes, who were chronically ill, or who were elderly found it increasingly difficult to afford private insurance.

▶ Government Financing

In 1984 at age 74 Rose Riveter developed colon cancer. She was now covered by Medicare, which had been enacted in 1965. Even so, her Medicare premium, hospital deductible expenses, physician copayments, short nursing home stay, and uncovered prescriptions cost her $2,700 the year she became ill with cancer.

Employment-based private health insurance grew rapidly in the 1950s, helping working people and their families to afford health care. But two groups in the population received little or no benefit: the poor and the elderly. The poor were usually unemployed or employed in jobs without the fringe benefit of health insurance; they could not afford insurance premiums. The elderly, who needed health care the most and whose premiums had been partially subsidized by community rating, were hard hit by the trend toward experience rating. In the late 1950s, less than 15% of the elderly had any health insurance (Harris, 1966). Only one program could provide affordable care for the poor and the elderly: tax-financed government health insurance.

Government entered the health care financing arena long before the 1960s through such public programs as municipal hospitals and dispensaries to care for the poor and through state-operated mental hospitals. But only with the 1965 enactment of Medicare (for the elderly) and Medicaid (for the poor) did public insurance payments for privately operated health services become a major feature of health care in the United States. Medicare Part A (Table 2–3) is a hospital insurance plan for the elderly financed largely through social security taxes from employers and employees. Medicare Part B (Table 2–4) insures the elderly for physician services and is paid for by federal taxes and monthly premiums from the beneficiaries. Medicare Part D, enacted in 2003, offers prescription drug coverage and is paid for by federal taxes and monthly premiums from beneficiaries. Medicaid (Table 2–5) is a program run by the states that is funded by federal and state taxes, which pays for the care of millions of low-income people. In 2017, Medicare and Medicaid expenditures totaled $706 and $582 billion, respectively (Martin et al., 2019). In 2018, the trustees of the Medicare program estimated that the Part A trust fund would be able to pay 100% of hospital costs until 2026, and thereafter – without new funding – would be able to pay only 80–90% of hospital costs through 2092 (Van de Water, 2018).

Medicare

With its large deductibles, copayments, and gaps in coverage, Medicare beneficiaries are in need of additional insurance. In 2016, 30% of beneficiaries had additional retiree coverage from their previous employment, 29% purchased supplemental private insurance, 22% were enrolled in both Medicare and Medicaid, and 19% had no additional coverage. Those beneficiaries with no additional coverage paid an average of $5,806 in out-of-pocket costs (Kaiser Family Foundation, 2019a).

The Medicare Modernization Act (MMA) of 2003 made two major changes in the Medicare program: the expansion of the role of private health plans (the Medicare Advantage program, Part C) and the establishment of a prescription drug benefit (Part D). In 2019, 20 million Medicare beneficiaries were enrolled in Medicare Advantage. Under the Medicare Advantage program, a beneficiary can elect to enroll in a private health plan contracting with Medicare. Medicare subsidizes the premium for that private health plan and the health plan pays hospitals, physicians, and other providers. Beneficiaries joining a Medicare Advantage plan sacrifice some freedom of choice of physician and hospital in return for lower out-of-pocket payments and

Table 2–3. Summary of Medicare Part A, 2019

Who is eligible?

Upon reaching the age of 65 years, people who are eligible for Social Security are automatically enrolled in Medicare Part A whether or not they are retired. A person who has paid into the Social Security system for 10 years and that person's spouse are eligible for Social Security. People who are not eligible for Social Security can enroll in Medicare Part A by paying a monthly premium.

People under the age of 65 years who are totally and permanently disabled may enroll in Medicare Part A after they have been receiving Social Security disability benefits for 24 months. People with amyotrophic lateral sclerosis (ALS) or end-stage renal disease requiring dialysis or a transplant are also eligible for Medicare Part A without a 2-year waiting period.

How is it financed?

Financing is through the Social Security system. Employers and employees each pay to Medicare 1.45% of wages and salaries. Self-employed people pay 2.9%. The 2010 Affordable Care Act increased the employee rate for higher-income taxpayers (incomes greater than $200,000 for individuals or $250,000 for couples) from 1.45% to 2.35%.

What services are covered?[a]

Services	Benefit	Medicare Pays
Hospitalization	First 60 days period[b]	All but a $1,364 deductible per benefit
	61st to 90th day[b]	All but $341/day
	91st to 150th day[c]	All but $682/day
	Beyond 90 days if lifetime reserve days are used up	Nothing
Skilled nursing facility	First 20 days	All
	21st to 100th day	All but $170.50/day
	Beyond 100 days	Nothing
Home health care	Medically necessary care for homebound people	100% for skilled care as defined by Medicare regulations
Hospice care	As long as a doctor certifies person suffers from a terminal illness	100% for most services, copays for outpatient drugs and coinsurance for inpatient respite care
Unskilled nursing home care	Care that is mainly custodial is not covered	Nothing

[a]For patients in Medicare Advantage plans, covered services and patient responsibility for payment changes based on the specifics of each Medicare Advantage plan.
[b]Part A benefits are provided by each benefit period rather than for each year. A benefit period begins when a beneficiary enters a hospital and ends 60 days after discharge from the hospital or from a skilled nursing facility.
[c]Beyond 90 days, Medicare pays for 60 additional days only once in a lifetime ("lifetime reserve days").

Table 2–4. Summary of Medicare Part B, 2019

Who is eligible?
People who are eligible for Medicare Part A who elect to pay the Medicare Part B premium of $135.50 per month. Some low-income persons can receive financial assistance with the premium. Higher-income beneficiaries (over $85,000 for individual, $170,000 for couple) have higher premiums related to income.

How is it financed?
Financing is in part by general federal revenues (personal income and other federal taxes) and in part by Part B monthly premiums.

What services are covered?[a]

Services	Benefit	Medicare Pays
Medical expenses Physician services Physical, occupational, and speech therapy Medical equipment Diagnostic tests (no coinsurance for laboratory services)	All medically necessary services	80% of approved amount after a $185 annual deductible
Preventive care	Pap smears; mammograms; colorectal/ prostate cancer, cardiovascular and diabetes screening; pneumococcal and influenza vaccinations; yearly physical examinations	Included in medical expenses, and for some services the deductible and copayment are waived
Outpatient medications	Partially covered under Medicare Part D	All except for premium, deductible, and coinsurance
Eye refractions, hearing aids, dental services	Not covered	Nothing

[a]For patients in Medicare Advantage plans, covered services and patient responsibility for payment change based on the specifics of each Medicare Advantage plan.

Table 2–5. Summary of Medicaid under the Affordable Care Act (ACA), 2019

Medicaid is a federal program administered by the states.

Eligibility
- **From 1965 through 2014**, Medicaid, while designed for low-income Americans, did not cover all poor people. In addition to being poor, Medicaid had required that people also meet "categorical" eligibility criteria such as being a young child, parent, pregnant, elderly, or disabled, leaving out nonpregnant adults without dependent children. Income eligibility for Medicaid varied by state; typically children were covered up to 100%, adults to 61%, and the elderly or disabled to 74% of the Federal Poverty Level.
- **In 2015, Medicaid under the ACA** varies widely between states participating in the Medicaid expansion and those not participating. For the latter states, the provisions summarized for the 1965 to 2014 period still apply. In participating states, all individuals with incomes up to 138% of the Federal Poverty Level are eligible for coverage, with no categorical eligibility criteria. To finance Medicaid expansion for the participating states, the federal government pays 100% of the costs of the newly eligible from 2014 to 2016, decreasing gradually to 90% in 2020 and beyond.
- Undocumented immigrants are not eligible for Medicaid.

State waivers
States can be granted waivers by the federal government to make changes in which services they provide to Medicaid recipients and whether recipients are required to receive the services through managed care plans.

that include Medicare Part D prescription drug coverage. In addition to their Part B premium, the average Medicare Advantage enrollee pays $34 per month to the health plan with half of enrollees paying no health plan premium. Medicare Advantage enrollees have lower out-of-pocket costs than traditional Medicare beneficiaries (Kaiser Family Foundation, 2018c).

In order to channel more patients into Medicare Advantage plans, the MMA provided generous payments to those plans, with the result that they initially cost the federal government 14% more than the government paid for health care services for similar Medicare beneficiaries in the traditional Part A and Part B programs. The ACA reduced payments to Medicare Advantage plans with the goal of saving the Medicare program $136 billion over the following 10 years. However in 2017, Medicare Advantage enrollees continued to cost the government more than beneficiaries in traditional Medicare (Brennan et al, 2018) even though Medicare Advantage enrollees are

are only allowed to receive care from health care providers connected with that plan. The average beneficiary in 2019 could choose among 24 Medicare Advantage plans (Kaiser Family Foundation, 2018b). In 2018, 58% of Medicare Advantage plans were provided by three huge insurance firms: UnitedHealthcare, Humana, and Anthem Blue Cross Blue Shield. Eighty-eight percent of Medicare Advantage enrollees are in plans healthier (Weil, 2019). Medicare Advantage plans have manipulated the payment system to get inappropriately high payments. The plans receive higher federal payments for patients who have a greater disease burden, measured by the Hierarchical Condition Categories (HCC) score. Plans commonly up-code diagnoses to raise their HCC scores and thereby inflate their payments. Audits of 37 plans found that all but two plans were overpaid, costing the Medicare program tens of billions of dollars (Schulte, 2019).

Medicare Part D provides partial coverage for prescription drugs with 73% financed through government revenues. Beneficiaries receive their Part D benefits from private health plans. In 2018, 43 million of the 60 million Medicare beneficiaries were enrolled in a Part D plan, 42% through their Medicare Advantage plans and 58% through stand-alone prescription drug plans. The Part D deductible in 2019 was $415 with 25% coinsurance up to $3,820 in total drug costs. Between $3,820 and $5,100 coinsurance for brand name drugs remained at 25% and for generic drugs, 37%. If total drug out of pocket costs exceed $5,100 during a year, the coinsurance drops to 5%. Part D plans often offer reduced deductibles and vary their copayments based on the cost of the drug (Kaiser Family Foundation, 2018d). Part D has been criticized because the proliferation of private drug plans is confusing to beneficiaries and the government is not allowed to negotiate with pharmaceutical companies for lower drug prices.

Medicaid

The Medicaid program is jointly administered by the federal and state governments. Prior to the ACA's Medicaid expansion, the federal government contributed between 50% and 76% of total Medicaid costs; the federal contribution being greater for states with lower per capita incomes. Although designed for low-income Americans, not all poor people have traditionally been eligible for Medicaid. Until enactment of the ACA, Medicaid required that people not only be poor but also meet "categorical" eligibility criteria such as being a young child, pregnant, elderly, or disabled.

The ACA (Table 2–5) eliminated the categorical eligibility criteria and required that beginning in 2014, states offer the program to all citizens and legal residents with income at or below 138% of the Federal

Poverty Level—$16,394 for an individual or $33,534 for a family of four in 2018. Undocumented immigrants were still excluded from federal funding. The ACA intended that all states expand Medicaid eligibility and provided states an incentive for expansion by having the federal government pay almost all the cost of the increased Medicaid enrollment (100% in 2014 to 2016, phased down to 90% in 2020 and thereafter). However, in June 2012, the Supreme Court ruled that the ACA's Medicaid expansion was optional for states. In April 2019, 36 states plus the District of Columbia had expanded Medicaid and three more states were planning to expand.

Medicaid now covers one in five people in the United States, making it the single largest health program in the nation. From 2000 to 2017, Medicaid expenditures rose from $200 billion to $582 billion. To slow down this expenditure growth, the federal government ceded to states enhanced control over Medicaid programs through Medicaid waivers, which allow states to make alterations in the scope of covered services, require Medicaid recipients to pay part of their costs, and obligate Medicaid recipients to enroll in managed care plans (see Chapter 4). In 2017, nearly two-thirds of Medicaid recipients were enrolled in managed care plans (Kaiser Family Foundation, 2018e). Because Medicaid pays primary care physicians an average of 66% of Medicare fees, about 30% of physicians limit the number of Medicaid patients they will see (Paradise, 2017).

During the Obama Administration, a number of states requested waivers that would restrict Medicaid eligibility but the federal government generally denied those waivers. In contrast, the Trump Administration has approved a number of restrictive Medicaid waivers such as the imposition of premiums and copayments which many families cannot afford. Thousands of recipients have been disenrolled for nonpayment of premiums. Thirteen states have requested waivers to require Medicaid recipients to work at least 20 hours per week; as of April 2019 seven of these have been approved (Kaiser Family Foundation, 2019b). The purpose of these waivers is to cut Medicaid costs by reducing the number of people on the program.

In 1997, the federal government created the Children's Health Insurance Program (CHIP), a companion program to Medicaid. CHIP covered children in families with incomes at or below 200% of the federal

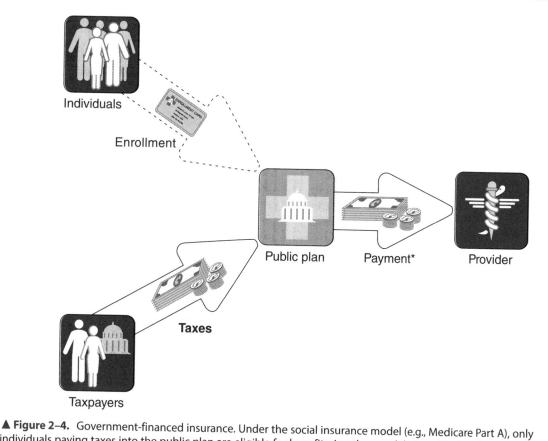

▲ **Figure 2–4.** Government-financed insurance. Under the social insurance model (e.g., Medicare Part A), only individuals paying taxes into the public plan are eligible for benefits. In other models (e.g., Medicaid), an individual's eligibility for benefits may not be directly linked to payment of taxes into the plan.
*Some public plans, for example Medicare Advantage, pay a private insurance intermediary that in turn pays providers.

poverty level, but above the Medicaid income eligibility level. In 2018, CHIP was reauthorized for children in families at or below 300% of the federal poverty level, with 6.6 million children enrolled in the program.

Government health insurance for the poor and the elderly added a new factor to the health care financing equation: the taxpayer (Fig. 2–4). With government-financed health plans, the taxpayer can interact with the health care consumer in two distinct ways:

1. The social insurance model, exemplified by Medicare, allows only those who have paid a certain amount of social security taxes to be eligible for Part A and only those who pay a monthly premium to receive benefits from Part B. As with private insurance, social insurance requires people to make a contribution in order to receive benefits.

2. The contrasting model is the Medicaid public assistance model, in which those who contribute (taxpayers) may not be eligible for benefits (Bodenheimer & Grumbach, 1992).

It must be remembered that private insurance contains a subsidy: redistribution of funds from the healthy to the sick. Tax-funded insurance has the same subsidy and usually adds another: redistribution of funds from upper- to lower-income groups. Under this double subsidy, exemplified by Medicare and Medicaid, healthy middle-income employees generally pay more in social security payments and other taxes than they receive in health services, whereas unemployed, disabled, and lower-income elderly persons tend to receive more in health services than they contribute in taxes.

The advent of government financing improved financial access to care for some people, but, in turn, aggravated the problem of rising costs. The federal government and state governments have responded by attempting to limit Medicare and Medicaid payments to physicians, hospitals, and managed care plans.

THE BURDEN OF FINANCING HEALTH CARE

Different methods of financing health care place different burdens on the various income levels of society. Payments are classified as **progressive** if they take a rising percentage of income as income increases, **regressive** if they take a falling percentage of income as income increases, and **proportional** if the ratio of payment to income is the same for all income classes (Pechman, 1985).

What principle should underlie the choice of revenue source for health care? A central purpose of the health care system is to maintain and improve the health of the nation's population. As discussed in Chapter 3, rates of mortality and disability are far higher for low-income people than for the wealthy. Burdening low-income families with high levels of payments for health care (i.e., regressive payments) reduces their disposable income, amplifies the ill effects of poverty, and thereby worsens their health. It makes little sense to finance a health care system—the purpose of which is to improve health—with payments that worsen health. Thus, regressive payments could be considered "unhealthy."

Rita Blue earns $10,000 per year for her family of four. She develops pneumonia, and her out-of-pocket health costs come to $1,000, 10% of her family income.

Cathy White earns $100,000 per year for her family of four. She develops pneumonia, and her out-of-pocket health costs come to $1,000, 1% of her family income.

Out-of-pocket payments are a regressive mode of financing. According to the 1987 National Medical Care Expenditure Survey, out-of-pocket payments took 12% of the income of families in the nation's lowest-income quintile, compared with 1.2% for families in the wealthiest 5% of the population (Bodenheimer & Sullivan, 1997). This pattern is confirmed by the 2000 Medical Expenditure Panel Survey (MEPS, 2005). Many economists and health policy experts would consider this regressive burden of payment as unfair. Aggravating the regressivity of out-of-pocket payments is the fact that lower-income people tend to be sicker and thus have more out-of-pocket payments than the wealthier and healthier.

Jim Hale is a young, healthy, self-employed accountant whose monthly income is $12,000, with a health insurance premium of $600, or 5% of his income.

Jack Hurt is a mine worker with black lung disease. His income is $2,700 per month, of which $900 (33%) goes for his health insurance. His experience-rated insurance premium is higher because he is in poor health.

Experience-rated private health insurance is a regressive method of financing health care because increased risk of illness tends to correlate with reduced income. If Jim Hale and Jack Hurt were enrolled in a community-rated plan, each with a premium of $600, they would respectively pay 5% and 22% of their incomes for health insurance. With community rating, the burden of payment is regressive, but less so than with experience rating. Most private insurance is not individually purchased but rather obtained through employment. How is the burden of employment-linked health insurance premiums distributed?

Jill is an assistant hospital administrator. To attract her to the job, the hospital offered her a package of salary plus health insurance of $8,600 per month. She chose to take $8,000 in salary, leaving the hospital to pay $600 for her health insurance.

Bill is a nurse's aide, whose union negotiated with the hospital for a total package of $4,600 per month; of this amount $4,000 is salary and $600 pays his health insurance premium.

Do Jill and Bill pay nothing for their health insurance? Not exactly. Employers generally agree on a total package of wages and fringe benefits; if Jill and Bill did not receive health insurance, their pay would probably go up by nearly $600 per month. That is why employer-paid health insurance premiums are generally considered deductions from wages or salary, and thus paid by the employee (Blumberg et al., 2007). For Jill, health insurance amounts to only 7% of her income, but for Bill it is 13%. In 2012, employer-sponsored health insurance premiums represented 58% of family income for the bottom 40% of American families compared with 4% for the top 5% (Blumenthal & Squires, 2014).

Larry Lowe earns $10,000 and pays $410 in federal and state income taxes, or 4.1% of his income.

Harold High earns $100,000 and pays $12,900 in income taxes, or 12.9% of his income.

The progressive income tax is the largest tax providing money for government-financed health care. Most other taxes are regressive (e.g., sales and property taxes), and the combined burden of all taxes that finance health care is roughly proportional (Pechman, 1985).

In 2017, 47% of health care expenditures were financed through out-of-pocket payments and premiums, which are regressive, while 43% was funded through government revenues (Martin et al., 2019), which are proportional. The sum total of health care financing is regressive. In 2013, medical expenses lowered the median income of the lowest income decile by 47.6% compared with 2.7% for the top decile (Christopher et al., 2018). Overall, the US health care system is financed in a manner that is unhealthy.

CONCLUSION

Neither Fred Farmer nor his great-grandson Ted had health insurance, but the modern-day Mr. Farmer's predicament differs drastically from that of his ancestor. Third-party financing of health care has fueled an expansive health care system that offers treatments unimaginable a century ago, but at tremendous expense.

Each of the four modes of financing health care developed historically as a solution to the inadequacy of the previous modes. Private insurance provided protection to patients against the unpredictable costs of medical care, as well as protection to providers of care against the unpredictable ability of patients to pay. But the private insurance solution created three new, interrelated problems:

1. The opportunity for health care providers to increase fees to insurers caused health services to become increasingly unaffordable for those with inadequate insurance or no insurance.

2. The employment-based nature of group insurance placed people who were unemployed, retired, or working part-time at a disadvantage for the purchase of insurance, and partially masked the true costs of insurance for employees who did receive health benefits at the workplace.

3. Competition inherent in a deregulated private insurance market gave rise to the practice of experience rating, which made insurance premiums unaffordable for many elderly people and other medically needy groups.

To solve these problems, government financing was required, but government financing fueled an even greater inflation in health care costs.

As each "solution" was introduced, health care financing improved for a time. But rising costs have jeopardized private and public coverage for many people and made services unaffordable even for people who are insured (Chapter 3). The problems of each financing mode and the problems created by each successive solution have accumulated into a complex crisis characterized by inadequate access for some and high costs for everyone.

REFERENCES

Aaron HJ. *Serious and Unstable Condition: Financing America's Health Care.* Washington, DC: Brookings Institution; 1991.

Arrow KJ. Uncertainty and the welfare economics of medical care. *Am Econ Rev.* 1963;53:941.

Blumberg LJ, et al. Setting a standard of affordability for health insurance coverage. *Health Affairs.* 2007;26:w463–473.

Blumenthal D, Squires D. Do health care costs fuel economic inequality in the United States? The Commonwealth Fund Blog. www.commonwealthfund.org/publications/blog/2014/sep/do-health-costs-fuel-inequality. Published September 9, 2014. Accessed September 19, 2019.

Bodenheimer T, Grumbach K. Financing universal health insurance: taxes, premiums, and the lessons of social insurance. *J Health Polit Policy Law.* 1992;17:439–462.

Bodenheimer T, Sullivan K. The logic of tax-based financing for health care. *Int J Health Serv.* 1997;27:409–425.

Brennan N, et al. Time to release Medicare Advantage claims data. *JAMA.* 2018;319:975–976.

Christopher AS, et al. The effects of household medical expenditures on income inequality in the United States. *Am J Public Health.* 2018;108:351–354.

Evans RG. *Strained Mercy*. Toronto: Butterworths; 1984.

Fein R. *Medical Care, Medical Costs*. Cambridge, MA: Harvard University Press; 1986.

Harris R. *A Sacred Trust*. New York, NY: New American Library; 1966.

Kaiser Family Foundation. Summary of the Affordable Care Act. 2013. http://kff.org/health-reform/fact-sheet/summary-of-the-affordable-care-act. Accessed September 19, 2019.

Kaiser Family Foundation. Employer Responsibility Under the Affordable Care Act. March 5, 2018a. https://www.kff.org/infographic/employer-responsibility-under-the-affordable-care-act/. Accessed September 19, 2019.

Kaiser Family Foundation. Medicare Advantage 2019 spotlight: first look. October, 2018b. https://www.kff.org/medicare/issue.../medicare-advantage-2019-spotlight-first-look/. Accessed September 19, 2019.

Kaiser Family Foundation. A dozen facts about Medicare Advantage. November 2018c. https://www.kff.org/medicare/issue.../a-dozen-facts-about-medicare-advantage-in-201. Accessed September 19, 2019.

Kaiser Family Foundation. An overview of the Medicare Part D prescription drug benefit. October 2018d. https://www.kff.org/medicare/.../an-overview-of-the-medicare-part-d-prescription-dru.... Accessed September 19, 2019.

Kaiser Family Foundation. Medicaid Managed Care Plans and access to care. March 2018e. files.kff.org/.../Report-Medicaid-Managed-Care-March-Plans-and-Access-to-Care. Accessed September 19, 2019.

Kaiser Family Foundation. An overview of Medicare. Issue brief. February 2019a. https://www.kff.org/medicare/issue-brief/an-overview-of-medicare/. Accessed September 19, 2019.

Kaiser Family Foundation. Medicaid waiver tracker. September 18, 2019b. https://www.kff.org/medicaid/.../medicaid-waiver-tracker-approved-and-pending-secti.... Accessed September 19, 2019.

Law SA. *Blue Cross: What Went Wrong?* New Haven, CT: Yale University Press; 1974.

Light DW. The practice and ethics of risk-rated health insurance. *JAMA*. 1992;267:2503–2508.

Martin AB et al. National health spending in 2017. *Health Affairs*. 2019;38:96–106.

Medical Expenditure Panel Survey. Statistical Brief #81: Concentration of health care expenditures in the U.S. civilian noninstitutionalized population. May 2005. https://meps.ahrq.gov › data_files › publications › stat81. Accessed September 19, 2019.

Paradise J. A large majority of physicians participate in Medicaid. Kaiser Family Foundation Data Note, May 10, 2017. https://www.kff.org/medicaid/.../data-note-a-large-majority-of-physicians-participate-i.... Accessed September 19, 2019.

Pechman JA. *Who Paid the Taxes, 1966–1985*. Washington, DC: Brookings Institution; 1985.

Schulte F. Medicare Advantage audits reveal pervasive overcharges. Updated 2019. https://publicintegrity.org/2016/08/29/20148/medicare-advantage-audits-reveal-pervasive-overcharges. Accessed September 19, 2019.

Starr P. *The Social Transformation of American Medicine*. New York, NY: Basic Books; 1982.

Van de Water PN. Medicare is not "bankrupt." Center on Budget and Policy Priorities, July 3, 2018. https://www.cbpp.org/research/health/medicare-is-not-bankrupt. Accessed September 19, 2019.

Weil AR. Physicians, Medicare, and more. *Health Affairs*. 2019;38:519.

Access to Health Care

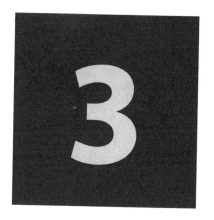

Access to health care is the ability to obtain health services when needed. Lack of adequate access for millions of people is a crisis in the United States.

Access to health care has two major components. First and most frequently discussed is the ability to pay. Second is the availability of health care personnel and facilities that are close to where people live, accessible by transportation, culturally acceptable, and capable of providing appropriate care in a timely manner and in a compatible language. The first and longest portion of this chapter dwells on financial barriers to care, specifically the access challenges faced by the *uninsured* and the *underinsured*. The second portion touches on nonfinancial barriers. The final segment explores the influences other than health care (in particular, socioeconomic status and race/ethnicity) that are important determinants of the health status of a population.

FINANCIAL BARRIERS TO HEALTH CARE

▶ Lack of Insurance

In 2018, Dan Coverless noticed that he was urinating a lot and feeling weak. He lived in South Carolina and earned $9,500 per year working part-time as a construction worker. Because South Carolina did not elect to participate in the Affordable Care Act's Medicaid expansion, Mr. Coverless was not eligible for Medicaid despite his low income. He also did not qualify for federal tax subsidies to purchase private insurance, which had annual premium costs of more than

half his income. His friend told him that his symptoms might mean that he had diabetes and that he should go see a doctor, but lacking health insurance, Mr. Coverless was afraid of the cost. Eight days later, his friend found him in a coma. He was hospitalized for diabetic ketoacidosis.

Health insurance coverage, whether public or private, is a key factor in making health care accessible. Despite gains in insurance coverage since enactment of the Affordable Care Act (ACA) in 2010, 28 million people in the United States in 2017 had no health insurance whatsoever (Fig. 3–1). *Forty-six percent of the population was covered by employer-based private insurance, 9% by individual private insurance, 17% by Medicare, and 19% by Medicaid, leaving 9% uninsured* (Table 3–1).

For many of the people in the United States, who do not have insurance, the unaffordability of health care is an insurmountable barrier. People lacking health insurance receive less care and have worse health outcomes than those with insurance. In 2017, 50% of uninsured adults, compared with 11% of those with private insurance, had no usual source of care; 24%, compared with 6% of those with private insurance, postponed seeking care due to cost, and 30%, compared with 4% for those with private insurance, went without needed care due to cost (Kaiser Family Foundation, 2018a). The uninsured suffer worse health outcomes than those with insurance. Compared with insured persons, the uninsured like Mr. Coverless have more avoidable hospitalizations, tend to be diagnosed at later stages of life-threatening

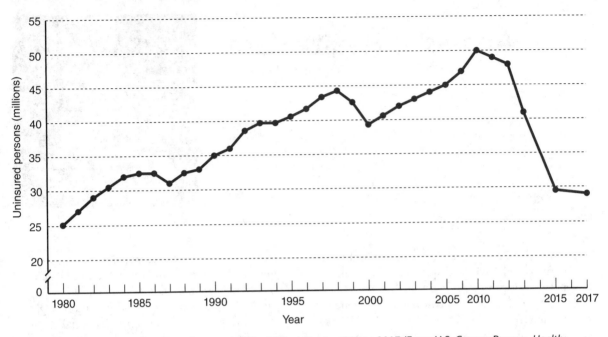

▲ **Figure 3–1.** Number of uninsured persons in the United States, 1980 to 2017 (From U.S. Census Bureau. *Health Insurance Coverage in the United States, 2017.* September 2018).

Table 3–1. Estimated principal source of health insurance, 2017

	Number of People (millions)	Population (%)
Medicare[a]	55	17
Medicaid	62	19
Employment-based private insurance	152	46
Individual private insurance	29	9
Uninsured	28	9
Total US population	326	100%

[a]For people with Medicare plus private insurance or Medicaid, Medicare is considered the principal source of insurance. The Medicaid and private insurance figures do not count Medicare beneficiaries who also have Medicaid or private insurance.
Source: Data extracted from U.S. Census Bureau: *Health Insurance Coverage* in the United States, 2017, September 2018; Claxton G, et al. Health benefits in 2018: modest growth in premiums, higher worker contributions at firms with more low-wage workers. *Health Aff (Millwood).* 2018;37:1892–1900.

illnesses, and are on average more seriously ill when hospitalized. Higher rates of cervical cancer and lower survival rates for breast cancer among the uninsured, compared with those with insurance, are associated with less access to cancer screenings (Ayanian et al., 2000). People without insurance have greater rates of uncontrolled hypertension, diabetes, and elevated cholesterol than those with insurance (Wilper et al., 2009). Most significantly, people who lack health insurance suffer a higher overall mortality rate than those with insurance (Woolhandler and Himmelstein, 2017). After adjusting for age, sex, education, poorer initial health status, and smoking, lack of insurance itself increases the risk of dying by 40% (Wilper et al., 2009).

Does Medicaid Make a Difference?

Medicaid, the federal and state public insurance plan, has made great strides in improving access to care for many low-income people. As a rule, people with Medicaid have a level of access to medical care that is intermediate between those without insurance and those with private insurance.

When Maria Buenasuerte became pregnant, her sister told her that she was eligible for Medicaid, which she obtained. She lived near a community health center and made an appointment the same week with a certified nurse midwife at the clinic for her prenatal intake. She had an uncomplicated pregnancy and delivered a healthy baby attended by her midwife and obstetrician at the local community hospital.

Concepcion Ortiz lived in a town of 25,000 persons. When she became pregnant, she enrolled in Medicaid. She called each private obstetrician in town but none would take Medicaid patients. The nearest community health center accepting Medicaid was 75 miles away and no one in Concepcion's family had a car. When she reached her sixth month, she became desperate.

Compared with uninsured people, those with Medicaid are more likely to have a regular source of medical care and are less likely to report delays in receiving care. For children enrolled in Medicaid, these access measures are comparable to the access reported for children with private insurance. Adults with Medicaid, although less likely than uninsured adults to report delays in seeking care, are still about twice as likely as privately insured adults to report delays (Kaiser Commission on Medicaid and the Uninsured, 2015). Similarly, when comparing specific services such as rates of immunizations, screening for breast and cervical cancer, hypertension and diabetes control, and timeliness of prenatal care, rates for people on Medicaid tend to fall between those of the uninsured and people with private insurance (Landon et al., 2007). A recent "natural experiment" occurred in Oregon in 2008, when the state implemented a lottery system to add a limited number of low income adults to the state's Medicaid program. Comparing outcomes over the subsequent 2 years among the patients who gained Medicaid through the lottery with similar patients who remained uninsured, those with Medicaid had better self-reported health, improved depression scores, more use of preventive services, and less financial stress than those who remained uninsured, but did not have better

control of diabetes and hypertension relative to the uninsured patients (Baicker et al., 2013). Counties in states that expanded Medicaid under the ACA have significantly reduced mortality than counties in non-expansion states (Allen and Sommers, 2019).

An access barrier faced by people covered by Medicaid is finding a physician. In most states, Medicaid pays physicians far less than does Medicare or private insurance with the result that many physicians limit the number of Medicaid patients they accept (see Chapter 2). Medicaid patients such as Maria Buenasuerte and Conception Ortiz often depend on community health centers for their care.

Who Are the Uninsured and Why Are They Uninsured?

Norris, a shipyard worker in Miami, was laid off in 2018 at age 55 and was unable to get another job. When he became unemployed and lost his employer-sponsored private insurance, he was ineligible for Medicaid because Florida had not expanded eligibility under the ACA and continued to limit Medicaid to adults who are parents of dependent children, older than 65, or disabled. Because his income is below the Federal Poverty Level, he is not eligible for ACA private insurance subsidies and is uninsured.

Morris has worked full-time for a corner grocery store in Jacksonville, Florida that employs five people. Morris once asked the owner whether the employees could receive health insurance, but the owner said it was too expensive to pay the insurance premium for Morris, his wife, and their daughter. Morris was excited when the ACA was passed and he learned that his family would be eligible for tax-subsidized private insurance in 2014. His excitement turned to chagrin when he found out that even with the subsidy, it would cost him $1,500 per month in premiums to enroll in a health plan that had a deductible below $5,000 per year. He decided to take his chances and pay the $900 ACA tax penalty and remain uninsured.

Morris's nephew Boris is an undocumented immigrant who delivers groceries at the same store. He is not eligible for ACA private insurance subsidies or Florida's Medicaid program.

The uninsured in 2017 included many low income individuals living in states not participating in Medicaid expansion, individuals opting out of the individual insurance mandate despite the tax penalty, individuals not enrolling in Medicaid even when eligible, and undocumented immigrants remaining ineligible for Medicaid and insurance subsidies. In 2017, 45% of uninsured adults said they were uninsured because premiums were too expensive; 77% of the uninsured had one or more full-time workers in the family (Kaiser Family Foundation, 2018a). Like Morris, the employed uninsured tended to be lower-wage workers at small firms. Twenty-five percent of the uninsured were unemployed, often with incomes below the poverty line but, like Norris, ineligible for Medicaid in many states.

Insurance coverage differs by race-ethnicity and socioeconomic status. In 2017, 6% of non-Latino whites were uninsured, compared with 11% of African Americans, 7% of Asians, and 16% of Latinos (Fig. 3–2). Fourteen percent of individuals with annual household incomes less than $25,000 were uninsured, compared with 4% of individuals with household incomes of $125,000 or more (Fig. 3–3) (U.S. Census Bureau, 2018).

▶ Underinsurance

Insurance coverage clearly makes a difference for access to care. But not all health insurance plans make health care affordable to individuals and families. Many people with insurance are underinsured, which means that their health insurance coverage has limitations that expose them to large amounts of out of pocket payments that can discourage access to needed services and saddle individuals with large medical bills. In 2007, 62% of bankruptcies in the United States were caused by inability to pay medical bills; 75% of these individuals had health insurance at the onset of their illness (Himmelstein et al., 2009). According to one commonly used framework, a person who is insured for an entire year and meets any of the following three criteria is considered underinsured: (1) out-of-pocket costs, excluding share of insurance premiums, equals 10% or more of income; (2) out-of-pocket costs, excluding premiums, equals 5% or more of income if low-income (<200% of poverty); or (3) deductibles equal 5% or more of income (Commonwealth Fund, 2017b). Based on this definition, between 2003 and 2016, the percent of insured adults ages 19–64 who were underinsured grew from 12% to 28%, amounting to 41 million people. For those below 200% of the Federal Poverty Level the underinsured rate was 44%. Almost half of the underinsured reported going without needed care in the past year because of cost (Commonwealth Fund, 2017a, 2017b).

There are two main reasons why even when they have health insurance, some people may face very high out of pocket expenses: (1) uncovered categories of services, and (2) high cost-sharing in the form of deductibles and copayments for covered services. (Table 3–2).

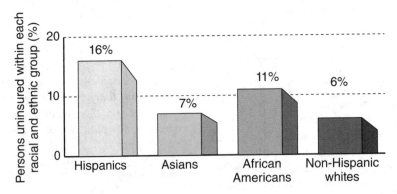

▲ **Figure 3–2.** Lack of health insurance by race and ethnicity in 2017 (From U.S. Census Bureau. *Health Insurance Coverage in the United States, 2017.* September 2018).

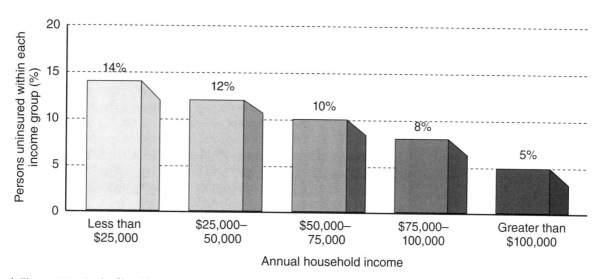

▲ **Figure 3–3.** Lack of health insurance by income in 2017 (From U.S. Census Bureau. *Health Insurance Coverage in the United States, 2017. September 2018*).

Table 3–2. Categories of underinsurance

1. Uncovered services
   Long-term care under Medicare
   Durable medical equipment under some insurance plans
   Caps on coverage such as limited physical therapy visits
   Restricted benefits from "limited benefits" insurance plans exempted from ACA requirements
2. Insurance deductibles and copayments

Uncovered Services

Victoria and Gus Pappas had $80,000 in the bank when Gus had a stroke. After his hospitalization, he was still paralyzed on the right side and unable to speak or swallow. After 18 months in the nursing home, most of the $80,000 was gone. At that point, Medicaid picked up the nursing home costs.

A glaring example of an uncovered category of service is the extremely limited benefits under Medicare for nursing home care and other long-term care expenses. As noted in Chapter 2, Medicare pays for a short duration of rehabilitative services at a long-term care facility following an acute hospitalization, but does not cover extended care. As a result, many elderly families

spend their life savings on long-term care, qualifying for Medicaid only after becoming impoverished (see Chapter 12).

Historically, private insurance varied widely from policy to policy in what services were covered, with some policies excluding maternity benefits, preventive care, mental health services, or other categories of services. Many plans also had a lifetime limit on the amount of total payments per insured person, often capped at $500,000. Individuals with severe forms of cancer or newborns with complications of prematurity would often reach the lifetime cap, exposing individuals and families to the entire costs of care after exhausting their insurance benefits. Many of the cases of bankruptcy due to medical expenses in the study cited above included insured individuals with costs exceeding lifetime caps. The ACA contained measures to limit many of these restrictions of covered services by private health plans, including prohibiting lifetime caps on payments. The ACA also required all private plans to meet a national standard for covered benefits which includes maternity care, family planning, and preventive services, among others. However, not all insurance plans cover equipment needed by people who are permanently or temporarily disabled, such as wheelchairs, hospital beds, or oxygen equipment.

Insurance Deductibles and Copayments

The terms deductible, copayment, and coinsurance were defined in Chapter 2 as different forms of cost-sharing. Cost-sharing is a prominent element of employment-based private insurance, the individual insurance plans offered through the federal and state "exchanges" established by the ACA, and Medicare.

Individual private insurance

Jim Underwood is a self-employed painter with diabetes and hypertension who purchased individual insurance on the Colorado ACA marketplace. Because he receives a government subsidy for his premiums he was able to afford a silver plan, but his annual deductible is $4,000 with a $20 copay for doctor visits and medications. He tries to take his four daily medications faithfully, but some months he lacks the funds to purchase refills.

Although the ACA reduced uncovered services, it had the opposite effect on cost-sharing by institutionalizing high deductible plans in the individual insurance market. People buying individual coverage choose among bronze, silver, gold, and platinum plans. Bronze plans have lower premiums and higher out-of-pocket costs, platinum plans have higher premiums and lower out-of-pocket costs. The average Bronze plan monthly premium in 2019 was $339 (increasing with age); with a federal subsidy the premium might cost only $70. The plan requires people to pay 40% of medical costs after the deductible is met. The average Bronze plan deductible in 2018 was $6,000 for an individual and $12,000 for a family. The average 2019 Silver plan monthly premium without subsidy was $452. The 2018 average Silver plan deductible was $4,000 for an individual and $8,000 for a family with a copay around $30 for primary care and $60 for a specialist visit. Eighty-five percent of people enrolling for insurance under the state and federal marketplaces chose Bronze or Silver plans. While individuals and families enrolling in ACA individual insurance are no longer *un*insured, most, like Jim Underwood, find themselves seriously *under*insured due to the high out-of-pocket costs required in Bronze and Silver plans.

Employment-based private insurance

High cost-sharing is not only a feature of individual insurance plans. For people receiving health insurance from their employer, 81% must pay an annual deductible; the average 2018 deductible for a single employee working at a large firm was $1,355 and $2,132 for workers at small firms. These are costs over and above the employee's share of the insurance premium. Since 2013 the average deductible for employed workers has increased by 53%. Most employed workers also pay an average of 19% of the cost of a hospital admission and a $25 copay for a primary care visit ($40 for a specialist visit). In addition, purchasing medications requires a copay (Fig. 3–4) (Claxton et al., 2018).

Heidi Bauer worked at a Swiss bakery which offered employees and their families only a high-deductible health plan with a savings option. The employer paid $10,000 for the premium and $1,500 for a medical savings account that Heidi and her family could use to assist with medical expenses. Heidi paid $6,000 for the premium and faced a deductible of $5,000 plus 40% of physician fees when she needed health care. She could use the $1,500 in the savings account to help get care for which she had to pay.

Some employers sponsor health savings accounts in an attempt to mitigate somewhat the financial burden employees bear under high deductible insurance plans. In 2018, 28% of employer-based health insurance plans were high-deductible plans with a savings option. Many employers, like Heidi's, offered only a high-deductible plan to their employees (Claxton et al., 2018). For small businesses like Heidi's, 50% of these plans had a deductible of $6,000 or more. The medical savings accounts that accompany these plans are funded by the employer; for small firms, employer contributions average about $1,500 with about 30% of firms paying nothing (Kaiser Family Foundation, 2017).

Medicare

Ferdinand Foote was covered by Medicare and had no supplemental private "Medigap" insurance or Medicaid coverage. He was hospitalized for peripheral vascular disease caused by diabetes and a nonhealing infected foot ulcer. He spent 4 days in the acute hospital and 1 month in the skilled nursing facility and made weekly physician visits

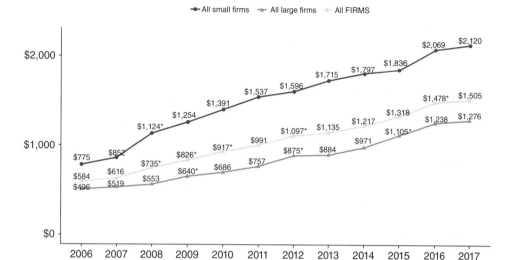

▲ Figure 3–4. Average general annual health plan deductible for single coverage, by firm size, 2006 to 2017. (From Kaiser Family Foundation and Health Research and Educational Trust. Employer Health Benefits 2017 Annual Survey. 2017. www.kff.org/health-costs/report/2017-employer-health-benefits-survey/.)

following his discharge. The costs of illness not covered by Medicare included a $1,364 deductible for acute hospital care, a $170.50 per day copayment for days 21 to 30 of the skilled nursing facility stay, a $185 physician deductible, and a 20% ($20) physician copayment per visit for 12 visits. The total came to $3,494, not including Mr. Foote's copayments under his Medicare Part D drug plan for the medications he was prescribed to take after leaving the hospital.

As discussed in Chapter 2, Medicare paid for only 58% of the average beneficiary's health care expenses in 2012. In 2013, average out of pocket sending by Medicare beneficiaries consumed 41% of their Social Security income. Half of Medicare beneficiaries in 2013 had an income below $26,200 (Kaiser Family Foundation, 2018b). In 2017, the average beneficiary in good health spent $7,600 out-of-pocket while average beneficiaries with a chronic disease such as diabetes or heart failure spent $10-12,000. These out of pocket expenses include premiums, deductibles, copayments, and uncovered services as explained in Chapter 2. Thus, Medicare beneficiaries without Medicare Advantage, supplemental insurance, or Medicaid (see Chapter 2) continue to have large out-of-pocket expenses that often limit their access to care.

The Effects of Underinsurance

Does underinsurance represent a serious barrier to the receipt of medical care? The Rand Health Insurance Experiment compared nonelderly individuals who had health insurance plans with no out-of-pocket costs and those who had plans with varying amounts of patient cost sharing (deductibles or copayments). The study found that cost sharing reduces the rate of ambulatory care use, especially among the poor, and that patients with cost-sharing plans demonstrate a reduction in both appropriate and inappropriate medical visits. For low-income adults, the cost-sharing groups received Pap smears 65% as often as the free-care group. Hypertensive adults in the cost-sharing groups had higher diastolic pressures, and children had higher rates of anemia and lower rates of immunization (Brook et al., 1983; Lohr et al., 1986; Lurie et al., 1987). In 2016, 52% of underinsured adults had at least one cost-related access problem, for example not seeing a doctor when sick; skipping a recommended test, treatment, or follow-up; not getting needed specialist care; or not filling a prescription (Commonwealth Fund, 2017b). Underinsured adolescents have lower rates of vaccination coverage than the fully insured (Smith et al., 2009). In 2012, 19% of Medicare beneficiaries over 65 experienced at least one cost-related access problem during the year—not seeing a doctor, not seeking recommended medical tests, not filling prescriptions, or skipping doses of pills (Cubanski and Boccuti, 2015). In summary, lack of comprehensive insurance reduces access to health care services and may contribute to poorer health outcomes.

► Trends in Insurance Coverage in the United States

Historically, trends in health insurance coverage in the United States in the modern era can be divided into three phases. The first phase, occurring between the 1930s and mid-1970s, saw a large increase in the proportion of Americans with health insurance due to the growth of employment-based private health insurance and the 1965 passage of Medicare and Medicaid. The second phase marks a reversal of this trend; between 1980 and 2010, the number of uninsured people in the United States grew from 25 to 50 million due to a sharp decrease in the number of people with private health insurance. The number of uninsured peaked in 2010—the year the ACA was signed into law—signifying the onset of the third phase in this historical trend (Fig. 3–1). The number of uninsured decreased from 50 to 28 million between 2010 and 2017 following implementation of the ACA's private insurance mandates and voluntary state Medicaid expansion (Carman et al., 2015; US Census Bureau, 2018).

Two key factors—increasing health care costs and a changing labor force—explain the rise in the number of uninsured that occurred in the second phase and gave impetus to enacting insurance expansion under the ACA that ushered in phase 3. From 2000 to 2018, employer-sponsored family health insurance premiums rose from $6,500 to $19,600. For individual employee coverage, the increase went from $2,500 to $6,900. Most employers shifted more of the cost of health insurance premiums and health services onto their employees, resulting in employees dropping health coverage because of unaffordability. In 2018 the average employee paid 29% of the employer-sponsored family premium and 18% of an individual premium; some paid as much as 42%. Low-income workers have been hit especially hard by the combination of rising insurance costs and declining employer

contributions as a share of total premium amount (Claxton et al., 2018).

Simultaneously, the economy in the United States has undergone a major transition. The number of highly paid, largely unionized, manufacturing workers with employer-sponsored health insurance has declined, and the workforce has shifted toward more low-wage, nonunionized service and clerical workers whose employers are less likely to provide insurance. Between 1960 and 2016, the percentage of workers in manufacturing decreased from 30% to 8% of all nonfarm workers while service sector employment rose from 65% to 80%. From 1957 to 2010, the percentage of workers with part-time jobs—generally without health benefits—increased from 12% to 20%.

These same factors have driven the growing prevalence of underinsurance among the insured. The rapidly rising cost of health insurance led employers to increase employee share of premium costs and to migrate to high deductible plans. The employee share of coverage is larger in small compared with large firms. Cost pressures influenced the decision to include high deductible Bronze and Silver plans in the ACA individual insurance marketplace. (We discuss health care costs in more detail in Chapter 8; in Chapter 14 we address how the United States is an international outlier in the proportion of residents without adequate insurance.)

The United States may be heading into a fourth historical phase with an uptick in the number of uninsured in 2017. The combination of relentless insurance premium increases, plus efforts by the Trump Administration and Congressional allies to undo the ACA, appear to be ushering in a new phase of rising uninsurance (Pear, 2019). As noted in Chapter 2, some states are also tightening eligibility for Medicaid, such as by imposing work requirements or premium payments.

The Instability of Health Insurance

Jean Irons worked for Bethlehem Steel as a clerk and her benefits included health insurance. Bethlehem Steel was bought by a global corporation and her plant moved to another country. In 2011 she found a job as a food service worker in a small restaurant. Her pay decreased by 35%, and the restaurant did not provide health insurance.

Sally Lewis worked as a receptionist in a physician's office. She received health insurance through her husband, who was a construction worker. They got divorced, she lost her health insurance, and her physician employer told her that he could not provide her with health insurance because of the cost.

John Childs was a single father caring for his 3-year old daughter in Arkansas. The state told him he needed to work to keep his Medicaid benefits, which was impossible because there were no jobs in town and he couldn't afford childcare. He lost his Medicaid and became uninsured.

When examining trends in the number of uninsured, it is important to understand that the number is dynamic. Individuals cycle through periods of having and losing insurance. One of the distinguishing features of the US approach to health care financing is not only the lack of universal coverage, but also the instability of coverage. The link of group private insurance with employment inevitably produces interruptions in coverage because of the unstable nature of employment. People who are laid off from their jobs or who leave jobs because of illness lose their insurance. Family members insured through the workplace of a spouse may lose their insurance in cases of divorce, job loss, or death of the working family member. Some sign up for individual insurance through the ACA but face higher deductibles and copays. The often transient nature of employment-linked insurance is compounded by difficulties in maintaining eligibility for Medicaid. Unemployed individuals who become employed may lose their Medicaid benefits even when their earnings are well below a living wage. The net result is that many people cycle in and out of the ranks of the uninsured every month.

NONFINANCIAL BARRIERS TO HEALTH CARE

Nonfinancial barriers to health care include inability to access care when needed, language, literacy, and cultural differences between patients and health caregivers, and factors of gender and race/ethnicity. Excellent discussions of these issues can be found in the book *Medical Management of Vulnerable and Underserved Patients* (King & Wheeler, 2016).

▶ Lack of Prompt Access

Medical practices often fail to provide their patients with access at the time when the patient needs care. This problem has worsened with the growing shortage of primary care physicians. In 2016, half of Americans reported that they were unable to obtain a same or next-day appointment when they needed it, and only 39% received after-hours care without going to the emergency department (Schneider et al., 2017).

▶ Access and Women's Health

Olga Madden is angry. Her male physician had not listened. He told her that her incontinence was from too many childbirths and that she would have to live with it. She had questions about the hormones he was prescribing, but he never seemed interested so she never asked. Ms. Madden calls her insurance plan and gets the names of two female physicians, a female physician assistant, and a nurse practitioner. Their receptionists tell her that none of them is accepting new patients; they are all too busy.

Access problems for women begin with finding a physician who provides women's health services. Forty-four percent of internists do not provide Pap smears (Cooper & Saraiya, 2014). Forty percent of reproductive age women have not been counseled on contraception with a care provider, 70% lack counseling on sexually transmitted infections, and 77% have not been counseled on domestic violence (Salganicoff et al., 2014). Contraceptive counseling is often provided with inadequate information and lack of patient-centered communication (Dehlendorf et al., 2014). Many women's health providers are poorly informed about emergency contraception and almost one in five practitioners are reluctant to provide this education to sexually active adolescents. Women who are poor, foreign born, or who are not high school graduates are less likely to learn about emergency contraception (American College of Obstetricians and Gynecologists, 2015).

In previous studies, women were more than twice as likely to report that their physician "talked down" to them or told them their problems were "all in their head" (Leiman et al., 1997). Even though more women than men die of cardiovascular disease in the United States each year, a large body of evidence has documented undertreatment and undertesting of women for cardiovascular disease, resulting in higher case fatality rates for women. Women are less likely than men to be diagnosed as having a heart attack (Bairey Merz, 2014).

While women have reduced access to certain kinds of care, an equally serious problem may be instances of inappropriate care. Studies have found that between 16% and 70% of hysterectomies are inappropriate and that 38% of women undergoing hysterectomy for benign indications were not counseled on alternative, nonsurgical treatments (Corona et al., 2015).

▶ Race/Ethnicity and Access to Health Care

Jose is suffering. The pain from his fractured femur is excruciating, and the emergency department physician has given him no pain medication. In the next room, Joe is resting comfortably. He has received 10 mg of morphine for his femur fracture.

At a California emergency department, 55% of Latino patients with extremity fractures received no pain medication compared with 26% of non-Latino whites. This marked difference in treatment was attributable not to insurance status but to ethnicity (Todd et al., 1993). African-American patients similarly received poorer pain control than whites (Todd et al., 2000).

Because a far higher proportion of minorities than whites is uninsured, has Medicaid coverage, or is poor, access problems are amplified for these groups. In 2016, African American, Latino, Asian, and American Indian adults were twice as likely as whites to report difficulty obtaining a timely medical appointment for illness or injury. Analyzing a group of quality measures in 2014–16, African Americans received worse care than whites for 40% of these quality measures and Latinos and American Indians received worse care than whites for about one-third of the indicators. While some inequities in access and quality, such as adolescent immunization rates, have decreased over the past 15 years, others have widened, such as disparities in blood pressure control among African Americans

relative to other groups (U.S. Agency for Healthcare Research and Quality, 2017). Overall, there has been a clear lack of progress on health equity over the past 25 years (Zimmerman and Anderson, 2019).

Neighborhoods that have high proportions of African-American or Latino residents have far fewer physicians practicing in these communities. African-American and Latino primary care physicians are more likely than white physicians to locate their practices in underserved communities (Komaromy et al., 1996; Marrast et al., 2014).

What explains these disparities in access to care across racial and ethnic groups that are not fully accounted for by differences in insurance coverage and socioeconomic status? Several hypotheses have been proposed. Cultural differences may exist in patients' beliefs about the value of medical care and attitudes toward seeking treatment for their symptoms. However, differences in patient preferences do not account for substantial amounts of the racial variations seen in cardiac surgery rates (Mayberry et al., 2000). Access barriers related to communication problems may be particularly acute for the subset of Latino patients for whom Spanish is the primary language. However, language issues do not fully account for access barriers faced by Latinos. In the study of emergency department pain medication cited previously, even Latinos who spoke English as their primary language were much less likely than non-Latino whites to receive pain medication.

Because many of these hypotheses do not satisfactorily explain the observed racial and ethnic disparities in access to care, an important consideration is whether racism may also contribute to these patterns (King & Wheeler, 2016). Medicine in the United States has not escaped the nation's legacy of institutionalized racism toward many minority groups. Many hospitals, including institutions in the North, were for much of the twentieth century either completely segregated or had segregated wards, with inferior facilities and services available to nonwhites. Explicit segregation policies persisted in many hospitals until a few decades ago. Racial barriers to entry into the medical profession gave rise to the establishment of historically black medical schools such as the Howard, Morehouse, and Meharry schools of medicine. Although such overt racism is a diminishing feature of medicine in the United States, more insidious forms of structural and implicit discrimination may continue to color the interactions between patients and their caregivers. For example, African American and other ethnic minority patients receive poorer interpersonal communication with physicians, including greater physician verbal dominance, less patient-centeredness, and shorter visits, compared with white patients (Martin et al., 2013).

THE RELATION BETWEEN HEALTH CARE AND HEALTH STATUS

Access to health care does not by itself guarantee good health. A complex array of factors, only one of which is health care, determines whether a person is healthy or not.

Ace Banks is 48, an executive vice president, with four grandparents who lived past 90 years of age and parents alive and well in their late 70s. Mr. Banks went to an Ivy League college where he was a star athlete. He has never seen a physician except for a sprained ankle.

Keith Cole is a coal miner who at age 48 developed pneumonia. He had excellent health insurance through his union and went to see the leading pulmonologist in the state. He was hospitalized but became less and less able to breathe because the pneumonia was severely complicated by black lung disease, which he contracted through his job. He received high-quality care in the intensive care unit at a fully insured cost of $195,000, but he died.

Bill Downes, an African-American man, knew that his father was killed by high blood pressure and his mother died of diabetes. Mr. Downes spent his childhood in poverty living with eight children at his grandmother's house. He had little to eat except what was provided at the school lunch program, a diet heavily laden with cheese and butter. To support the family, he left school at age 15 and got a job. At age 24, he was diagnosed with high blood pressure and diabetes. He did not smoke and was meticulous in following the diet prescribed by his physician. He had private health insurance through his job as a security guard and was cared for by a professor of medicine at the medical school. In spite of excellent medical care, his glucose and cholesterol levels and blood pressure were

difficult to control, and he developed retinopathy, kidney failure, and coronary heart disease. At age 48, he collapsed at work and died of a heart attack.

Health Status and Income

The gap between the rich and the poor has widened markedly in the United States. The top 10% of earners received 50% of the nation's total income in 2017 compared with 33% in 1965 (Saez, 2019). The top 10% also control three-quarters of all the wealth in the United States (Khullar and Chokshi, 2018). Household income for the average family has stagnated (Khullar and Chokshi, 2018). As the stories of Ace Banks, Keith Cole, and Bill Downes suggest, the health of an individual or a population is influenced less by medical care than by broad socioeconomic factors such as income and education (Braveman & Gottlieb, 2014). People in the United States with incomes above four times the poverty level live on average 7 years longer than those with incomes below the poverty level (Table 3–3). In 2014, life expectancy for 40-year-old men was 10 years greater for those in the top income quartile than those in the bottom quartile; for women the difference was 6 years (Chetty et al., 2016). Poor adults are five times more likely to report being in poor or fair health than those with incomes above 400% of the federal poverty level. Low-income Americans have higher rates of physical limitation and of heart disease, stroke, and diabetes. Middle aged persons in the highest quintile of wealth had a

Table 3–3. Income, race, and life expectancy in years (at age 25)[a]

Race	Income as Percent of Federal Poverty Level (FPL)			
	≤100% FPL	101–200% FPL	201–400% FPL	≥401% FPL
Black	45.5	48.0	50.7	52.6
White	49.0	51.4	53.8	55.8

[a]Life expectancy in years indicates the average additional years of life expected for individuals in each group at age 25 and is calculated from data in the National Mortality Longitudinal Survey, 1988–1998 as reported in Braveman PA et al. Socioeconomic disparities in health in the United States: What the patterns tell us. *Am J Public Health.* 2010;100:S186–S196.

5% chance of dying and 15% chance of becoming disabled over the next decade compared with those in the lowest wealth quintile who had a 17% chance of dying and 48% chance of becoming disabled (Khullar and Chokshi, 2018). Age-adjusted male cancer mortality is 43% greater for men below the federal poverty level (FPL) than for those above 600% of FPL; for women the disparity is 26%. Fifty-eight percent of people in the highest income decile survive their cancer for at least 12 years compared with 39% for those in the lowest income decile (Singh and Jemal, 2017).

▶ Health Status and Race

African Americans experience worse health than white Americans. Life expectancy is lower for African Americans than for whites (Table 3–4). In 2017, infant mortality rates among African Americans were more than double those for whites (Table 3–5). Mortality rates for African Americans exceed those for whites for 7 of the 10 leading causes of death in the United States, including the most common killers in the US population—heart disease, strokes, and cancer (Table 3–6) (U.S. Department of Health and Human Services, 2017). African-American men between 45 and 54 years of age have three times the mortality rate from stroke caused by hypertension than white men of the same age group (U.S. Department of Health and Human Services, 2013). Although the incidence of breast cancer is lower in African-American women

Table 3–4. Life expectancy at birth in years

In 1950	Women	Men
White	72.2	66.5
African American	62.9	59.1
In 2012		
White	81.2	76.5
African American	78.1	71.9
In 2016		
White	81.0	76.1
African American	77.9	71.5

Source: US Department of Health and Human Services. *Health United States* 2017. www.cdc.gov.

Table 3–5. Infant mortality, 2015 (per 1,000 live births)

White, non-Latino	4.90
African American	11.25
Latino	4.96
Asian or Pacific Islander	4.08
American Indian or Alaska Native	8.58

Source: US Department of Health and Human Services. *Health United States* 2017. www.cdc.gov.

Table 3–6. Age-adjusted death rates per 100,000 population, 2016

	White	African American
Malignant neoplasms (cancer)	156.6	177.9
Coronary heart disease	94.8	108.3
Stroke	36.1	50.5

Source: US Department of Health and Human Services. *Health United States* 2017. www.cdc.gov.

than in white women, in African-American women this disease is diagnosed at a more advanced stage of illness, and thus they are more likely to die of breast cancer (U.S. Agency for Healthcare Research and Quality, 2014). American Indians are another ethnic group with far poorer health than that of whites; the American Indian infant mortality rate is 75% higher than the rate of whites; and diabetes mortality is 360% that of whites (U.S. Department of Health and Human Services, 2017; Cho et al., 2014).

Latinos and Asians and Pacific Islanders are minority groups characterized by great diversity. Health status varies widely between Cuban Americans, who tend to be more affluent, and poor Mexican American migrant farm workers, as well as between Japanese families, who are more likely to be middle class, and Laotians, many of whom live in poverty. Compared with whites, Latinos have markedly higher death rates for diabetes. Overall, Latinos have lower age-adjusted mortality rates than whites because of less cardiovascular disease and cancer. Asians in the United States have lower death rates than whites (U.S. Department of Health and Human Services, 2013).

Some of the differences in mortality rates of African Americans and American Indians compared with whites are related to the higher rates of poverty among these minority groups. In 2017, the white poverty rate was 8% compared with 20% for African Americans, 24% for Latinos, and 22% for American Indians (Kaiser Family Foundation, 2019). However, even compared with whites in the same income class, African Americans as a group have inferior health status. Although mortality rates decline with rising income among both African Americans and whites, at any given income level, the mortality rate for African Americans is consistently higher than the rate for whites (Table 3–3). Thus, social factors and stresses related to race itself seem to contribute to the relatively poorer health of African Americans in addition to factors as lower income. The inferior health outcomes among African Americans, such as higher mortality rates for heart disease, cancer, and stroke, are also in part explained by the lower rate of access to health services among this group.

If lower income is associated with poorer health, and if Latinos tend to be poorer than non-Latino whites in the United States, then why do Latinos have overall lower mortality rates than non-Latino whites? The question is debated and may be related to foreign-born people having lower mortality rates than people born in the United States at the same level of income (Barcellos et al., 2012; Goel et al., 2004). This phenomenon is often referred to as the "healthy immigrant" effect. If this is the case, mortality rates for Latinos may rise as a higher proportion of their population is born in the United States.

CONCLUSION

Health outcomes are determined by multiple factors. Social determinants powerfully influence health status; yet health care and public health interventions are also important. The advent of effective medications to treat HIV infection dramatically improved life expectancy and quality of life for millions of people across the globe. From 1970 to 2016, age-adjusted death rates in the United States from stroke decreased by over 150%—a successful result of hypertension diagnosis and treatment (U.S. Department of Health and Human Services, 2017). Early prenatal care can prevent low–birth-weight and infant deaths. The health care system provides patients with chronic disease welcome relief from pain and suffering and helps them to cope with their illnesses. In the United States, having no insurance or being underinsured makes health care unaffordable to many people and inhibits their ability to access care when needed. Access to health care does not guarantee good health, but without such access, health is certain to suffer.

REFERENCES

Agency for Healthcare Quality and Research. 2014. National Healthcare Quality and Disparities Report. Available at www.rootcausecoalition.org/wp-content/uploads/2017/07/2014-National-Healthcare-Quality-and-Disparities-Report.pdf. Accessed November 11, 2019.

Agency for Healthcare Quality and Research. 2017. National Healthcare Quality and Disparities Report. Available at https://www.ahrq.gov/research/findings/nhqrdr/nhqdr17/index.html. Accessed September 20, 2019.

Allen H, Sommers BD. Medicaid expansion and health. *JAMA*. 2019, September 6.

American College of Obstetricians and Gynecologists. Emergency Contraception. Practice Bulletin 152, 2015. Available at www.acog.org/-/media/Practice-Bulletins/Committee-on-Practice-Bulletins----Gynecology/Public/pb152. Accessed September 20, 2019.

Ayanian JZ, et al. Unmet needs of uninsured adults in the United States. *JAMA*. 2000;284:2061–2069.

Baicker K, et al. The Oregon experiment—effects of Medicaid on clinical outcomes. *N Engl J Med*. 2013;368:1713–1722.

Bairey Merz CN. Sex, death and the diagnosis gap. *Circulation*. 2014;130:740–742.

Barcellos SH, et al. Undiagnosed disease, especially diabetes, casts doubt on some of reported health "advantage" of recent Mexican immigrants. *Health Aff (Millwood)*. 2012;31:2727–2737.

Braveman P, Gottlieb L. The social determinants of health: it's time to consider the causes of the causes. *Public Health Rep*. 2014;129(suppl 2):19–31.

Brook RH, et al. Does free care improve adults' health? Results from a randomized controlled trial. *N Engl J Med*. 1983;309:1426–1434.

Carman KG, et al. Trends in health insurance enrollment, 2013–15. *Health Aff (Millwood)*. 2015;34:1044–1048.

Chetty R, et al. The association between income and life expectancy in the United States, 2001–2004. *JAMA*. 2016;316:1750–1766.

Cho P, et al. Diabetes-related mortality among American Indians and Alaska Natives, 1990–2009. *Am J Public Health*. 2014;104:S496–S503.

Claxton G, et al. Health benefits in 2018: modest growth in premiums, higher worker contributions at firms with more low-wage workers. *Health Aff (Millwood)*. 2018;37:1892–1900.

Commonwealth Fund. Underinsured rate increased sharply in 2016. October 2017a. Available at www.commonwealthfund.org/.../underinsured-rate-increased-sharply-2016-mo. Accessed September 20, 2019.

Commonwealth Fund. How well does insurance coverage protect consumers from health care costs? November 2017b. Available at www.commonwealthfund.org/publications/issue-briefs/2017/oct/how-well-does-insurance-coverage-protect-consumers-health-care. Accessed September 20, 2019.

Cooper CP, Saraiya M. Opting out of cervical cancer screening. *Am J Prev Med*. 2014;47:315–319.

Corona LE, et al. Use of other treatments before hysterectomy for benign conditions in a statewide hospital collaborative. *Am J Obstet Gynecol*. 2015;212:304.e1–e7.

Cubanski J, Boccuti C. Medicare coverage, affordability, and access. *Generations*. 2015;39:26–34.

Dehlendorf C, et al. Contraceptive counseling: best practices to ensure quality communication and enable effective contraceptive use. *Clin Obstet Gynecol*. 2014;57:659–673.

Goel MS, et al. Obesity among US immigrant subgroups by duration of residence. *JAMA*. 2004;292:2860–2867.

Himmelstein DU, et al. Medical bankruptcy in the United States, 2007. Results of a national study. *Am J Med*. 2009;122:741–746.

Kaiser Commission on Medicaid and the Uninsured. *Medicaid Moving Forward*. Kaiser Family Foundation; 2015. Available at www.kff.org/health-reform/issue-brief/medicaid-moving-forward/. Accessed September 20, 2019.

Kaiser Family Foundation. *Poverty Rate by Race/Ethnicity*. 2019. Available at https://www.kff.org/other/state-indicator/poverty-rate-by-raceethnicity/?currentTimeframe=0&sortModel=%7B%22colId%22:%22Location%22,%22sort%22:%22asc%22%7D. Accessed September 20, 2019.

Kaiser Family Foundation and Health Research and Educational Trust. *Employer Health Benefits*. 2017. Available at www.kff.org/health-costs/report/2017-employer-health-benefits-survey/. Accessed September 20, 2019.

Kaiser Family Foundation. *Key Facts about the Uninsured Population*. December 2018a. Available at www.kff.org/uninsured/fact-sheet/key-facts-about-the-uninsured-population/. Accessed September 20, 2019.

Kaiser Family Foundation. *Medicare Beneficiaries' Out-of-Pocket Health Care Spending as a Share of Income Now and Projections for the Future*. January 26, 2018b. Available at www.kff.org/medicare/report/medicare-beneficiaries-out-of-pocket-health-care-spending-as-a-share-of-income-now-and-projections-for-the-future/. Accessed September 20, 2019.

Khullar D, Chokshi DA. Health, income and poverty: where we are and what could help. Health Affairs Policy Brief, October 4, 2018.

King TE, Wheeler MB. *Medical Management of Vulnerable and Underserved Patients*. New York, NY: McGraw-Hill; 2016.

Komaromy M, et al. The role of black and Hispanic physicians in providing health care for underserved populations. *N Engl J Med*. 1996;334:1305–1310.

Landon BE, et al. Quality of care in Medicaid managed care and commercial health plans. *JAMA*. 2007;298:1674–1681.

Leiman JM, et al. *Selected Facts on U.S. Women's Health: A Chart Book*. New York: The Commonwealth Fund; 1997.

Lohr KN, et al. Use of medical care in the Rand Health Insurance Experiment. Diagnosis-and service-specific analyses in a randomized controlled trial. *Med Care*. 1986;24(suppl 9):S1–S87.

Lurie N, et al. Preventive care: Do we practice what we preach? *Am J Public Health*. 1987;77:801–804.

Marrast LM, et al. Minority physicians' role in the care of underserved patients: diversifying the physician workforce may be key in addressing health disparities. *JAMA Int Med*. 2014;174:289–291.

Martin KD, et al. Physician communication behaviors and trust among black and white patients with hypertension. *Med Care*. 2013;51:151–157.

Mayberry RM, et al. Racial and ethnic differences in access to medical care. *Med Care Res Rev*. 2000;57(suppl 1):108–145.

Pear R. Trump officials broaden attack on health law, arguing courts should repeal all of it. *New York Times*, March 25, 2019.

Saez E. Striking it richer: the evolution of top incomes in the United States. UC Berkeley, 2019. https://eml.berkeley.edu › ~saez › saez-UStopincomes-2017. Accessed September 20, 2019.

Salganicoff, et al. *Women and Health Care in the Early Years of the Affordable Care Act*. Kaiser Family Foundation; 2014. Available at www.kff.org/womens-health-policy/report/women-and-health-care-in-the-early-years-of-the-aca-key-findings-from-the-2013-kaiser-womens-health-survey/. Accessed September 20, 2019.

Schneider EC, et al. Mirror, Mirror 2017: International Comparison Reflects Flaws and Opportunities for Better U.S.

Health Care. Commonwealth Fund, July 2017. Available at www.commonwealthfund.org/.../fund.../mirror-mirror-2017-international-com. Accessed September 20, 2019.

Singh GK, Jemal A. Socioeconomic and racial/ethnic disparities in cancer mortality, incidence, and survival in the United States, 1950–2014. *J Environ Public Health.* 2017;2017:2819372.

Smith PJ, et al. Underinsurance and adolescent immunization delivery in the United States. *Pediatrics.* 2009;124(suppl 5):S515–S521.

Todd KH, et al. Ethnicity as a risk factor for inadequate emergency department analgesia. *JAMA.* 1993;269:1537–1539.

Todd KH, et al. Ethnicity and analgesic practice. *Ann Emerg Med.* 2000;35:11–16.

U.S. Census Bureau. *Health Insurance Coverage in the United States, 2017.* September 2018. Available at www.census.gov/library/publications/2018/demo/p60-264.html. Accessed September 20, 2019.

U.S. Department of Health and Human Services. *Health United States, 2013.* Available at https://www.cdc.gov/nchs/data/hus/hus12.pdf. Accessed September 20, 2019.

Wilper AP, et al. Hypertension, diabetes, and elevated cholesterol among insured and uninsured U.S. adults. *Health Aff (Millwood).* 2009;28:1151–1159.

Woolhandler S, Himmelstein DU. The relationship of health insurance and mortality: is lack of insurance deadly? *Ann Intern Med.* 2017;167:424–431.

Zimmerman FJ, Anderson NW. Trends in health equity in the United States by race/ethnicity and income, 1993 – 2017. *JAMA Netw Open.* 2019;2(6):e196386.

Paying Health Care Providers

Chapter 2 described the different modes of financing health care: out-of-pocket payments, individual health insurance, employment-based health insurance, and government financing. Each of these mechanisms attempted to solve the problem of unaffordable care for certain groups, but each "solution" in turn created new problems by stimulating rapid rises in health care costs. One of the factors contributing to this inflation was the payment of physicians and hospitals by insurance companies and government programs. Currently, new methods of payment are being tried to lower the growth rate in health care costs.

Dr. Mary Young has recently finished her family medicine residency and joined a small group practice, PrimaryCare. On her first day, she has the following experiences with health care financing: her first patient is insured by Blue Shield; PrimaryCare is paid a fee for the physician encounter and for the electrocardiogram (ECG) performed. Dr. Young's second patient requires the same services, for which PrimaryCare receives no payment but is forwarded $30 for each month that the patient is enrolled in the practice. In the afternoon, a hospital utilization review physician calls Dr. Young, explains the diagnosis-related group (DRG) payment system, and suggests that she send home a patient hospitalized with pneumonia. In the evening, she goes to the emergency department, where she has agreed to work two shifts per week for $200 per hour. She was also delighted to read her email and find a notification of an automatic deposit in her bank account for providing high-quality care for her PrimaryCare patients.

During the course of a typical day, some physicians will be involved with four or five distinct types of payment. This chapter will describe the different ways in which physicians and hospitals are paid. Although payment has many facets, from the setting of prices to the processing of claims, this discussion will focus on one of its most basic elements: establishing the unit of payment. This basic principle must be grasped before one can understand the key concept of physician-borne risk.

UNITS OF PAYMENT

Methods of payment can be placed along a continuum that extends from the least to the most aggregated unit. The methods range from the simplest (one fee for one service rendered) to the most complex (one payment for many types of services rendered), with many variations in between (Table 4–1).

▶ Definitions of Methods of Payment

Fee-for-Service Payment

The unit of payment is the visit or procedure. The physician or hospital is paid a fee for each office visit, ECG, intravenous fluid, or other service or supply provided. This is the only form of payment that is based on individual components of health care. All other payment modes aggregate or group together several services into one unit of payment.

Table 4–1. Units of payment

	Least Aggregated Procedure	Day	Episode of Illness	Patient	Most Aggregated Time
Physician	Fee-for-service	—	Surgical or obstetric fee Physician DRG	Capitation	Salary
Hospital	Fee-for-service	Per diem	Hospital DRG	Capitation	Global budget

DRG, diagnosis-related group.

Episode-Based Payment

The physician or hospital is paid one sum for all services delivered during one illness or surgical procedure.

Per Diem Payments to Hospitals

The hospital is paid for all services delivered to a patient during 1 day in the hospital.

Capitation Payment

One payment is made for each patient's care during a month or year.

Payment for All Services Delivered to All Patients within a Certain Time Period

This includes global budget payment of hospitals and salaried payment of physicians.

▶ Managed Care Plans

Traditionally physicians and hospitals have been paid on a fee-for-service basis. The development of managed care plans introduced changes in the methods by which hospitals and physicians are paid, largely for the purpose of controlling costs. Managed care is discussed in more detail in Chapter 6; in this chapter, only those aspects needed to understand physician and hospital payment will be considered.

There are three major forms of managed care: fee-for-service practice with utilization review, preferred provider organizations (PPOs), and health maintenance organizations (HMOs).

Fee-for-Service Payment with Utilization Review

This is the traditional type of payment, with the addition that the third-party payer (whether private insurance company or government agency) assumes the power to authorize or deny payment for expensive medical interventions such as hospital admissions, extra hospital days, and surgeries.

Preferred Provider Organization Payment

With PPO insurance products, insurers contract with a limited number of physicians and hospitals who agree to care for patients, usually on a discounted fee-for-service or, for hospitals, a per diem basis, with utilization review (the insurer authorizing or denying payment for services deemed unnecessary). Patients with a PPO plan pay a much higher share of the cost when using physicians or hospitals outside the "preferred" network.

Health Maintenance Organization Payment

Patients with HMO insurance are required (except in emergencies) to receive their care from physicians and hospitals within that HMO. The types of HMOs are discussed in Chapter 6. Some HMOs pay physicians and hospitals by more highly bundled units of payment (e.g., capitation or salary).

METHODS OF PHYSICIAN PAYMENT

▶ Payment per Procedure: Fee-for-Service

Roy Singleton, a patient of Dr. Weisman, is seen for recent onset of diabetes. Dr. Weisman spends 20 minutes performing an examination, finger-stick blood glucose test, urinalysis, and ECG. Each service has a fee set by Dr. Weisman: $100 for a visit, $10 for a finger-stick glucose test, $10 for a urinalysis, and $30 for an ECG. Because Mr. Singleton is uninsured, Dr. Weisman reduces the total bill from $150 to $100.

In 2018, Dr. Lenz, an ophthalmologist, requested that Dr. Weisman do a medical consultation for Gertrude Rales, who developed congestive heart failure and arrhythmias following cataract surgery. Dr. Weisman took 90 minutes to perform the consultation and was paid $120 by Medicare. Dr. Lenz had spent 90 minutes on the surgery plus pre- and postoperative care and received $900 from Medicare.

Melissa High, a Medicaid recipient, makes three visits to Dr. Weisman for hypertension. He bills Medicaid $120 for one complex visit and $60 each for two follow-up visits. Under the state's Medicaid fee schedule he is paid $30 per visit. Medicaid does not allow Dr. Weisman to bill Ms. High for the balance of his fees.

Dr. Weisman contracted with Blue Cross to care for its PPO patients at 70% of his normal fee. Rick Payne, a PPO patient, comes in with a severe headache and is found to have left arm weakness and hyperreflexia. Dr. Weisman is paid $84 for a complex visit. Before a magnetic resonance imaging (MRI) scan can be ordered, the PPO must be asked for authorization.

Traditionally, private physicians have been paid by patients and insurers through the fee-for-service mechanism. Physicians may discount their fees for uninsured or other patients in financial need. Private insurers, as well as Medicare and Medicaid in the early years, usually paid physicians according to the usual, customary, and reasonable (UCR) system, which allowed physicians a great deal of latitude in setting fees. As cost containment became more of a priority, the UCR approach to fees was largely supplanted by payer-determined fee schedules. An example of this is Melissa High's three visits, which incurred charges of $240 of which Medicaid paid only $90 ($30 per visit).

In the early 1990s, Medicare moved to a fee schedule determined by a resource-based relative-value scale (RBRVS). With this system, fees (which vary by geographic area) are set for each service by estimating the time, mental effort and judgment, technical skill, physical effort, and stress typically related to that service (Bodenheimer et al., 2007). The RBRVS system made a somewhat feeble attempt to correct the bias of physician payment that has historically paid for surgical and other procedures at a far higher rate than primary care and cognitive services; however, this bias persists. In 2018, primary care physician (PCP) Dr. Weisman received $120 for 90 minutes of his time while specialist Dr. Lenz received $900 for 90 minutes.

PPO-managed care plans often pay contracted physicians on a discounted fee-for-service basis and require prior authorization for expensive procedures.

With fee-for-service payments, physicians have an economic incentive to perform more services because more services bring in more payments (see Chapter 10). The fee-for-service incentive to provide more services has contributed to the rapid rise in health care costs in the United States (Relman, 2007; National Commission on Physician Payment Reform, 2013). Despite payment reform efforts since the 1980s, 95% of physician office payments in 2013 remained fee-for-service (Zuvekas & Cohen, 2016).

Payment per Episode of Illness

Dr. Nick Belli removes Tom Stone's gallbladder and is paid $1,300 by Blue Cross. Besides performing the cholecystectomy, Dr. Belli sees Mr. Stone three times in the hospital and twice in his office for postoperative visits. Because surgery is paid by means of a global fee, Dr. Belli may not bill separately for the visits, which are included in his $1,300 cholecystectomy fee.

Joan Cluster has had type 2 diabetes for 8 years with no complications or other illnesses. Dr. Violet Sweet used to bill diabetes patients a fee for each visit but is now practicing in a bundled payment pilot. She receives one payment for taking care of Ms. Cluster's diabetes for 1 year.

Surgeons usually receive a single payment for several services (the surgery itself and postoperative care) that have been grouped together, and obstetricians are paid in a similar manner for a delivery plus pre- and postnatal care. This bundling together of payments is often referred to as payment at the unit of the case or episode (Bundled payments, 2018).

With payment by episode, surgeons have an economic incentive to limit the number of postoperative visits because they do not receive extra payment for extra visits. On the other hand, they continue to have an incentive to perform more surgeries, as with the traditional fee-for-service system.

The Important Concept of Risk

At this point, it is helpful to introduce the concept of risk. Risk refers to the potential to lose money, earn less money, or spend more time without additional payment on a transaction. With the traditional fee-for-service system, the party paying the bill (insurance company, government agency, or patient) absorbs all the risk; if Dr. Weisman sees Rick Payne 10 times rather than five times for his headaches, Blue Cross pays more money and Mr. Payne spends more in copayments. Bundling of services transfers a *portion* of the risk from the payer to the physician; if Dr. Belli sees Tom Stone 10 times rather than five times for follow-up after cholecystectomy, he does not receive any additional money. However, Blue Cross is also partially at risk; if more Blue Cross enrollees require gallbladder surgery, Blue Cross is responsible for more $1,300 payments. As a general rule, the more services aggregated into one payment, the larger the share of financial risk that is shifted from payer to provider.

Payment per Patient: Capitation

Capitation payments (per capita payments or payments "by the head") are monthly payments made to a physician for each patient signed up to receive care from that physician—generally a primary care physician. The essence of capitation is a shift in financial risk from insurers to providers. Under fee-for-service, patients who require expensive health services cost their health plan more than they pay the plan in insurance premiums; the insurer is at risk and loses money. Physicians and hospitals who provide the care earn more money for treating ill people. In a 180-degree role reversal, capitation shifts financial risk from insurance plan to providers. An HMO that pays physicians via capitation has little to fear in the short run from patients who become ill. The HMO pays a fixed sum no matter how many services are provided. The providers, in contrast, earn no additional money yet spend a great deal of time and incur large office and hospital expenditures to care

for people who are sick. On the other hand, providers may financially benefit from having relatively healthy patients who use few services.

Certain methods have been developed to mitigate the financial risk associated with capitation payment. One method involves reintroducing fee-for-service payments for specified services. Such types of services provided but not covered within the capitation payment are called *carve-outs*; their payment is "carved out" of the capitation payment and paid separately. For example, immunizations and minor surgical procedures may be carved out and paid on a fee-for-service basis.

A common method of managing risk is called "risk-adjusted capitation." For physicians paid by capitation, patients with greater health care needs require a great deal more time without any additional payment, creating an incentive to sign up healthy patients and avoid those who are sick. Risk-adjusted capitation provides higher monthly payments for elderly patients and for those with chronic illnesses. Precisely how to risk-adjust is a topic of debate; some feel that adjusting by age and gender is sufficient, others add diagnoses or number of medications, and recent proposals would include socioeconomic status (Juhnke et al., 2016; National Quality Forum, 2017).

Capitation may control costs by providing an alternative to the inflationary tendencies of fee-for-service payment. In addition, capitation has been advocated for its potential beneficial influence on the organization of care. Capitation payments require patients to register with a physician or group of physicians. The clear enumeration of the population of patients in a primary care practice offers advantages for monitoring appropriate use of services and planning for these patients' needs. Capitation also allows for more flexibility at the practice level in how to most effectively and efficiently organize and deliver services. For example, fee-for-service typically only pays for an in-person visit with a physician; under capitation payment, a physician could substitute "virtual visits" such as e-mail and telephone contacts for in-person visits for following up on blood pressure or diabetes control, or delegate routine preventive care tasks to nurses or medical assistants in the practice, without experiencing a financial disincentive for these alternative ways of delivering care. Capitation also explicitly defines—in advance—the amount of money available to care for an enrolled population of patients, providing a better framework for rational allocation of resources and innovation in developing better modes of delivering services. For a large group of PCPs, the sheer size of the aggregated capitation payments provides clout and flexibility over how to best arrange ancillary and specialty services.

Capitation with Two-Tiered Structures

Jennifer is a young woman in England with strep throat; her general practitioner, Dr. Walter Liston, sees her and prescribes antibiotics. Jennifer pays no money at the time of the visit and receives no bill. Dr. Liston is paid the British equivalent of $12 per month to care for Jennifer, no matter how many times she requires care. When Jennifer develops appendicitis and requires an x-ray and surgical consultation, Dr. Liston sends her to the local hospital for these services; payment for these referral services is incorporated into the hospital's operating budget paid for separately by the National Health Service.

British System—Capitation payments to physicians in the United States are complicated, as will shortly be seen. But in the United Kingdom, they have traditionally been simple (see Chapter 14). Under the traditional British National Health Service, each person enrolls with a general practitioner, who becomes the PCP. For each person on the general practitioner's list, the physician receives a monthly capitation payment. The more patients on the list, the more money the physician earns. Patients are required to route all non-emergency medical needs through the general practitioner "gatekeeper," who makes referrals for specialist services or hospital care. Patients can freely change from one general practitioner to another. This simple arrangement, illustrated in Figure 4–1, is referred to as a two-tiered capitation structure. One tier is the health plan (the government in the case of the United Kingdom) and the other tier the individual PCP or several physicians in group practice.

United States System—In the United States, capitation payment is associated with HMO plans and not with traditional or PPO insurance. Some HMO plans have two-tiered structures, with HMOs paying capitation fees directly to PCPs (Fig. 4–1). However, capitation payment in US-managed care organizations often involves a three-tiered structure.

Capitation with Three-Tiered Structures

In three-tiered structures, HMOs do not pay capitation fees directly to individual physicians or small group practices, but instead rely on an intermediary administrative structure for processing these payments (Robinson & Casalino, 1995). In one variety of such three-tiered structures (Fig. 4–2), physicians remain in their own private offices but join together into physician groups called independent practice associations (IPAs).

George is enrolled through his employer in SmartCare, an HMO plan of Smart Insurance Company. SmartCare has contracted with DoctorFriendly IPA, which provides physician services for its enrollees in the area where George lives. George has chosen to receive his care from Dr. Bunch, a PCP affiliated with DoctorFriendly IPA. SmartCare pays the IPA a $70 monthly capitation fee on George's behalf for all physician and related outpatient services. DoctorFriendly IPA in turn pays Dr. Bunch an $18 monthly capitation fee to serve as George's primary care physician.

George develops symptoms of urinary obstruction consistent with benign prostatic hyperplasia. Dr. Bunch orders some laboratory tests and refers George to a urologist for cystoscopy. The laboratory and the urologist bill the IPA on a fee-for-service basis. At the end of the year, the IPA has money left over in this diagnostic and specialist services risk pool and distributes some of this surplus revenue to its physicians as a bonus.

Sorting out the flow of payments and nature of risk-sharing becomes difficult in this type of three-tiered capitation structure. In most three-tiered HMO plans,

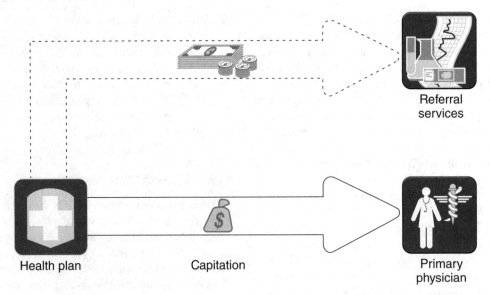

▲ **Figure 4–1.** Two-tiered capitated payment structures. The health plan pays the primary care physician by capitation and pays for referral services (e.g., x-rays and specialist consultations) through a different payment stream.

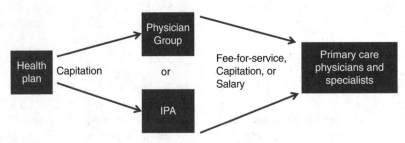

▲ **Figure 4–2.** Three-tiered capitation payment structures. The health plan pays a capitation payment to a physician group or independent practice association (IPA), which in turn pays primary care and specialist physicians fee-for-service, capitation, or salary.

the financial risk for diagnostic and specialist services is borne by the overall IPA organization and spread among the participating physicians in the IPA. In the 1980s and 1990s, IPAs often provided financial incentives to PCPs to limit the use of diagnostic and specialist services by returning to these physicians any surplus funds that remain at the end of the year. This method of compensation was known as capitation-plus-bonus payment. The less frequent the use of diagnostic and

specialist services, the higher the year-end bonus for IPA physician gatekeepers. This arrangement came under criticism as representing a conflict of interest for PCPs because their personal income was increased by denying diagnostic and specialty services to their patients (Rodwin, 1993). More recently, some managed care organizations have begun to tie bonus payments to quality measures—"pay for performance"—rather than to cost control (see Chapter 10).

Payment per Time: Salary

Dr. Joyce Parto is employed as a salaried obstetrician-gynecologist by a large medical group affiliated with a local hospital. She considers the financial security and lack of business worries in her current work setting an improvement over the stresses she faced as a solo fee-for-service practitioner before joining the physician group. However, she has some concerns that the other obstetricians are allowing the hospital's obstetric residents to manage most of the deliveries during the night, and wonders if the lack of financial incentives to attend deliveries may be partly to blame. She is also annoyed by the bureaucratic hoops she has to jump through to cancel an afternoon clinic to attend her son's school play.

In contrast with traditional private physicians, physicians in the public sector (municipal, Veterans Health Administration and military hospitals, state mental hospitals) and in community clinics are usually paid by salary (Fig. 4–3). Salaried practice aggregates payment for all services delivered during a month or year into one lump sum. The growth of physicians working as employees of medical groups, community health centers, and hospitals (see Chapter 6) has brought salaried practice to the private sector, sometimes with a salary-plus-bonus arrangement.

Physicians paid purely by salary bear little if any individual financial risk; the employer, whether a medical group or community health center, is at risk if expenses are too high. To manage risk, administrators may place constraints on their physician employees, such as scheduling them for a high volume of patient visits. Salaried physicians are at risk of not getting extra pay for extra work hours. For a physician paid an annual salary without allowances for overtime pay, a high volume of complex patient visits may turn an 8-hour day into a 12-hour day with no increase in income. Some organizations offer bonuses to salaried physicians if their patients receive high-quality, low-cost care (see pay-for-performance, below), or index a large portion of the salary to the physician's individual clinical productivity.

METHODS OF HOSPITAL PAYMENT

Payment per Procedure: Fee-for-Service

Kwin Mock Wong is hospitalized for a bleeding ulcer. At the end of his 4-day stay, the hospital sends a $48,000 seven-page itemized hospital bill to Blue Cross, Mr. Wong's insurer.

In the past, insurance companies made fee-for-service payments to private hospitals based on the principle of "reasonable cost," a system under which hospitals had a great deal of influence in determining the level of payment. Because the American Hospital Association and Blue Cross played a large role in writing payment regulations for Medicare, that program initially paid hospitals according to a similar reasonable cost formula (Law, 1974). More recently, private and public payers concerned with cost containment have begun to question hospital charges and negotiate lower payments, or to shift financial risk toward the hospitals by using per diem, DRG, or capitation payments.

Payment per Day: Per Diem

John Johnson, a patient with PPO insurance with a severe headache, is admitted to the hospital. During his 3-day stay, he undergoes MRI scanning, lumbar puncture, and cerebral arteriography, procedures that are all costly to the hospital in terms of personnel and supplies. The hospital receives $6,000, or $2,000 per day from the PPO plan; Mr. Johnson's stay costs the hospital $8,200 in expenses.

Tom Thompson, in the same PPO, is admitted for congestive heart failure. He receives intravenous furosemide for 3 days and his condition improves. Diagnostic testing is limited to a chest x-ray, ECG, and basic blood work. The hospital receives $6,000; the cost to the hospital is $5,200.

Many insurance companies and Medicaid plans contract with hospitals for per diem payments rather than paying a fee for each itemized service (room charge, MRI, arteriogram, chest x-ray, and ECG). The hospital receives a lump sum for each day the patient is in the hospital. The insurer may send a utilization review

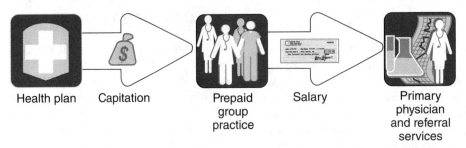

▲ Figure 4–3. Salaried payment. A prepaid group practice receives capitation payments from the health plan and then pays its physicians by salary.

nurse to the hospital to review the charts of its patients, and if the nurse decides that a patient is not acutely ill, the insurance plan may stop paying for additional days.

Per diem payments represent a bundling of all services provided for one patient on a particular day into one payment. With traditional fee-for-service payment, if the hospital performs several expensive diagnostic studies, it makes more money because it charges for each study, whereas with per diem payment the hospital receives no additional money for expensive procedures. Per diem bundling of services into one fee removes the hospital's financial incentive because it loses, rather than profits, by performing expensive studies.

With per diem payment, the insurer continues to be at risk for the number of days a patient stays in the hospital because it must pay for each additional day. However, the hospital is at risk for the number of services performed on any given day because it incurs more costs without additional payment when it provides more services. It is in the insurer's interest to conduct utilization reviews to reduce the number of hospital days, but the insurer is less concerned about how many services are performed within each day; that fiscal concern has been transferred to the hospital.

▶ Payment per Episode of Hospitalization: Diagnosis-Related Groups

Bill is a 67-year-old man who enters the hospital for acute pulmonary edema. He is treated with furosemide and oxygen in the emergency room, spends 36 hours in the hospital, and is discharged. The cost to the hospital is $5,200. The hospital receives a $7,000 DRG payment from Medicare.

Will is an 82-year-old man who enters the hospital for acute pulmonary edema. In spite of repeated treatments with furosemide, ACE inhibitors, and nitrates, he remains in heart failure. He requires oxygen, telemetry, daily blood tests, several chest x-rays, electrocardiograms, and an echocardiogram, and is finally discharged on the ninth hospital day. His hospital stay costs $23,000 and the hospital receives $7,000 from Medicare.

The DRG method of payment for Medicare patients started in 1983. Rather than pay hospitals on a fee-for-service basis, Medicare pays a lump sum for each hospital admission, with the size of the payment dependent on the patient's diagnoses. The DRG system has gone one step further than per diem payments in bundling services into one payment. While per diem payment lumps together all services performed during 1 day, DRG payment lumps together all services performed during one acute care hospital episode.

With the DRG system, the Medicare program is at risk for the number of admissions, but the hospital is at risk for the length of hospital stay and the resources used during the hospital stay. Medicare has no financial interest in the length of stay, which (except in unusually long "outlier" stays) does not affect Medicare's payment. In contrast, the hospital has an acute interest in the length of stay and in the number of expensive procedures performed; a long, costly hospitalization such as Will's produces a financial loss for the hospital, whereas a short stay yields a profit. Hospitals therefore conduct internal utilization review to reduce the costs incurred by Medicare patients.

Payment per Patient: Capitation

Jane is enrolled in Blue Cross HMO, which contracts with Upscale Hospital to care for Jane if she requires hospitalization. Upscale receives $80 per month as a capitation fee for each patient enrolled in the HMO. Jane is healthy, and during the 36 months that she is an HMO member, the hospital receives $2,880, even though Jane never sets foot in the hospital.

Wayne is also enrolled in Blue Cross HMO. Twenty-four months following his enrollment, he develops leukemia and in the following 12 months he spends 8 weeks in Upscale Hospital at a cost of $282,000. Upscale receives a total of $2,880 (the $80 capitation fee per month for 36 months) for Wayne's care.

With capitation payment, hospitals are at risk for admissions, length of stay, and resources used; in other words, hospitals bear all the risk and the insurer, usually an HMO, bears no risk. Capitation payment to hospitals is uncommon in the United States.

Payment per Institution: Global Budget

Don Samuels, a member of the Kaiser Health Plan, suffers a sudden overwhelming headache and is hospitalized for 1 week at Kaiser Hospital in Oakland, California, for an acute cerebral hemorrhage. He goes into a coma and dies. No hospital bill is generated as a result of Mr. Samuels' admission, and no capitation payments are made from any insurance plan to the hospital.

Kaiser Health Plan is a large integrated delivery system that in some regions of the United States operates its own hospitals. Kaiser hospitals are paid by the Kaiser Health Plan through a global budget: a fixed payment is made for all hospital services for 1 year. Global budgets are also used in Veterans Health Administration and Department of Defense hospitals in the United States, as well as being a standard payment method in Canada and many European nations. In managed care parlance, one might say that the hospital is entirely at risk because no matter how many patients are admitted and how many expensive services are performed,

the hospital must figure out how to stay within its fixed budget. Global budgets represent the most extensive bundling of services: Every service performed on every patient during 1 year is aggregated into one payment.

VALUE-BASED PAYMENT AND PAYMENT REFORM

The health system is witnessing a flurry of new approaches to paying physicians and hospitals. The National Commission on Physician Payment Reform (2013) called for fundamental changes, including the eventual elimination of fee-for-service payment in favor of payment that rewards value (i.e., high quality at reasonable cost) rather than volume. A number of "value-based" payment models are currently in use.

Pay-for-Performance

One of the most basic reforms is paying not just for units of service—whether they be visits, hospital episodes, or hours of work—but for how well physicians and other providers perform in delivering those services. Many public and private payers are supplementing the basic mode of payment with bonus payments to physicians and hospitals that achieve a specified high level of performance on certain measures such as preventive care services, diabetes care, patient experience, and cost reduction (James, 2012; Mendelson et al., 2017). In the United States, these payments tend to be small relative to the dominant payment mechanisms of fee-for-service for physicians and per diem or DRGs for hospitals. Pay-for-performance is discussed further in Chapter 10.

Bundled Payments

The term "bundled payment" has taken on a specific meaning under Medicare payment reform. Under this model, Medicare not only bundles payments into more aggregated units using an episode-based rather than fee-for-service method; the physician and hospital payments are also bundled together into a single payment. An example is bundled payment for a joint replacement. Medicare negotiates with a hospital and the members of its medical staff involved in joint replacements (orthopedic surgeons, anesthesiologists, and others) to agree on a total payment for the joint replacement services, set at a level somewhat below what Medicare estimates it has paid for those services to the same groups of providers under fee-for-service. Bundled payment provides an incentive for the hospital and its medical staff to collaborate to eliminate unnecessary costs, such as by selecting a limited number of joint prostheses and negotiating lower prices with supply vendors for those prostheses, resulting in savings to Medicare and higher earnings for the hospital and physicians. The hospital and physicians share the risk of potentially losing money relative to the traditional payment model if they cannot control the average total cost for joint replacements. Also, bundled payments typically place the hospital and physicians at financial risk for postacute care expenses, such as outpatient physical therapy and a postoperative stay in a skilled nursing facility, since Medicare defines the episode as lasting at least 30 days after the date of surgery, and often 90 days (Ryan, 2018). Medicare launched bundled payment programs in 2013 on a voluntary basis and now has more than 25 conditions for which hospitals and physicians can elect to be paid using this method; Medicare plans to make bundled payment a mandatory payment method for several of these conditions (Bundled payments, 2018).

▶ Care Coordination Payments

Medicare and some private insurers are paying some primary care practices through a blended model that adds a small capitation payment to the main fee-for-service payment to provide resources and incentives for better management of patients with chronic conditions. For example, a primary care practice caring for 100 patients with diabetes might receive $40 per diabetes patient per month, and use those funds to hire a health coach to help patients control their diabetes.

▶ Accountable Care Organizations

The term "accountable care organization" was introduced in 2006 by Elliott Fisher. Since that time, more than one thousand ACOs have sprung up around the United States, involving both public and private payers (Muhlestein et al., 2018).

In 2013, Northeast Hospital System organized the NewCare ACO to participate in the Medicare ACO program. To form NewCare ACO, Northeast brought together both hospital-owned and independent physician practices, laboratories, imaging centers, and home care agencies in its suburban town. The physician members of NewCare cared for 10,000 Medicare beneficiaries. In the year prior to the ACO's formation, those 10,000 patients cost Medicare an average of $10,000 per patient, a total of $100 million. Based on typical annual health care cost inflation of 5%, Medicare estimated that those same patients would cost $105 million in 2013. Under the ACO contract with Medicare, if NewCare held total Medicare costs for those 10,000 patients in 2013 below $103 million, NewCare would retain half of every dollar saved by Medicare below that $103 million target. Medicare would still pay NewCare constituent providers in the usual way: DRGs for hospitals and fee-for-service for physicians. However, all payments would be tracked against the shared-savings target to determine at the end of the year if NewCare would receive a supplemental payment from Medicare for achieving the threshold cost reductions. To ensure that patients would not suffer from cost-saving measures compromising access and quality, Medicare would not share the savings with NewCare unless NewCare achieved certain quality benchmarks. Medicare expenses in 2013 for NewCare patients wound up to be $101 million and NewCare hit its quality benchmarks. Medicare paid NewCare a $1 million shared saving bonus, which NewCare distributed equally to Northeast Hospital and the physician members of NewCare.

ACO payment models try to make fee-for-service payments to physicians and per diem or episode payments to hospitals function more like a globally budgeted payment model. While retaining the basic disaggregated payments, ACOs create an overall budget target that puts physicians and hospitals at financial risk for overall expenditures. In the case of NewCare, the risk was exclusively "upside" risk, meaning that NewCare could share in savings if it was successful in holding down costs but was not at financial risk if its Medicare expenditures exceeded the budget target ("downside" risk). Medicare ACO models provide an opportunity for physician and hospital organizations to retain a greater share of the upside risk if they are willing to also assume some downside risk and pay money back to Medicare if total costs exceed a threshold target. Similar to bundled payment, the ACO payment model provides an incentive for physicians, hospitals, and other involved providers to collaborate in eliminating wasteful spending. ACO models typically include an element of pay for performance insofar as provider organizations are only eligible for shared savings bonuses if they achieve quality targets. ACOs are discussed in more detail in Chapters 6 and 9.

CONCLUSION

The push for cost containment has changed in two fundamental ways how physicians and hospitals are paid:

1. Whereas levels of payment were formerly set largely by providers themselves (reasonable cost reimbursement for hospitals and usual, customary, and reasonable fees for physicians), payment levels are increasingly determined by negotiation between payers and providers or by fee schedules set by payers.
2. Private insurers, Medicare, and Medicaid are gradually replacing fee-for-service payment, which encourages use of more services, with more aggregated payment mechanisms that shift financial risk away from payers toward physicians and hospitals in an effort to control costs.

While fee-for-service encourages expensive overtreatment (Relman, 2007), payments that place physicians and hospitals at risk raise concerns about restricting needed care. Although the perfect payment method that strikes the right balance between economic incentives for overtreatment and undertreatment remains elusive (Casalino, 1992), payers continue to experiment by blending units of payment and reforming payment models to achieve the right recipe for producing high quality, affordable care.

REFERENCES

Bodenheimer T, et al. The primary care-specialty income gap: why it matters. *Ann Intern Med.* 2007;146:301–306.

Bundled payments. NEJM Catalyst, February 28, 2018. https://catalyst.nejm.org/what-are-bundled-payments/. Accessed September 20, 2019.

Casalino LP. Balancing incentives: how should physicians be reimbursed? *JAMA.* 1992;267:403–405.

James J. Pay-for-Performance. Health Affairs Health Policy Brief, October 11, 2012.

Juhnke C, et al. A review of methods of risk adjustment and their use in integrated healthcare systems. *Intern J Integrated Care.* 2016;16(4):4.

Law SA. *Blue Cross: What Went Wrong?* New Haven, CT: Yale University Press; 1974.

Mendelson A, et al. The effects of pay-for-performance programs on health, health care use, and processes of care. *Ann Intern Med.* 2017;166:341–353.

Muhlestein D, et al. Recent progress in the value journey: growth of ACOs and value-based payment in 2018. Health Affairs blog, August 14, 2018. www.healthaffairs.org/do/10.1377/hblog20180810.481968/full.

National Commission on Physician Payment Reform, March 2013. http://physicianpaymentcommission.org/. Accessed September 20, 2019.

National Quality Forum. Evaluation of the NQF trial period for risk adjustment for social risk factors. July 18, 2017. www.qualityforum.org/Projects/s-z/SES_Trial_Period/Final_Report.aspx.

Relman A. *Second Opinion: Rescuing America's Health Care.* New York, NY: Public Affairs; 2007.

Robinson JC, Casalino LP. The growth of medical groups paid through capitation in California. *N Engl J Med.* 1995;333:1684–1687.

Rodwin MA. *Medicine, Money, and Morals: Physicians' Conflicts of Interest.* New York, NY: Oxford University Press; 1993.

Ryan AM. Medicare bundled payment programs for joint replacement. *JAMA.* 2018;320:877–879.

Zuvekas SH, Cohen JW. Fee-for-service, while much maligned, remains the dominant payment method for physician visits. *Health Aff (Millwood).* 2016;35:411–414.

How Health Care Is Organized—I: Primary, Secondary, and Tertiary Care

In 1989, Frank Hope developed Acquired Immune Deficiency Syndrome (AIDS) and was in and out of the hospital with debilitating infections. Yet he remained hopeful that a scientific breakthrough would give him a chance. By 1995, with the discovery of life-saving protease inhibitors, his wish had come true. In Frank's mind, these types of scientific discoveries attest to the wonders of the US health care system. Frank's grandson attends a day care program. Ruby, a 3-year-old girl in the program, was recently hospitalized for a severe asthma attack complicated by pneumococcal pneumonia. She spent 2 weeks in a pediatric intensive care unit, including several days on a respirator. Ruby's mother works full time as a bus driver while raising three children. She has comprehensive private health insurance through her job but finds it difficult to keep track of all her children's immunization schedules and to find a physician's office that offers convenient appointment times. She takes Ruby to an evening-hours urgent care center when Ruby has some wheezing but never sees the same physician twice. Ruby never received all her pneumococcal vaccinations or consistent prescription of a steroid inhaler to prevent a severe asthma attack. Ruby's mother blames herself for her child's hospitalization.

People in the United States rightfully take pride in the technologic accomplishments of their health care system. Innovations in biomedical science have almost eradicated such scourges as polio, and measles. Yet for all its successes, the health care system also has its failures. In cases such as Ruby's, the failure to prevent a severe asthma flare-up is not related to financial barriers, but rather reflects organizational problems, particularly in the delivery of primary care services.

The organizational task facing all health care systems is one of "assuring that the right patient receives the right service at the right time and in the right place" (Rodwin, 1984). An additional criterion could be "… and by the right caregiver." The fragmented care Ruby received for her asthma is an example of this challenge. Who is responsible for planning and ensuring that every child receives the right services at the right time? Can an urgent care center or an in-store clinic at Walmart designed for episodic needs be held accountable for providing comprehensive care to all patients passing through its doors? Should parents be expected to make appointments for routine visits at medical offices and clinics, or should clinics actively assume the responsibility to ensure that all their patients receive the chronic and preventive services they need when they need them? What is the proper balance between intensive care units that provide life-saving services to critically ill patients and primary care services geared toward less dramatic medical and preventive needs?

The previous chapters have emphasized financial transactions in the health care system. In this chapter and the following one, the organization of the health care system will be the main focus. While a heated debate persists on how to improve financial access to care, less emphasis is given to the question "access to what?" In this chapter, organizational systems will be viewed through a wide-angle lens, examining such broad concepts as the relationship between primary, secondary, and tertiary levels of care, and the influence of the biomedical paradigm and medical professionalism in shaping US health care delivery. In Chapter 6, a zoom lens will be used to focus on specific organizational models that have appeared (often only to disappear) in this country over the past century.

MODELS OF ORGANIZING CARE

▶ Primary, Secondary, and Tertiary Care

One concept is essential in understanding the topography of any health care system: the organization of care into primary, secondary, and tertiary levels. In the Lord Dawson Report, an influential British study written in 1920, Dawson (1975) proposed that each of the three levels of care should correspond with certain unique patient needs.

1. Primary care involves common health problems (e.g., sore throats, diabetes, arthritis, depression, or hypertension) and preventive measures (e.g., vaccinations or mammograms) that account for 80% to 90% of visits to a physician or other caregiver.
2. Secondary care involves problems that require more specialized clinical expertise such as hospital care for a patient with acute renal failure.
3. Tertiary care, which lies at the apex of the organizational pyramid, involves the management of rare disorders such as pituitary tumors and congenital malformations.

Two contrasting approaches can be used to organize a health care system around these levels of care: (1) the carefully structured Dawson model of regionalized health care and (2) a more free-flowing model.

1. One approach uses the Dawson model as a scaffold for a highly structured system. This model is based on the concept of regionalization: the organization and coordination of all health resources and services within a defined area (Bodenheimer, 1969). In a regionalized system, different types of personnel and facilities are assigned to distinct tiers in the primary, secondary, and tertiary levels, and the flow of patients across levels occurs in an orderly, regulated fashion. This model emphasizes the primary

care base and a population-oriented framework for health planning.
2. An alternative model allows for more fluid roles for caregivers, and more free-flowing movement of patients across all levels of care. This model tends to place a higher value on services at the tertiary care apex than at the primary care base.

Although most health care systems embody elements of both models, some gravitate closer to one polarity or the other. The traditional British National Health Service (NHS) and some large integrated delivery systems in the United States resemble the regionalized approach, while US health care as a whole follows the more dispersed format.

▶ The Regionalized Model: The Traditional British National Health Service

Basil, a 60-year-old man living in a London suburb, is registered with Dr. Prime, a general practitioner in his neighborhood. Basil goes to Dr. Prime for most of his health problems, including hay fever, back spasms, and hypertension. One day, he experiences numbness and weakness in his face and arm. By the time Dr. Prime examines him later that day, the symptoms have resolved. Suspecting that Basil has had a transient ischemic attack, Dr. Prime prescribes aspirin and refers him to the neurologist at the local hospital, where a carotid artery sonogram reveals high-grade carotid stenosis. Dr. Prime and the neurologist agree that Basil should make an appointment at a London teaching hospital with a vascular surgeon specializing in head and neck surgery. The surgeon recommends that Basil undergo carotid endarterectomy on an elective basis to prevent a major stroke. Basil returns to Dr. Prime to discuss this recommendation and inquires whether the operation could be performed at a local hospital closer to home. Dr. Prime informs him that only a handful of London hospitals are equipped to perform this type of specialized operation. Basil schedules his operation in London and several months later has an uncomplicated carotid endarterectomy. Following the operation, he returns to Dr. Prime for his ongoing care.

The British NHS traditionally typified a relatively regimented primary–secondary–tertiary care structure (Fig. 5–1).

1. For physician services, the primary care level is virtually the exclusive domain of general practitioners (commonly referred to as GPs), who practice in small- to medium-sized groups and whose main responsibility is ambulatory care. About half of all physicians in the United Kingdom are GPs.
2. The secondary tier of care is occupied by physicians in such specialties as internal medicine, pediatrics, neurology, psychiatry, obstetrics and gynecology, and general surgery. These physicians are located at hospital-based clinics and serve as consultants for outpatient referrals from GPs, in turn routing most patients back to GPs for ongoing care needs. Secondary-level physicians also provide care to hospitalized patients.
3. Tertiary care subspecialists such as cardiac surgeons, immunologists, and pediatric hematologists are located at a few tertiary care medical centers.

Hospital planning followed the same regionalized logic as physician services. District hospitals were local facilities equipped for basic inpatient services. Regional tertiary care medical centers handled highly specialized inpatient care needs.

Planning of physician and hospital resources within the traditional NHS occurred with a population focus. GP groups provided care to a base population of 5,000 to 50,000 persons, depending on the number of GPs in the practice. District hospitals had a catchment area population of 50,000 to 500,000, while tertiary care hospitals served as referral centers for a population of 500,000 to 5 million (Fry, 1980).

While this regionalized structure has recently become more fluid (Chapter 14), patient flow still moves in a stepwise fashion across the different tiers. Except in emergency situations, all patients are first seen by a GP, who may then steer patients toward more specialized levels of care through a formal process of referral. Patients may not directly refer themselves to a specialist.

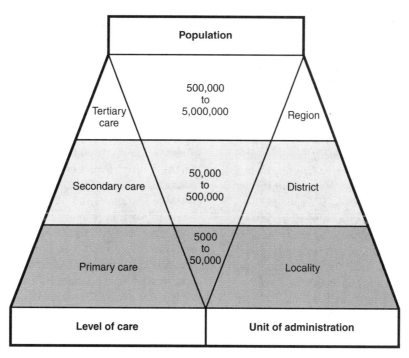

▲ **Figure 5–1.** Organization of services under the traditional National Health Service model in the United Kingdom. Care is organized into distinct levels corresponding to specific functions, roles, administrative units, and population bases.

While nonphysician health professionals, such as nurses, play an integral role in staffing hospitals at the secondary and tertiary care levels, especially noteworthy is the NHS' multidisciplinary approach to primary care. GPs work in close collaboration with practice nurses (similar to nurse practitioners in the United States), home health visitors, public health nurses, and midwives (who attend most deliveries in the United Kingdom). Such teamwork, along with accountability for a defined population of enrolled patients and universal health care coverage, helps to avert such problems as missed childhood vaccinations. Public health nurses visit all homes in the first weeks after a birth to provide education and assist with scheduling of initial GP appointments. A national vaccination tracking system notifies parents about each scheduled vaccination and alerts GPs and public health nurses if a child has not appeared at the appointed time. As a result, more than 90% of British preschool children receive a full series of immunizations.

A number of other nations, ranging from industrialized countries in Scandinavia to developing nations in Latin America, have adopted a similar approach to organizing health services. In low-income nations, the primary care tier relies more on community health educators and other types of public health personnel than on physicians.

▶ ### The Dispersed Model: Traditional US Health Care Organization

Polly Seymour, a 55-year-old woman with private health insurance who lives in the United States, sees several different physicians for a variety of problems: a dermatologist for eczema, a gastroenterologist for recurrent heartburn, and an orthopedist for tendinitis in her shoulder. She may ask her gastroenterologist to treat a few general medical problems, such as borderline diabetes. On occasion, she has gone to the nearby hospital emergency department for treatment of urinary tract infections. One day, Polly feels a lump in her breast and consults a gynecologist. She is referred to a surgeon for biopsy, which indicates cancer. After discussing treatment options with Polly, the surgeon performs a lumpectomy and refers her to an oncologist and radiation therapy specialist for further therapy. She receives all these treatments at a local hospital, a short distance from her home.

The US health care system has had a far less structured approach to levels of care than the British NHS. In contrast to the stepwise flow of patient referrals in the United Kingdom, insured patients in the United States, such as Polly Seymour, have traditionally been able to refer themselves and enter the system directly at any level. While many patients in the United Kingdom have a primary care physician (PCP) to initially evaluate all their problems, many people in the United States have become accustomed to taking their symptoms directly to the specialist of their choice.

One unique aspect of the US approach to primary care has been to broaden the role of internists and pediatricians. While general internists and general pediatricians in the United Kingdom and most European nations serve principally as referral physicians in the secondary tier, their US counterparts share in providing primary care. Moreover, the overlapping roles among "generalists" in the United States (family physicians, general internists, and general pediatricians) are not limited to the outpatient sector. PCPs in the United States have assumed a number of secondary care functions by providing substantial amounts of inpatient care. Only recently has the United States moved toward the European model that removes inpatient care from the domain of some PCPs and assigns this work to "hospitalists"—physicians who exclusively practice within the hospital (Wachter & Goldman, 1996; Goroll & Hunt, 2015).

Including general internists and general pediatricians in addition to family physicians, the total supply of PCPs amounts to 28% of all physicians in the United States, a number well below the 50% or more found in the United Kingdom (Association of American Medical Colleges, 2019). In contrast to physicians, nurse practitioners and physician assistants are more likely to work in primary care settings, and by 2025 will constitute 41% of the primary care practitioner workforce (Auerbach et al., 2013).

US hospitals are not constrained by rigid secondary and tertiary care boundaries. Instead of a pyramidal system featuring a large number of general community hospitals at the base and a limited number of tertiary care referral centers at the apex, hospitals in the United States each aspire to offer the latest in specialized care. In most urban areas, for example, several hospitals compete with each other to perform open heart surgery, organ transplants, radiation therapy, and high-risk obstetric procedures. The resulting structure resembles a diamond more than a pyramid, with a small number of hospitals (mostly rural) that lack specialized units at the base, a small number of elite university medical centers providing highly super-specialized referral services at the apex, and the bulk of hospitals providing a wide range of secondary and tertiary services in the middle.

Which Model Is Right?

Critics of the US health care system find fault with its "top-heavy" specialist and tertiary care orientation and lack of organizational coherence. Analyses of health care in the United States over many decades abound with such descriptions as "a nonsystem with millions of independent, uncoordinated, separately motivated moving parts," "fragmentation, chaos, and disarray," and "uncontrolled growth and pluralism verging on anarchy" (Somers, 1972; Halvorson & Isham, 2003). The high cost of health care has been attributed in part to this organizational disarray. Quality of care may also suffer. For example, when many hospitals each perform small numbers of surgical procedures such as coronary artery bypass grafts, mortality rates are higher than when such procedures are regionalized in a few higher-volume centers (Gonzalez et al., 2014).

Defenders of the dispersed model reply that pluralism is a virtue, promoting flexibility and convenience in the availability of facilities and personnel. In this view, the emphasis on specialization and technology is compatible with values and expectations in the United States, with patients placing a high premium on direct access to specialists and tertiary care services, and on autonomy in selecting caregivers of their choice for a particular health care need. Similarly, the desire for the latest in-hospital technology available at a convenient distance from home competes with plans to regionalize tertiary care services at a limited number of hospitals.

Balancing the Different Levels of Care

Dr. Billie Ruben completed her residency training in internal medicine at a major university medical center. Like most of her fellow residents, she went on to pursue subspecialty training, in her case gastroenterology. Dr. Ruben chose this career after caring for a young woman who developed irreversible liver failure from autoimmune hepatitis. After a nerve-racking, touch-and-go effort to secure a donor liver, transplantation was performed and the patient made a complete recovery.

Upon completion of her training, Dr. Ruben joined a growing subspecialty practice at Atlantic Heights Hospital, a successful private hospital in the city. Even though the metropolitan area of 2 million people already has two liver transplant units, Atlantic Heights has just opened a third such unit, feeling that its reputation for excellence depends on delivering tertiary care services at the cutting edge of biomedical innovation. In her first 6 months at the hospital, Dr. Ruben participates in the care of only two patients requiring liver transplantation. Most of her patients seek care for chronic, often ill-defined digestive problems. As Dr. Ruben begins seeing these patients on a regular basis, she starts to give preventive care and treat nongastrointestinal problems such as hypertension and diabetes. At times she wishes she had experienced more general medicine during her training.

Advocates of a stronger role for primary care in the United States believe that it is too important to be considered an afterthought in health planning. In this view, overemphasis on the tertiary care apex of the pyramid creates a system in which health care resources are not well matched to the prevalence and incidence of health problems in a community. In an article entitled "The Ecology of Medical Care" published more than 5 decades ago, Kerr White recorded the monthly prevalence of illness for a general population of 1,000 adults (White et al., 1961). In this group, 750 experienced one or more illnesses or injuries during the month. Of these patients, 250 visited a physician at least once during the month, nine were admitted to a hospital, and only one was referred to a university medical center. Dr. White voiced concern that the training of health care professionals at tertiary care–oriented academic medical centers gave trainees like Dr. Billie Ruben an unrepresentative view of the health care needs of the community. Updating Kerr White's findings, Larry Green found precisely the same patterns 4 decades later (Fig. 5–2) (Green et al., 2001).

The ecological framework uses a population-based approach: For a defined population in the community,

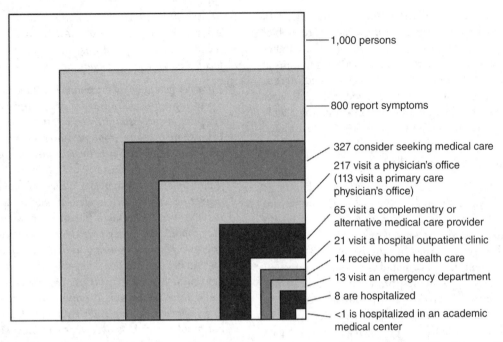

- ___ 1,000 persons
- ___ 800 report symptoms
- ___ 327 consider seeking medical care
- 217 visit a physician's office (113 visit a primary care physician's office)
- 65 visit a complementry or alternative medical care provider
- 21 visit a hospital outpatient clinic
- 14 receive home health care
- 13 visit an emergency department
- 8 are hospitalized
- <1 is hospitalized in an academic medical center

▲ **Figure 5–2.** Monthly prevalence of illness in the community and the roles of various sources of health care. Each box represents a subgroup of the largest box, which comprises 1,000 persons. Data are for persons of all ages. (From Green LA, et al. The ecology of medical care revisited. *N Engl J Med.* 2001;344:2021.)

what is the incidence and prevalence of disease and health care needs and patterns of care seeking? This framework confirms the adage that "common disorders commonly occur and rare ones rarely happen" (Fry, 1980). The dominant pathology in an unselected population consists of minor ailments, chronic conditions such as hypertension and arthritis, and an array of behavioral conditions ranging from children with attention deficit and hyperactivity disorder to adults with depression and substance use disorders to elders with cognitive decline. The incidence of new cancers is relatively rare, and only a handful of patients manifest complex syndromes such as multiple sclerosis. This is very different from the pattern of disease viewed from the reference point of an emergency department or intensive care unit, where distinct subsets of patients are encountered.

The ecological framework does not imply that most health care resources should be devoted to primary care. The minority of patients with severe conditions requiring secondary or tertiary care will command a much larger share of health care resources per capita

than the majority of people with less dramatic health care needs. Treating a patient with liver failure costs a great deal more than treating a patient for hypertension. Even in the United Kingdom, where the 50% of physicians who are GPs provide the majority of ambulatory care, expenditures on their services account for about 10% of the overall NHS budget. In the United States, the percentage of the budget spent on primary care is even lower. Thus, the pyramidal shape shown in Figure 5–1 better represents the distribution of health care problems in a community than the apportionment of health care expenditures. While almost all industrialized nations devote a dominant share of health care resources to secondary and tertiary care, the ecologic view reminds us that most people have health care needs at the primary care level.

▶ **The Functions and Value of Primary Care**

Dr. O. Titus Wells has cared for all four of Bruce and Wendy Smith's children. As a family physician whose practice includes obstetrics, Dr. Wells attended the births of all but one of the children. The Smiths' 18-month-old daughter Ginny has had many ear infections. Even though this is a common problem, Dr. Wells finds that it presents a real medical challenge. Sometimes examination of Ginny's ears indicates a raging infection and at other times shows the presence of middle ear fluid, which may or may not represent a bona fide bacterial infection. He tries to reserve antibiotics for clear-cut cases of severe bacterial otitis. He feels it is important that he be the one to examine Ginny's ears because her eardrums never look entirely normal and he knows what degree of change is suspicious for a genuinely new infection.

When Ginny is 2 years old, Dr. Wells recommends to the Smiths that she see an otolaryngologist and audiologist to check for hearing loss and language impairment. The audiograms show modest diminution of hearing in one ear. The otolaryngologist informs the Smiths that ear tubes are an option. At Ginny's return visit with Dr. Wells, he discusses the pros and cons of tube placement with the Smiths. He also uses the visit as an opportunity to encourage Mrs. Smith to quit smoking, mentioning that research has shown that exposure to tobacco smoke may predispose children to ear infections.

Barbara Starfield, a foremost scholar in the field of primary care, conceptualized the key tasks of primary care as (1) first contact care, (2) continuity, (3) comprehensiveness, and (4) coordination. Dr. Wells' care of the Smith family illustrates these essential features of primary care. He is the *first-contact* physician performing the initial evaluation when Ginny or other family members develop symptoms of illness. *Continuity* refers to sustaining a patient–caregiver relationship over time. Dr. Wells' familiarity with Ginny's condition helps him to better discern an acute infection. *Comprehensiveness* consists of the ability to manage a wide range of health care needs, in contrast with specialty care, which focuses on a particular organ system or procedural service. Dr. Wells' comprehensive, family-oriented care makes him aware that Mrs. Smith's smoking cessation program is an important part of his treatment plan for Ginny. *Coordination* builds upon longitudinality. Through referral and follow-up, the primary care provider integrates services delivered by other caregivers.

These tasks performed by Dr. Wells meet the standard definition of primary care: "Primary care is the provision of integrated, accessible health care services by clinicians who are accountable for addressing a large majority of personal health care needs, developing sustained partnerships with patients, and practicing in the context of family and community" (Institute of Medicine, 1996).

A functional approach helps characterize which health care professionals truly fill the primary care niche. Among physicians in the United States, family physicians, general internists, and general pediatricians typically provide first contact, longitudinal, comprehensive, coordinated care. Emergency medicine physicians provide first contact care that may be relatively comprehensive for acute problems, but they do not provide continuity of care or coordinate care for patients on an ongoing basis. Some obstetrician-gynecologists provide first contact and longitudinal care, but usually only for reproductive health conditions; it is the rare obstetrician-gynecologist who is trained and inclined to comprehensively care for the majority of a woman's health needs throughout the lifespan. Similarly, a patient with kidney failure or a patient with cancer may have a strong continuity of care relationship with a nephrologist or an oncologist, but these medical subspecialists rarely assume responsibility for comprehensive care of clinical problems outside of their specialty area or coordinate most ancillary and referral services.

In addition to physicians, many generalist nurse practitioners and physician assistants in the United States deliver the four key Starfield functions and serve as primary care clinicians for their patients. A study of 23,704 patient visits to 1,139 practitioners demonstrated comparable quality of care for patients treated by PCPs, nurse practitioners, and physician assistants (Kurtzman and Barnow, 2017).

Studies have found that the core elements of good primary care advance the "triple aim" of health system improvement: better patient experiences, better patient outcomes, and lower costs (Starfield, 1998; Bodenheimer & Grumbach, 2007; Friedberg et al., 2010). For example, continuity of care is associated with greater patient satisfaction, higher use of preventive services, reductions in hospitalizations, and lower costs (Saultz & Albedaiwi, 2004; Saultz & Lochner,

2005). Care that is comprehensive, provided by family physicians, is associated with a 10% to 15% reduction in Medicare expenditures per beneficiary (Bazemore et al., 2015). Persons whose care meets a primary care–oriented model have better perceived access to care, are more likely to receive recommended preventive services, are more likely to adhere to treatment, and are more satisfied with their care (Bindman et al., 1996; Stewart et al., 1997; Safran et al., 1998). International comparisons have indicated that nations with a greater primary care orientation tend to have more satisfied patients and better performance on health indicators such as infant mortality, life expectancy, and total health expenditures (Starfield et al., 2005). Similar observations have been made comparing regions in the United States (Starfield et al., 2005). In an analysis of quality and cost of care across states for Medicare beneficiaries, Baicker and Chandra (2004) found that states with more PCPs per capita had lower per capita Medicare costs and higher quality. States with more specialists per capita had lower quality and higher per capita Medicare expenditures. An United States analysis by county showed that greater PCP supply was associated an increase in life expectancy and lower cardiovascular, cancer, and respiratory mortality from 2005 to 2015 (Basu et al., 2019).

▶ Care Coordination and "Gatekeeping"

Polly Seymour, described earlier in the chapter, feels terrible. Every time she eats, she feels nauseated and vomits frequently. She has lost 8 lb, and her oncologist is worried that her breast cancer has spread. She undergoes blood tests, an abdominal CT scan, and a bone scan, all of which are normal. She returns to her gastroenterologist, who tells her to stop the ibuprofen she has been taking for tendinitis. Her problem persists, and the gastroenterologist performs an endoscopy, which shows mild gastric irritation. A month has passed, $3,000 has been spent, and Polly continues to vomit.

Polly's friend Martha recommends a nurse practitioner who has been caring for Martha for many years and who, in Martha's view, seems to spend more time talking with patients than do many physicians. Polly makes an appointment with the nurse

practitioner, Sara Steward. Ms. Steward takes a complete history, which reveals that Polly is taking tamoxifen for her breast cancer and that she began to take aspirin after stopping the ibuprofen. Ms. Steward explains that either of these medications can cause vomiting and suggests that they be stopped for a week. Polly returns in a week, her nausea and vomiting resolved. Ms. Steward then consults with Polly's oncologist, and together they decide to restart the tamoxifen but not the aspirin. Polly becomes nauseated again, but eventually begins to feel well and gains weight while taking a reduced dose of tamoxifen. In the future, Ms. Steward handles Polly's medical problems, referring her to specialty physicians when needed, and making sure that the advice of one consultant does not interfere with the therapy of another specialist.

A concept that incorporates many of the elements of primary care is that of the primary care provider as gatekeeper. Gatekeeping took on pejorative connotations in the heyday of managed care, when, as described in Chapter 4, some types of financial arrangements with PCPs provided incentives for them to "shut the gate" in order to limit specialist referrals, diagnostic tests, and other services (Grumbach et al., 1998). A more accurate designation of the role of the PCP in helping patients navigate the complexities of the health care system is that of coordinator of care (Bodenheimer et al., 1999). Stories such as Polly's demonstrate the importance of having a generalist care coordinator who can advocate on behalf of his or her patients and work in partnership with patients to integrate an array of services involving multiple providers to avoid duplication of services, enhance patient safety, and care for the whole person.

▶ The Patient-Centered Medical Home

Dr. Retro is counting the days until he can retire from his solo practice of general internal medicine. He feels overwhelmed most days. The next available appointment in his office is in 10 weeks, and patients call every day frustrated about lack of access. A health plan just sent him a quality report card indicating that many diabetic patients in his practice have not achieved the targeted levels of control of their blood sugar, blood pressure, and lipids. He is also behind in keeping his patients up to date on their mammograms and colorectal cancer screening. Many days he has trouble finding information in the thick paper medical records about when his patients last received their preventive care services or diabetic tests. He never has time to take his daughter to her soccer games. He was hoping to recruit a new internal medicine residency graduate to take over his practice, but most young internists in his region are pursuing more highly paid careers in subspecialties.

Dr. Avantgard has always embraced innovation. When she read a book about new primary care practice models (Bodenheimer & Grumbach, 2007), she proposed to her three physician and two nurse practitioner partners that their primary care practice become a Patient Centered Medical Home. Dr. Avantgard starts by revamping the scheduling system to a "same-day" appointment system, where 50% of appointment slots are left unbooked until the day prior so that patients can call and be guaranteed a same day or next day appointment. Despite her partners' concerns about being overrun with patient appointments, the new scheduling system results in the same number of patients being seen each day, but with happier patients who are delighted to be able to get prompt access to care. The practice buys an electronic medical record system and uses the EMR to develop registries of all the patients in the practice due for preventive and chronic care services. Dr. Avantgard and her associates train their medical assistants to use the EMR, along with standing orders, to proactively order mammograms and blood lipid tests when due and to administer vaccinations and screen for depression during patient intake at medical visits. Now that many of the routine preventive and chronic care tasks are being capably handled by other staff, Dr. Avantgard and her clinician colleagues have more time during office visits to focus on the problems patients want to talk with them about. With the quality indicators and patient satisfaction scores for the practice rising to the top decile of scores for practitioners in the region, Dr. Avantgard plans to start negotiations with several health plans to add a monthly care coordination payment to the current fee-for-service payments, so that the practice can be compensated for the hours spent on care coordination outside of office visits.

By the turn of the 21st century, primary care in the United States had reached a critical juncture and alarms sounded about an "impending collapse of primary care medicine" (American College of Physicians, 2006; Bodenheimer, 2006). Primary care clinicians like Dr. Retro struggled to meet patient demands for accessible, comprehensive, well-coordinated care. Many gaps in quality existed, and care often fell short of being patient centered. PCPs were demoralized by outmoded practice models ill-equipped to meet the demands of modern-day primary care and an ever-widening gap between their take-home pay and the escalating earnings of specialists. In the face of these challenges, decreasing numbers of US medical school graduates selected careers in primary care and many policy analysts concluded that the nation faced a major shortage of PCPs (Bodenheimer & Pham, 2010; Petterson et al., 2015).

In response to this crisis, the four major professional organizations representing the nation's PCPs—the American Academy of Family Physicians, American College of Physicians, American Academy of Pediatrics, and American Osteopathic Association—came together in 2007 and issued a report on a common vision for reform of primary care. The *Joint Principles of a Patient-Centered Medical Home* has served as a rallying point for building a broad movement to revitalize primary care in the United States (Grundy et al., 2010). A more inclusive group with consumer advocates and representatives from nursing and other professions in addition to physicians updated the medical home concept in 2018 in the *Shared Principles of Primary Care* (Epperly et al., 2019).

The term "medical home" dates back to 1967, when it was first used by the American Academy of Pediatrics to describe the notion of a primary care practice that would coordinate care for children with complex needs. Contemporary frameworks begin by reaffirming Starfield's fundamental functions of primary care and build on those principles by calling for greater attention to patient-centeredness, such as the type of same-day scheduling methods adopted by Dr. Avantgard; implementation of innovative practice models, such

Table 5–1. "Old" and "new" model primary care: some elements of transforming a practice into a patient-centered medical home

Traditional Model	Patient-Centered Medical Home
My patients are those who make appointments to see me	Our patients are those who are registered in our medical home
Care is determined by today's problem and time available today	Care is determined by a proactive plan to meet health needs, with or without visits
Care varies by scheduled time and memory or skill of the doctor	Care is standardized according to evidence-based guidelines
I know I deliver high-quality care because I'm well trained	We measure our quality and make rapid changes to improve it
Patients are responsible for coordinating their own care	A prepared team of professionals works with all patients to coordinate care
It's up to the patients to tell us what happened to them	We track tests and consultations, and follow-up after ED and hospital care
Clinic operations center on meeting the doctor's needs	An interdisciplinary team works at the top of our licenses to serve patients

Source: Adapted with permission from F. Daniel Duffy, MD, MACP, Senior Associate Dean for Academics, University of Oklahoma School of Community Medicine.

as Dr. Avantgard's development of team-care models that reengineer workflows and tasks; and changes in physician payment, such as blending fee-for-service with partial capitation and quality incentives. Another perspective on the patient-centered medical home is shown in Table 5–1.

The Affordable Care Act set in motion several programs to support patient-centered medical home reforms, such as the Medicare Comprehensive Primary Care Initiative (Peikes et al., 2018). Organizations such as the National Committee on Quality Assurance (NCQA) created a checklist of requirements for grading practices applying to be recognized as patient-centered medical homes. Groups facilitating comprehensive reengineering of primary care practices issued road-maps to transformation, such as the Building Blocks of High-Performing Primary Care (Bodenheimer et al., 2014) and the Change Concepts of the Safety

Net Medical Home Initiative (Wagner et al., 2012). Evaluation of the first wave of practices and systems implementing patient-centered medical home reforms have demonstrated mixed results in quality of care improvement and health care cost reduction (Sinaiko et al., 2017; Peikes et al., 2018).

FORCES DRIVING THE ORGANIZATION OF HEALTH CARE IN THE UNITED STATES

▶ The Biomedical Model

The growth of the dispersed mode of health care delivery in the United States was shaped by several forces. One factor was the preeminence of the biomedical model among medical educators. An influential national study, the Flexner report of 1906, led to consolidation of medical training in academically oriented medical schools (Starr, 1982). These academic centers embraced the biomedical paradigm that was the legacy of such renowned 19th-century European microbiologists as Pasteur and Koch. The antimicrobial model engendered the faith that every illness has a discrete, ultimately knowable cause and that "magic bullets" can be crafted to eradicate these sources of disease. Physicians were trained to master pathophysiologic changes within a particular organ system, leading to the development of specialization (Luce & Byyny, 1979).

Advocates of a larger role for generalism and primary care in US health care have not so much rejected the concepts of scientific medicine and professional specialism as they have attempted to broaden the interpretation of these terms. They have called for a more integrated scientific approach to understanding health and illness that incorporates information about the individual's psychosocial experiences and family, cultural, and environmental context as well as physiologic and anatomic constitution (Engel, 1977). The attempt to more rigorously define the scientific and clinical basis of generalism contributed to the emergence of family medicine in the 1969 as a specialty discipline in its own right, and the 1-year general practice internship was replaced by a 3-year residency program and specialty board certification.

▶ Financial Incentives

A second and related factor influencing the structure of health care was the financial incentive for physician

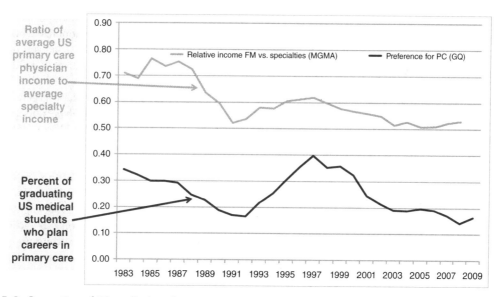

▲ Figure 5–3. Proportion of US medical students entering primary care strongly tracks relative incomes of primary care physicians. The figure shows trends over time in the average income of primary care physicians relative to specialist physicians in the United States, and in the percentage of graduating medical students in the United States planning on entering careers in primary care. In 1990, when the average primary care physician income was about half that of specialists, fewer than 20% of graduating students planned to enter primary care fields. By 1997, when primary care physician incomes had risen to more than 60% that of specialists, the proportion of graduating students entering primary care had increased in a parallel direction with 40% of graduates planning to enter primary care fields in 1997. Both relative incomes and intentions to enter primary care decreased after 1997. (From the Council on Graduate Medical Education. *Twentieth Report: Advancing Primary Care,* December 2010. www.hrsa.gov/advisorycommittees/bhpradvisory/cogme/Reports/twentiethreport.pdf. Accessed October 4, 2019.)

specialization and hospital expansion, which played out in a number of ways.

1. Insurance benefits first offered by Blue Cross covered hospital costs but not physician visits and other outpatient services.

2. As physician services came to be covered later under Blue Shield and other plans, a growing differential in payment between generalist and specialist physicians developed. New technologic and other procedures often required considerable physician time when first introduced, and higher fees were justified for these procedures. But as the procedures became routine, fees remained high, while the time and effort required to perform them declined (Starr, 1982); this resulted in an increasing disparity in income between PCPs and specialists (Bodenheimer et al., 2007). In the mid-1980s, the average PCP's income

was 75% of the average specialist's income; by 2006, PCP income had dropped to only 50% of specialists' income (Council of Graduate Medical Education, 2010). As Figure 5–3 shows, the percentage of graduating medical students planning to enter careers in primary care tracks the PCP-specialist income gap closely, with the proportion of students entering primary care decreasing as the earnings of PCPs relative to specialists declines.

3. Federal involvement in health care financing further fueled the expansion of hospital care and specialization. The Hill–Burton Hospital Construction Act of 1946 allocated billions of dollars between 1946 and 1971 for expansion of hospital capacity rather than development of ambulatory services (Starr, 1982). The enactment of Medicare and Medicaid in 1965 perpetuated the private insurance tradition of higher payment for procedurally oriented specialists

than for generalists. Medicare further encouraged specialization through its policy of extra payments to hospitals to cover costs associated with residency training. Linking Medicare teaching payments to the hospital sector added yet another bias against community-based primary care training.

The growth of hospitals and medical specialization was intertwined. As medical practice became more specialized and dependent on technology, the site of care increasingly shifted from the patient's home or physician's office to the hospital. The emphasis on acute hospital care had an effect on the nursing profession comparable to that on physicians. World War I was a watershed period in the transition of nursing from a community-based to a hospital-based orientation. During the war, US military hospitals overseas were much heralded for their success in treating acute war injuries. At the war's conclusion, the nation rallied behind a policy of boosting the civilian hospital sector. According to Rosemary Stevens (1989),

> Before the war, public-health nursing was the elite area; nurses had been instrumental in the campaigns against tuberculosis and for infant welfare. In contrast, the war emphasized the supremacy and glamour of hospitals . . . nurses, like physicians, were trained—and ready—to perform in an increasingly specialized, acute-care medical environment rather than to expand their interests in social medicine and public health.

▶ Professionalism

The final factor accounting for the organizational evolution of US health care delivery was the nature of control over health planning. The United States is unique in its relative laxity of public regulation of health care resources. In most industrialized nations, governments wield considerable control over health planning through measures such as regulation of hospital capacity and technology, allocation of the number of residency training positions in generalist and specialist fields, and coordination of public health with medical care. In the United States, the government has provided much of the financing for health care, but without an attendant degree of administrative control. The Hill–Burton program, for example, did not make grants for

hospital construction contingent upon any rigorous community-wide plan for regionalized hospital services. Medicare funding for physician training did not stipulate any particular distribution of residency positions according to specialty.

With government controls kept largely at bay, the professional "sovereignty" of physicians emerged as the preeminent authority in health care (Starr, 1982). Societies grant certain occupations special status as "professions" because of the unique knowledge and skill required of members of the profession, and the expectation that this knowledge and skill will be applied beneficially (Friedson, 1970; Light & Levine, 1988). Professionalism thus involves a social contract; in return for the privilege of autonomy, physicians bear the responsibility for acting as the patient's agent, and the profession must regulate itself to preserve the public trust.

Their professional status vested physicians with special authority to guide the development of the US health care system. As described in Chapter 2, third-party payment for physician services was established with physician control of the initial Blue Shield insurance plans. Physician judgment about the need for technology and greater inpatient capacity drove the expansion of hospital facilities.

What was the nature of the profession that so heavily influenced the development of the US health care organization? It was a profession that, because of the primacy of the biomedical paradigm and the nature of financial incentives, was weighted toward hospital and specialty care. Small wonder that US health care has emphasized its tertiary care apex over its primary care base. In Chapter 16, we discuss the shifting power relationships in health care that are challenging the professional dominance of physicians.

CONCLUSION

Jeff leaves a town forum at the local medical center feeling confused. It featured two speakers, one of whom criticized the medical center as being out of touch with the community's needs, and the other of whom defended the center's contributions to society. Jeff found the first speaker very convincing about the need to pay more attention to primary care, prevention, and public health. He had never had a regular primary care physician, and the idea of having a family physician appealed to him. He was equally impressed by the second speaker, whose account of how research at the medical center had led to life-saving treatment of children with a hereditary blood disorder was very moving, and whose description of the hospital's plan for a new imaging center was spellbinding. Jeff felt that if he ever became seriously ill, he would certainly want all the specialized services the medical center had to offer.

The professional model and the biomedical paradigm are responsible for many of the successes of the US health care system. The biomedical model has instilled respect for the scientific method and curtailed medical quackery. Professionalism has directed physicians to serve as agents acting in their patients' best interests and has made the practice of medicine more than just another business. Expansion of hospital facilities has meant that people with health insurance have had convenient access to tertiary care services and new technology and the expertise and availability of a wide variety of specialists. In many circumstances, the system is well organized to deliver the "right care." For a patient in cardiogenic shock, the right place to be is an intensive care unit; for a patient with a detached retina, an ophthalmologist's office is the right place to be.

However, there is widespread concern that despite the benefits of biomedical science and medical professionalism, the US health care system is precariously off balance. A model of excellence focused on specialization, technology, and curative medicine has led to relative inattention to basic primary care services, including such needs as disease prevention and supportive care for patients with chronic and incurable ailments. The value placed on autonomy for health care professionals and institutions has contributed to fragmentation of care. A system that prizes specialists who focus on organ systems and researchers who concentrate on genomics has bred apprehension that health care has somehow lost sight of the whole person and the whole community. The net result is a system structured to perform miraculous feats for individuals who are ill, but at great expense and often without satisfactorily attending to the full spectrum of health care needs of the entire population. During the 2009 debate

in Congress leading up to the passage of the Affordable Care Act, one of the harshest critiques of the status quo in US health care came not from a Congressional Democrat, but from Senator Orrin Hatch, the senior Republican Senator from Utah. At a hearing on health reform, Senator Hatch said, "The US is first in providing rescue care, but this care has little or no impact on the general population. We must put more focus on primary care and preventive medicine" (Grundy et al., 2010).

REFERENCES

American College of Physicians. *The impending collapse of primary care medicine and its implications for the state of the nation's health care.* January 30, 2006. Available at https://www.acponline.org/acp_policy/policies/impending_collapse_of_primary_care_medicine_and_its_implications_for_the_state_of_the_nations_health_care_2006.pdf. Accessed October 4.

Association of American Medical Colleges. The complexities of physician supply and demand: projections from 2017 to 2032. Washington, DC; 2019. Association of American Medical Colleges › workforce-studies › reports. Accessed October 4, 2019.

Auerbach DI, et al. Nurse-managed health centers and patient-centered medical homes could mitigate expected primary care physician shortage. *Health Aff (Millwood).* 2013;32:1933–1941.

Baicker K, Chandra A. Medicare spending, the physician workforce, and beneficiaries' quality of care. *Health Aff (Millwood).* 2004:W4-184–197.

Basu S, et al. Association of primary care physician supply with population mortality in the United States, 2005 – 2015. *JAMA Intern Med.* 2019;179:506–514.

Bazemore A, et al. More comprehensive care among family physicians is associated with lower costs and fewer hospitalizations. *Ann Fam Med.* 2015;13:206–213.

Bindman AB, et al. Primary care and receipt of preventive services. *J Gen Intern Med.* 1996;11:269–276.

Bodenheimer T. Regional medical programs: no road to regionalization. *Med Care Rev.* 1969;26:1125–1166.

Bodenheimer T. Primary care—will it survive? *N Engl J Med.* 2006;355:861–864.

Bodenheimer T, Grumbach K. *Improving Primary Care. Strategies and Tools for a Better Practice.* New York, NY: McGraw-Hill; 2007.

Bodenheimer T, Pham HH. Primary care: current problems and proposed solutions. *Health Aff (Millwood).* 2010;29:799–805.

Bodenheimer T, et al. Primary care physicians should be coordinators, not gatekeepers. *JAMA*. 1999;281(21): 2045–2049.

Bodenheimer T, et al. The primary care-specialty income gap: why it matters. *Ann Intern Med*. 2007;146:301–306.

Bodenheimer T, et al. The 10 building blocks of high-performing primary care. *Ann Fam Med*. 2014;12:166–171.

Council on Graduate Medical Education. Twentieth report: advancing primary care, December 2010. Available at www.hrsa.gov/advisorycommittees/bhpradvisory/cogme/Reports/twentiethreport.pdf. Accessed October 4, 2019.

Dawson W. Interim report on the future provision of medical and allied services. In: Saward EW, ed. *The Regionalization of Personal Health Services*. London, England: Prodist; 1975.

Engel GL. The need for a new medical model: a challenge for biomedicine. *Science*. 1977;196:129–136.

Epperly T, et al. The shared principles of primary care: a multistakeholder initiative to find a common voice. *Fam Med*. 2019;52:179–184.

Friedberg MW, et al. Primary care: a critical review of the evidence on quality and costs of health care. *Health Aff (Millwood)*. 2010;29:766–772.

Friedson E. *Professional Dominance: The Social Structure of Medicine*. Atherton, CA: Atherton Publishing; 1970.

Fry J. Primary care. In: Fry J, ed. *Primary Care*. London, England: William Heinemann; 1980.

Gonzalez AA, et al. Understanding the volume-outcome effect in cardiovascular surgery: the role of failure to rescue. *JAMA Surg*. 2014;149:119–123.

Goroll AH, Hunt DP. Bridging the hospitalist-primary care divide through collaborative care. *N Engl J Med*. 2015;372:308–309.

Green LA, et al. The ecology of medical care revisited. *N Engl J Med*. 2001;344:2021–2025.

Grumbach K, et al. Primary care physicians' experience of financial incentives in managed care systems. *N Engl J Med*. 1998;339:1516–1521.

Grundy P, et al. The multi-stakeholder movement for primary care renewal and reform. *Health Affairs*. 2010;29:791–798.

Halvorson GC, Isham GJ. *Epidemic of Care*. San Francisco, CA: Jossey-Bass; 2003.

Institute of Medicine. *Primary Care: America's Health in a New Era*. Washington, DC: National Academies Press; 1996. Available at www.ncbi.nlm.nih.gov/pubmed/25121221. Accessed October 4, 2019.

Kurtzman E, Barnow BS. A comparison of nurse practitioners, physician assistants, and primary care physicians'

patterns of practice and quality of care in health centers. *Medical Care*. 2017;55:615–622.

Light D, Levine S. The changing character of the medical profession: a theoretical overview. *Milbank Mem Fund Q*. 1988;66:10–32.

Luce JM, Byyny RL. The evolution of medical specialism. *Perspect Biol Med*. 1979;22:377–389.

Peikes D, et al. The comprehensive primary care initiative: effects on spending, quality, patients, and physicians. *Health Aff (Millwood)*. 2018;37:890–899.

Petterson SM, et al. Estimating the residency expansion required to avoid projected primary care physician shortages by 2035. *Ann Fam Med*. 2015;13:107–114.

Rodwin VG. *The Health Planning Predicament*. Berkeley, CA: University of California Press; 1984.

Safran DG, et al. Linking primary care performance to outcomes of care. *J Fam Pract*. 1998;47:213–220.

Saultz JW, Albedaiwi W. Interpersonal continuity of care and patient satisfaction: a critical review. *Ann Fam Med*. 2004;2:445–451.

Saultz JW, Lochner J. Interpersonal continuity of care and care outcomes: a critical review. *Ann Fam Med*. 2005;3: 159–166.

Sinaiko AD, et al. Synthesis of research on patient-centered medical homes brings systematic differences into relief. *Health Aff (Millwood)*. 2017;36:500–508.

Somers AR. Who's in charge here? Alice searches for a king in Mediland. *N Engl J Med*. 1972;287:849–855.

Starfield B. *Primary Care*. New York, NY: Oxford University Press; 1998.

Starfield B, et al. Contribution of primary care to health systems and health. *Milbank Q*. 2005;83:457–502.

Starr P. *The Social Transformation of American Medicine*. New York, NY: Basic Books; 1982.

Stevens R. *In Sickness and in Wealth: American Hospitals in the Twentieth Century*. New York, NY: Basic Books; 1989.

Stewart AL, et al. Primary care and patient perceptions of access to care. *J Fam Pract*. 1997;44:177–185.

Wachter RM, Goldman L. The emerging role of "hospitalists" in the American health care system. *N Engl J Med*. 1996;335:514–517.

Wagner EH, et al. The changes involved in patient-centered medical home transformation. *Prim Care*. 2012;39: 241–259.

White KL, et al. The ecology of medical care. *N Engl J Med*. 1961;265:885–892.

How Health Care Is Organized—II: Health Delivery Systems

The last chapter explored general principles of health care organization, including levels of care, regionalization, physician and other practitioner roles, and patient flow through the system. This chapter looks at actual structures of medical practice.

The traditional dispersed model of the US medical practice has been referred to as a "cottage industry" of independent private physicians working as solo practitioners or in small groups. By 2020, a major change was evident, with small organizations either banding together to form large enterprises, or being swallowed up by health care giants. The dispersed model is evolving into a more consolidated model of health care delivery.

THE TRADITIONAL STRUCTURE OF MEDICAL CARE

Physicians and Hospitals

Dr. Harvey Commoner finished his residency in general surgery in 1976. For the next 30 years, he and another surgeon practiced medicine together in a middle-class suburb near St. Peter's Hospital, a nonprofit church-affiliated institution. Dr. Commoner received most of his cases from family physicians and internists on the St. Peter's medical staff. By 1996, the number of surgeons operating at St. Peter's had grown. Because Dr. Commoner was not getting enough cases, he and his partner joined the medical staff of Top Dollar Hospital, a for-profit facility 3 miles away, and University Hospital downtown. On an average morning,

Dr. Commoner drove to all three hospitals to perform operations or to do postoperative rounds on his patients. The afternoon was spent seeing patients in his office. He was on call every other night and weekend.

Dr. Commoner was active on the St. Peter's medical staff executive committee, where he frequently proposed that the hospital purchase new radiology and operating room equipment needed to keep up with advances in surgery. Because the hospital received more than 1 million dollars each year for providing care to Dr. Commoner's patients, and because Dr. Commoner had the option of admitting his patients to Top Dollar or University, the St. Peter's administration usually purchased the items that Dr. Commoner recommended. The Top Dollar Hospital administrator did likewise.

During the period when Dr. Commoner was practicing, most medical care was delivered by fee-for-service private physicians in solo or small group practices. Most hospitals were private nonprofit institutions, sometimes affiliated with a religious organization, occasionally with a medical school, often run by an independent board of trustees composed of prominent people in the community. Most physicians in traditional fee-for-service practice were not employees of any hospital, but joined one or several hospital medical staffs, thereby gaining the privilege of admitting patients to the hospital and at times acquiring the responsibility to assist the hospital through work on medical staff committees or by caring for emergency department patients who have no physician.

For many years, physicians were the dominant power in the hospital because physicians admit the patients, and hospitals without patients have no income. Because physicians were free to admit their patients to more than one hospital, the implicit threat to take their patients elsewhere gave them influence. Under traditional fee-for-service medicine, physicians used informal referral networks, often involving other physicians on the same hospital medical staff. In metropolitan areas with a high ratio of physician specialists to population, referrals could become a critical economic issue. Most surgeons obtained their cases by referral from primary care physicians (PCPs) or medical specialists; surgeons like Dr. Commoner who were not readily available when called soon found their case load drying up.

THE SEEDS OF NEW MEDICAL CARE STRUCTURES

The dispersed structure of fee-for-service private practice was not always the dominant model in the United States. When modern medical care took root in the first half of the 20th century, a variety of structures blossomed. Among these were multispecialty group practices, community health centers, and prepaid group practices. Some of these flourished but then wilted, while others became the seeds from which the emerging health care system of the 21st century is germinating.

▶ Multispecialty Group Practice

In 1905, Dr. Geraldine Giemsa joined the department of pathology at the Mayo Clinic. The clinic, led by the brothers William and Charles Mayo, was becoming a nationally renowned referral center for surgery and was recruiting pathologists, microbiologists, and other specialized diagnosticians to support the work of the clinic's surgeons. Dr. Giemsa received a salary and became an employee of the group practice. With time, she became a senior partner and part owner of the Mayo Clinic.

Together with their father, the Mayo brothers, general practitioners skilled at surgical techniques, formed a group practice in the small town of Rochester, MN, in the 1890s. As the brothers' reputation for excellence grew, the practice added surgeons and physicians in laboratory-oriented specialties. By 1929, the Mayo Clinic had more than 375 physicians and 900 support staff and eventually opened its own hospitals (Starr, 1982). Although the clinic paid its physician staff by salary, the clinic itself billed patients, and later insurance plans, on a fee-for-service basis. The Mayo Clinic was the inspiration for other group practices that developed in the United States, such as the Menninger Clinic in Topeka, KS, and the Palo Alto Medical Foundation in California. These clinics were owned and administered by physicians in various specialties—hence the common use of the term *multispecialty group practice* to describe this organizational model. The multispecialty group practices brought a large number of physicians together under one roof to deliver care.

By formally integrating specialists into a single clinic structure, group practice attempted to promote a collaborative style of care in which colleagues shared responsibility for the care of patients. Critics warned that large practice structures would subject patients to an impersonal style of care and jeopardize the intimate patient–physician relationship possible in a solo or small group setting.

In 1932, the blue ribbon Committee on the Costs of Medical Care recommended that the delivery of care be organized around large group practices (Starr, 1982). The eight private practice physicians on the committee dissented from the recommendations, roundly criticizing the sections on group practice. An editorial in the *Journal of the American Medical Association* was scathing in its attack on the committee's majority report:

> *The physicians of this country must not be misled by utopian fantasies of a form of medical practice, which would equalize all physicians by placing them in groups under one administration. The public will find to its cost, as it has elsewhere, that such schemes do not answer that hidden desire in each human breast for human kindliness, human forbearance, and human understanding. It is better for the American people that most of their illnesses be treated by their own physicians rather than by industries, corporations, or clinics.* (The Committee on the Costs of Medical Care, 1932)

Several multispecialty group practices flourished during the period between the world wars, and to this day remain among the most highly regarded systems of care in the United States. Yet multispecialty group practice did not become the dominant organizational structure, in part due to resistance by professional societies. In addition, as hospitals assumed a central role in medical care, group practice lost some of its unique attractions. Hospitals could provide the ancillary services physicians needed for the increasingly specialized and technology-dependent work of medicine. Hospitals also served as an organizational focus for the informal referral networks that developed among private physicians in independent practice.

▶ Community Health Centers

A far-reaching alternative to private medical practice is the community health center, emphasizing primary and preventive care and striving to take responsibility for the health status of the community served by the health center. An early 20th-century example of such an institution was the Greater Community Association at Creston, Iowa. The association brought together civic, religious, education, and health care groups in a coordinated system centered on the community hospital serving a six-county area with 100,000 residents. The plan placed its greatest emphasis on preventive care and public health measures administered by public health nurses. In describing the association, Kepford (1919) wrote:

The motto of the Greater Community Association is "Service." Among the principles of the hospital management are the precept that it shall be a long way from the threshold of the hospital to the operating room . . . . We have a hospital that makes no attempt to pattern after the great city institutions, but is organized to meet the needs of a rural neighborhood. The Greater Community Association has been taught to regard the hospital as a repair shop, necessary only where preventive medicine has failed.

In 1928, Sherry Kidd joined the Frontier Nursing Service in Appalachia as a nurse midwife. For $5 per year, families could enroll in the service and receive pregnancy-related care. Sherry

was responsible for all enrolled families within a 100-mile radius. She referred patients with complications to an obstetrician in Lexington, KY, the service's physician consultant.

Another pioneering model, the Frontier Nursing Service was established by Mary Breckinridge, an English-trained midwife, in 1925 (Dye, 1983). Breckinridge designed the service to meet the needs of a poor rural area in Kentucky that lacked basic medical and obstetric care and suffered from high rates of maternal and infant mortality. The Frontier Nursing Service shared many features of the Creston model: regionalized services planned on a geographic basis to serve rural populations with an emphasis on primary care and health education. Like the Creston system, the service relied on nurses to provide primary care, with physicians reserved for secondary medical services.

These rural programs had their urban counterparts in health centers that focused on maternal and child health services during the early 1900s (Stoeckle & Candib, 1969; Rothman, 1978), typically serving low-income, immigrant populations. The clinics primarily served populations in low-income districts in large cities and were often involved with large immigrant populations. As in the rural systems, public health nurses played a central role in health education, nutrition, and sanitation. Both the urban and rural models of community health centers waned during the middle years of this century. Public health nursing declined in prestige as hospitals became the center of activity for nursing education and practice (Stevens, 1989). A team model of nurses working in collaboration with physicians withered under a system of hierarchical professional roles.

The community health center model was revived in 1965 by the federal Office of Economic Opportunity's "War on Poverty." The program's goals included the combining of comprehensive medical care and public health to improve the health status of defined low-income communities, the building of multidisciplinary teams to provide health services, and participation in the governance of the health centers by community members.

Dr. Franklin Jefferson was professor of hematology at a prestigious medical school. His distinguished career was based on laboratory research, teaching, and subspecialty medical practice, with a focus on sickle cell anemia. Dr. Jefferson felt that his work was serving his community, but that he would like to do more. In 1965, with the advent of the federal neighborhood health center program, he left his laboratory in the hands of a well-trained assistant and began to talk with community leaders in the poor neighborhood that surrounded the medical school. After a year, the trust that developed between Dr. Jefferson and members of the neighborhood bore fruit in a decision to approach the medical school dean about a joint medical school–community application for funds to create a neighborhood health center. Two years later, the center opened its doors, with Dr. Jefferson as its first medical director.

By the early 1980s, 800 federally funded community health centers were in operation, administered by governing boards that included patients of the health center. Many of the centers trained community members as outreach workers, who became members of health care teams that included public health nurses, physicians, mental health workers, and health educators. Some health centers strived to meld clinical services with public health activities in programs of community-oriented primary care. For example, the rural health center in Mound Bayou, Mississippi, helped organize a cooperative farm to improve nutrition in the county, dig wells to supply safe drinking water, and train community residents to become health care professionals (Geiger, 2016). By improving the ambulatory care of low-income patients, the centers were able to reduce hospitalization and emergency department visits by their patients. Community health centers also had some success in improving community health status, particularly by reducing infant and neonatal mortality rates among African Americans (Geiger, 1984). In 2018, nearly 1,300 community health centers at 11,000 sites were serving over 28 million people, most uninsured or covered by Medicaid (National Association of Community Health Centers , 2018).

▶ Prepaid Group Practice and Health Maintenance Organizations

One alternative to small office-based, fee-for-service practice became the major challenge to that traditional model: prepaid group practice.

In 1929, the Ross–Loos Clinic began to provide medical services for employees of the Los Angeles Department of Water and Power on a prepaid basis. By 1935, the clinic had enrolled 37,000 employees and their dependents, who each paid $2 per month for a specified list of services. Also in 1929, an idealistic physician, Dr. Michael Shadid, organized a medical cooperative in Elk City, OK, based on four principles: group practice, prepayment, preventive medicine, and control by the patients, who were members of the cooperative. In the late forties, more than a hundred rural health cooperatives were founded, many in Texas, but they faded away, partly from the stiff opposition of organized medicine. In the 1950s, another version of the consumer-managed prepaid group practice sprang up in Appalachia, where the United Mine Workers established union-run group practice clinics, each receiving a budget from the union-controlled medical care fund. A few years later in Seattle, Group Health Cooperative of Puget Sound acquired its own hospital, began to grow, and by the mid-1970s had 200,000 subscribers, a fifth of the Seattle-area population. In 1947, the Health Insurance Plan of New York opened its doors, operating 22 group practices; within 10 years, its enrollment approached 500,000 (Starr, 1982).

Rather than preserving a separation between insurance plans and the providers of care, these prepaid group practice models meld the financing and delivery of care into a single organizational structure. Paying a premium for health insurance coverage in this approach does not just mean that a third-party payer will pay for some or all the costs of care delivered by independent practitioners. Rather, the premium serves to directly purchase, in advance, health services from a particular system of care. In addition to the prepayment component, care is delivered by a large group of practitioners working under a common administrative structure—the "group practice" aspect of prepaid group practice.

The most successful of the prepaid group practices that emerged in the 1930s and 1940s was Kaiser Permanente. In 1938, a surgeon named Sidney Garfield began providing prepaid medical services for industrialist Henry J. Kaiser's employees working at the Grand Coulee Dam in Washington State. Rather than receiving a salary from Kaiser, Garfield was prepaid a fixed sum per employee, a precursor to modern capitation payment. Kaiser transported this concept to 200,000 workers in his shipyards and steel mills on the West Coast during World War II (Garfield, 1970; Starr, 1982). In this way, company-sponsored medical care in a remote area gave birth to today's largest alternative to fee-for-service practice. Kaiser opened its doors to the general public after World War II. In 2017, Kaiser was present in eight states plus Washington, DC, with 12.2 million patients enrolled.

Prepaid group practices were renamed "health maintenance organizations" in the 1970s, with the term *health maintenance* designed to suggest that these systems would place more emphasis on preventive care than had the traditional medical model. We will return later in the chapter to discuss how health maintenance organizations (HMOs) have taken on a new meaning separate from the prepaid group practice model. But first, we will use the Kaiser Permanente organization to introduce the key concepts of *vertical* and *horizontal* *integration*.

VERTICAL AND HORIZONTAL INTEGRATION

▶ Kaiser Permanente

Maria Fuentes was a professor at the University of California. She and her family belonged to the Kaiser Health Plan, and the university paid her family's premium. Professor Fuentes had once fractured her clavicle, for which she went to the urgent care clinic at Kaiser Hospital in Oakland; otherwise, she had not used Kaiser's facilities. Professor Fuentes' wife suffered from rheumatoid arthritis; her regular physician was a salaried rheumatologist at the Permanente Medical Clinic, the group practice in which Kaiser physicians work. One of the Fuentes' sons, Juanito, had been in an automobile accident a year earlier near a town 90 miles away from home. He had been taken to a local emergency department and released; Kaiser had paid the bill because no Kaiser facility was available in the town. Three days after returning home, Juanito developed a severe headache and became drowsy; he was taken to the urgent care clinic, received a CT scan, and was found to have a subdural hematoma. He was immediately transported to Kaiser's regional neurosurgery center in Redwood City, CA, where he underwent surgery to evacuate the hematoma.

Dr. Roberta Short had mixed feelings about working at Kaiser. She liked the salary and the paucity of administrative tasks. She particularly liked working in the same building with other internists and specialists, providing the opportunity for discussions on diagnostic and therapeutic problems. However, she was not happy about the large number of patients she was scheduled to see. Overall, Dr. Short felt that the Kaiser system worked well but perhaps needed more physicians per enrolled patient.

Kaiser Permanente is the largest of the nation's prepaid group practices, consisting of three interlocking administrative units: Kaiser Foundation Health Plan, which performs the functions of health insurer, Kaiser Foundation Hospitals, and Permanente Medical Groups, the physician organizations that provide medical services to Kaiser members under a capitated contract with the Health Plan.

This organizational model has come to be known as vertical integration. *Vertical integration* refers to consolidating under one organizational roof and common ownership all levels of care, from primary to tertiary care, and the facilities and staff necessary to provide this full spectrum of care (Fig. 6–1). Although structures differ somewhat across Kaiser's regions, most Kaiser Permanente units own their hospitals and clinics, hire the nurses, pharmacists, and other personnel staffing these facilities, and contract with a single large group practice (Permanente) to exclusively serve patients covered by the Kaiser health plan. The Kaiser Permanente health system differs from traditional fee-for-service models in how it pays physicians (salary) and hospitals (global budget). The prepaid group practice structure contrasts with solo, independent private practice.

Kaiser Permanente is also *horizontally integrated.* Horizontal integration refers to consolidation of health care units providing the same type of services. As noted above, one division of Kaiser Permanente is its Foundation Hospitals; Kaiser hospitals in a region operate under common ownership and management rather than as autonomous facilities. Horizontal integration of hospitals has allowed Kaiser to regionalize

Vertically integrated system

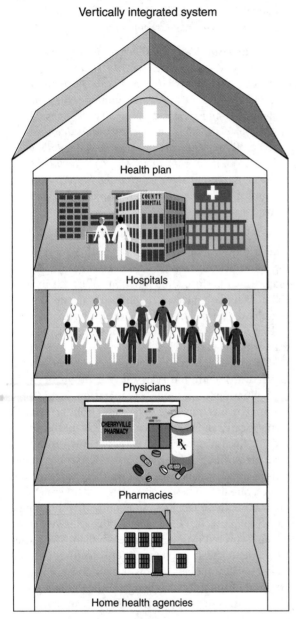

▲ Figure 6–1. Vertical integration consolidates health services under one organizational roof.

tertiary care services at a select number of specialized centers. For example, Northern California Kaiser has centralized neurosurgical care at only two hospitals, in contrast to dispersed models in which competing independent hospitals often duplicate many of the same specialized services. Similarly, the Permanente Medical Group represents horizontal integration of physicians and other health professionals. This approach has given Kaiser Permanente considerable control of its internal workforce policy, resulting in the Permanente Medical Group having a greater proportion of PCPs than the overall US workforce and incorporating nurse practitioners and physician assistants into the primary care team. Many observers consider this ability to coherently plan and regionalize services to a defined population to be a strength of vertically and horizontally integrated systems. Structural integration also facilitates functional integration in patient care, such as by having a shared electronic medical record used throughout the organization. The prepaid nature of enrollment in the Kaiser plan permits Kaiser to orient its care more toward a population health model.

▶ The Rise of Other Models of Integrated Health Systems

Ollie Gopoly, CEO of California Health, smiled as he reviewed the hospital system's year-end financial report. Fifteen years ago, Ollie was CEO of an independent hospital that was rapidly going from profitable to running in the red as Kaiser gained ever-increasing market share in the region. Ollie realized that the only way to compete was to become more horizontally organized. His first step was to orchestrate a merger with another two local hospitals. Over the ensuing years, the hospital partnership acquired six other hospitals in the region, created a new hospital corporation, California Health, that named Ollie as CEO, and implemented an integrated model with a shared electronic medical record. California Health was now second only to Kaiser in the volume of hospital care in the region. Because of its size, it was able to negotiate higher payment rates with health insurance plans and discounts on the supplies and equipment it purchased. This year's financial performance had generated a substantial positive margin that would allow Ollie to take the next step in his strategic plan: acquiring physician practices.

The greatest growth in integrated models in the past two decades has come not from organizations replicating the Kaiser Permanente model but through consolidation of hospitals into large horizontal systems. Hospitals across the nation have engaged in a process of mergers and acquisitions to create regional systems. Examples of non-profit systems are Sutter Health in California, Carilion Health System in Virginia, Carolinas Health Care System (now known as Atrium Health), and Banner Health in Arizona. Several for-profit horizontal hospital systems such as Tenet and HCA have a national scope. This consolidation was motivated in part by a desire to achieve the functional benefits and economies of scale of horizontal integration. But another powerful motivator was achieving a stronger bargaining position in the health care marketplace. This trend has raised concerns about hospitals consolidating so much market share as to become oligopolies that function in an anti-competitive manner to drive up hospital prices (we discuss this issue more in Chapter 16).

The first stage of horizontal consolidation of hospitals into regional health systems has been followed by a second stage of becoming more vertically integrated, principally by purchasing physician practices and converting physicians from independent small business owners to employees of the hospital or of a hospital-sponsored medical group. Despite the admonitions of the dissenting *JAMA* editorialists in 1932 who warned physicians not to be "misled by utopian fantasies" of group practice, a tipping point has occurred in the 21st Century, with the health care cottage industry giving way to larger organizations for delivering care. From 2002 to 2008, the percentage of medical practices that are doctor-owned fell from 70% to 48% while the percentage owned by hospitals grew from 24% to 50% (Kocher & Sahni, 2011) (Fig. 6–2). Most new residency graduates are eschewing the tradition of becoming autonomous proprietors of their own private practices and entering employed positions, seeking "regular paychecks instead of shopkeeper risks" (Harris, 2011). Several of these regional delivery systems, such as Sutter Health and Banner Health, have added the final element of vertical integration—operating their own health insurance plan. However, unlike Kaiser Permanente, none of these regional systems relies exclusively on its own health plan; all also contract with other private plans for the majority of their privately insured patients.

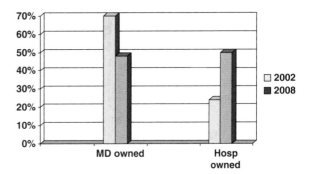

▲ **Figure 6–2.** Ownership of medical practices. (From Kocher R, Sahni NR. Hospitals race to employ physicians—the logic behind a money-losing proposition. *N Engl J Med.* 2011;364:1790–1793.)

VIRTUAL INTEGRATION

We have contrasted the traditional dispersed model of US health care with the growing integration that is occurring. Despite the accelerating consolidation of hospitals and physicians into larger systems, many health care stakeholders remain interested in a third way that brings some of the functional benefits of integration while retaining some of the independence of traditional practice. An example is how a group of physicians in California organized themselves many years ago to create an alternative to the Kaiser Permanente model.

Network Models

In 1954, the medical society in San Joaquin County, CA, fretted about the possibility of Kaiser moving into the county. Patients might go to the lower cost Kaiser, and physicians' incomes would fall. An idea was born: to compete with Kaiser, the San Joaquin Foundation for Medical Care was set up as a network of physicians in independent private practice to contract as a group with employers for a monthly payment per enrollee; the Foundation would then pay the physicians on a discounted fee-for-service basis and conduct utilization review to discourage overtreatment (Starr, 1982). It was hoped that the plan would reduce the costs to employers, who would choose the Foundation rather than Kaiser. This "network model" of horizontal integration spread widely

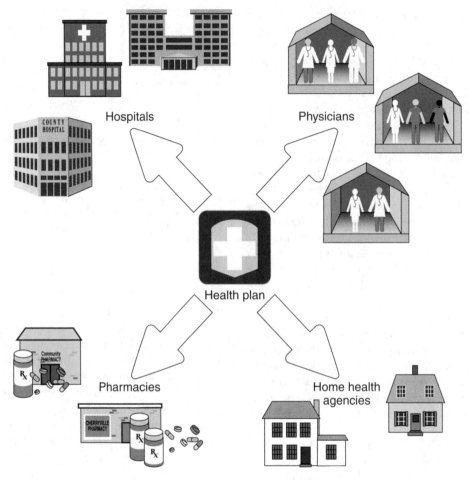

▲ Figure 6–3. Virtual integration involves contractual links between HMOs and physician groups, hospitals, and other provider units.

in California as Independent Practice Associations (IPAs) brought together doctors in their private offices to gain more favorable contracts with insurance companies. In the three-tiered payment model described in Chapter 4, insurers pay the IPA which in turn pays its physicians.

This approach of weaving together autonomous physician practices in an IPA in turn engendered a network HMO model of loose vertical integration that became the alternative to the tightly integrated prepaid group practice model. Like the prepaid group practice HMO model, the network HMO model differs from traditional insurance in that the insurance plan only pays for services provided by those physicians and hospitals that participate in the HMO plan—often referred to as a "narrow network" of providers. However, unlike the prepaid group practice model, these providers are not owned or employed by a single organized health delivery system. As shown in Figure 6–3, the network HMO model consists of contractual links between HMO health insurance plans and individual physicians, IPAs, multispecialty medical groups, hospitals, and other provider units, rather than the "everything-under-one-roof" model of the prepaid group practice model of vertical integration. Even when network HMOs contract with large hospital-based regional health systems with employed physician groups, they almost always also have contracts with other hospitals and physicians that are not part of the regional systems. Unlike the "monogamous" arrangement between the Kaiser health plan, Kaiser hospitals, and Permanente medical group, under network HMO models hospitals and physicians can establish contractual relationships with many different insurance plans. Observers have dubbed the network model of organization "virtual integration," signifying an integration of services based on contractual relationships rather than unitary ownership (Robinson & Casalino, 1996).

An even looser provider network configuration occurs under Preferred Provider Organization (PPO) health plan products. In response to the reluctance of many patients to be locked into a narrow network of physicians and hospitals in HMO plans, PPO plans have a "preferred" network of physicians and hospitals but allow patients to use physicians and hospitals that are not in the network, with the stipulation that patients pay a higher share of the cost out of pocket when they use non-network physicians and hospitals. Physicians joining the PPO network agree to accept discounted fees from the health plan with the hope that being listed as a "preferred" provider will attract more patients to their practice. Unlike HMO plans, PPO plans use fee for service payment and do not require patients to select a PCP for their medical home. PPO enrollment was 163 million in 2016, compared with HMO enrollment of 92 million (MCOL, 2016).

Both network model HMOs and PPOs are considered forms of "managed care." But do these types of managed care truly represent more integrated forms of care delivery? PPOs do not change how care is organized and are simply a minor variation of fee-for-service insurance products. Network HMOs drive a modest degree of change in care organization; they establish a tighter relationship between patients and primary care clinicians and often use capitated payment that emphasizes population health-oriented care. Network HMOs that contract with IPAs rather than directly with individual physicians may also encourage "virtual group practice."

Although IPAs initially did little more than to act as brokers between physicians and HMOs, over time IPAs have taken on a larger portion of financial risk for care (see Chapter 4), become more active in attempting to control costs, and assumed responsibility for authorizing utilization of services, profiling physicians' practice patterns, and facilitating quality improvement efforts.

The various permutations of horizontal and vertical integration are shown in Table 6–1.

▶ Accountable Care Organizations

As described in Chapter 4, an Accountable Care Organization (ACO) is defined as "a provider-led organization whose mission is to manage the full continuum of care and be accountable for the overall costs and quality of care for a defined population" (Rittenhouse et al., 2009). The Affordable Care Act authorized Medicare to initiate an ACO program beginning in 2012 (Gold, 2015). Private insurance plans and large employers also contract with provider organizations to form ACOs. In 2018, 53% of ACO contracts were private, 37% Medicare, and 10% Medicaid. In early 2018, ACOs covered 32.7 million people in all 50 states (Figure 6–4) (Muhlestein et al., 2018). ACOs span a spectrum of organizational structures. Provider groups form ACOs in order to be able to participate in a reformed payment model that places physicians and hospitals at shared financial risk with the payer for a global budgetary target for a population of patients. Chapters 4 and 9 provide additional details about risk sharing under ACO payment models. Payers do not prescribe the exact organizational form an ACO may take; ACOs may include tight structures such as vertically integrated delivery systems and looser federations of independent hospitals and physician networks. But even for the more loosely organized ACOs, the shared savings payment approach pushes them toward a more integrated model of care.

This movement is evident for ACOs participating in the Medicare Shared Savings Program. Medicare's traditional payment model—fee-for-service for physicians and DRGs for hospitals—reinforced a dispersed model, providing little incentive for physicians and hospitals to collaborate to achieve Medicare's quality and cost control goals or embrace a population health

Table 6–1. Varieties of health system integration

	Physicians	Hospitals	Insurance Plan	Organizational Model	Examples
Horizontally loosely integrated medical group	✓	−	−	Independent practice association	Hill Physicians Medical Group
Horizontally tightly integrated medical group	✓	−	−	Integrated multispecialty medical group	Palo Alto Medical Foundation
Horizontally integrated hospital system	+/−	✓	+/−	Regional or national hospital system	Sutter Health, Tenet Health*
Vertically and horizontally tightly-integrated delivery system	✓	✓	+/−	Regional health system	Atrium Health, Baylor Scott & White, University of Pittsburgh Medical Center
Vertically and horizontally loosely integrated system	✓	✓	✓	HMO Network model	Anthem Blue Cross HMO's provider network
Vertically and horizontally tightly integrated system	✓	✓	✓	Prepaid group practice model HMO	Kaiser Permanente

✓, essential component.

−, not a component.

+/−, optional component; usually a subsidiary element if present.

*Over time, these initially horizontally integrated systems added vertical integration; i.e., after several hospitals merged into hospital systems, the hospital systems began to add physician groups either by owning them or contracting with them, thereby becoming a health system rather than only a hospital system.

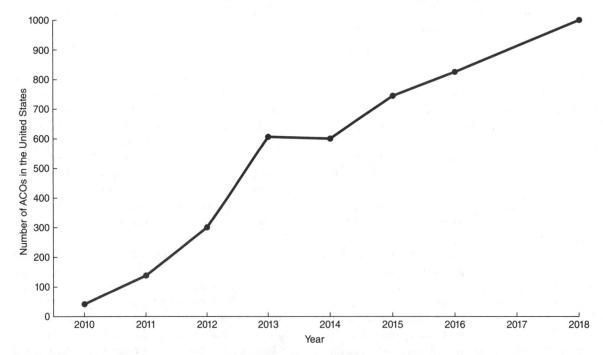

▲ **Figure 6–4.** Number of ACO contracts in the United States, 2012–2018. (From Muhlestein D, et al. Recent progress in the value journey: growth of ACOs and value-based payment in 2018. *HealthAffairs blog*, August 14, 2018.)

approach. A few important things change when providers form an ACO, even though the underlying payment method remains fee-for-service and DRGs:

1. When physicians share financial risk with other physicians, and physicians share risk with hospitals, they are all motivated to work together to achieve common performance goals. By forming an ACO, providers—even if remaining in dispersed practice settings and ownerships—agree to collaborate on achieving operational goals, such as by creating outpatient teams of nurses and social workers to assist clinicians in managing the care of patients with costly illnesses to avoid unnecessary hospitalizations, requiring greater clinical and data integration than occurs under the dispersed organizational model. Integration is also promoted by the policy that shared savings for ACOs are contingent on improvements in quality of care. ACOs have made quality gains (Song and Fisher, 2016), in part by changing physician attitudes to foster the idea that good ambulatory care can often avoid an expensive specialty referral or hospitalization (de Lisle et al., 2017).

2. Because the global payment target is applied to a defined group of Medicare beneficiaries, it moves ACOs toward a population health model. Although the Medicare Shared Savings Program stops short of compelling Medicare beneficiaries to formally register with a primary care gatekeeper or medical group and does not restrict beneficiaries' use of providers outside the ACO's physician and hospital network, it does establish a "soft" form of patient empanelment known as "attribution." Medicare attributes beneficiaries to physicians and hospitals based on where a beneficiary has chosen to receive the plurality of his or her care. If Medicare claims show that a patient received the plurality of care from the physicians in a particular ACO, then that patient is included in the population of Medicare beneficiaries used for measuring the ACO's performance on cost and quality targets. Medicare reinforces this population health approach by requiring ACOs to have a minimum number of PCPs in their network, and by specifying cost and quality performance metrics that heavily depend on high performing primary care.

One key difference between the Medicare Shared Savings Program and Medicare Advantage (the Medicare HMO option discussed in Chapter 2) is the role of insurance companies. Medicare Advantage involves Medicare contracting with insurance plans that operate as HMOs, including both network and prepaid group practice model HMOs. The Medicare Shared Savings Program is a direct financial relationship between Medicare and provider organizations without a private insurance plan intermediary.

COMPARING STRUCTURALLY AND VIRTUALLY INTEGRATED MODELS

▶ From Medical Homes to Medical Neighborhoods

In Chapter 5, we introduced the concept of medical homes. Much of the current chapter can be described as the attempt to create well-functioning medical neighborhoods. The medical *neighborhood* is a term coined by Fisher to describe the constellation of services, providers, and organizations in a health system that contributes to the care of a population of patients (Fisher, 2008). The primary care medical home resides in the medical neighborhood and the medical neighborhood also includes the secondary, tertiary, community, and related services needed by different patients at different times to meet their comprehensive health care needs. High-performing health care requires both excellent medical homes and excellent medical neighborhoods (Rittenhouse et al., 2009; Huang and Rosenthal, 2014). The distinguishing feature of a hospitable medical neighborhood is care that is functionally integrated, but not necessarily structurally integrated along the lines of vertically integrated systems like Kaiser. According to one definition, "Integrated health care starts with good primary care and refers to the delivery of comprehensive health care services that are well coordinated with good communication among providers; includes informed and involved patients; and leads to high-quality, cost-effective care. At the center of integrated health care delivery is a high-performing primary care provider who can serve as a medical home for patients" (Aetna Foundation, 2010).

Organizations that are structurally integrated have the potential to provide care that is functionally integrated. These organizations have assets such as multispecialty groups, a unified electronic medical record, interdisciplinary health care teams, and a quality improvement infrastructure equipped to promote care coordination and the free flow of information among all providers involved in a patient's care. One of the ongoing challenges in the United States is whether virtually integrated health systems can achieve the degree of functional integration needed to deliver more effective and efficient care and overcome what we cited in Chapter 5 as the "fragmentation, chaos, and disarray" that has long plagued the US health system. One approach to functional integration is the negotiation of service agreements between primary care and specialty practices that define the expectations of referrals between the two offices and clarifies common issues such as urgent access to the consultant and timely exchange of information (Safford, 2018).

▶ Evidence on the Relative Performance of Structurally and Virtually Integrated Models

Does greater organizational integration result in a more functionally integrated medical neighborhood and better patient care? Research suggests that more integrated organizational models have their advantages. Integrated medical groups perform better than IPAs in delivering up-to-date preventive care such as mammograms and Pap tests (Mehrotra et al., 2006). Patients are more satisfied with integrated HMOs such as Kaiser than with network-model HMOs. Compared with physicians in IPAs or those not affiliated with any network, physicians in prepaid group practices report greater adoption of tools for chronic illness care (Rittenhouse et al., 2004). Overall, a strong association exists between integrated health care delivery organizations and quality of care (Hwang et al., 2013).

The dispersed model does appear to have one important strength from the patient perspective, which is the satisfaction that comes from receiving care from a small practice where patients have a sense that clinicians and staff know them personally. Patient satisfaction is higher when care is received in small offices rather than larger clinic structures (Rubin et al., 1993). People value having a familiar receptionist at the end of the line when they call about a child with a fever rather than experiencing the frustration of navigating impersonal clinic switchboard operators and voicemail systems—what has been described as the "chain store" persona of some large delivery systems (Mechanic, 1976). Patients whose regular source of care is a small primary care practice with one to two physicians are less likely than patients cared for by larger practices to have preventable hospital admissions, such as admissions for poorly controlled asthma and heart failure, suggesting that the personal touch of a small office may confer meaningful advantages in access and quality to avert deterioration of chronic conditions (Casalino et al., 2014).

CONCLUSION

Will the rapid organizational changes occurring in health care in the United States result in a higher-quality, more affordable health system? Will patients be cared for at the proper level of care—primary, secondary, and tertiary? Will the flow of patients among these levels be constructed in an orderly way within each geographic region—a regionalized structure? Will a sufficient number of primary care providers—generalist physicians, physician assistants, and nurse practitioners—be available so that everyone in the United States can have a regular source of primary care that allows for continuity and coordination of care? Will HMOs, ACOs, and other organizations require their physicians to take responsibility for the health of their enrolled population, or will physicians be content to care only for whoever walks in the door? What is an ideal health delivery system? Different people would have different answers. One vision is a system in which people choose their own primary care clinicians in modest-sized, decentralized, prepaid group practices that would be linked to community hospitals, including specialists' offices providing secondary care. Difficult cases could be referred to the academic tertiary care center in the region. In the primary care practices, teams of health caregivers would endeavor to provide medical care to those people seeking attention, and would also concern themselves with the health status of the entire population served by the practice.

REFERENCES

Aetna Foundation. Program Areas: Specifics, 2010. Available at http://www.aetna.com/about-aetna-insurance/aetna-foundation/aetna-grants/program-area-specifics.html. Accessed October 5, 2019.

Casalino LP, et al. Small primary care physician practices have low rates of preventable hospital admissions. *Health Aff (Millwood)*. 2014;33:1680–1688.

Committee on the Costs of Medical Care. Editorial. *JAMA*. 1932;99:1950.

de Lisle K, et al. The 2017 ACO survey: what do current trends tell us about the future of accountable care? *HealthAffairs* blog. October 4, 2017.

Dye NS. Mary Breckinridge, the Frontier Nursing Service and the introduction of nurse-midwifery in the United States. *Bull Hist Med*. 1983;57:485–507.

Fisher ES. Building a medical neighborhood for the medical home. *N Engl J Med*. 2008;359:1202–1205.

Garfield SR. The delivery of medical care. *Sci Am*. 1970;222:15–23.

Geiger HJ. The first community health center in Mississippi: communities empowering themselves. *Am J Pub Health*. 2016;106:1738–1740.

Geiger HJ. Community health centers: health care as an instrument of social change. In: Sidel VW, Sidel R, eds. *Reforming Medicine*. New York, NY: Pantheon Books; 1984.

Gold J. Accountable Care Organizations, explained. Kaiser Health News, September 14, 2015. Available at http://kaiserhealthnews.org/news/aco-accountable-care-organization-faq/. Accessed October 5, 2019.

Harris G. More doctors giving up private practice and family physicians can't give away solo practice. *New York Times*. March 25 and April 22, 2011.

Huang X, Rosenthal MB. Transforming specialty practice—the patient-centered medical neighborhood. *N Engl J Med*. 2014;370:1376–1379.

Hwang W, et al. Effects of integrated delivery system on cost and quality. *Am J Manag Care*. 2013;19:e175–e184.

Kepford AE. The Greater Community Association at Creston, Iowa. *Mod Hosp*. 1919;12:342.

Kocher R, Sahni NR. Hospitals race to employ physicians—the logic behind a money-losing proposition. *N Engl J Med*. 2011;364:1790–1793.

MCOL. Current national managed care enrollment. 2016. Available at www.mcol.com/current_enrollment. Accessed October 5, 2019.

Mechanic D. *The Growth of Bureaucratic Medicine*. New York, NY: John Wiley & Sons; 1976.

Mehrotra A, et al. Do integrated medical groups provide higher-quality medical care than individual practice associations? *Ann Intern Med*. 2006;145:826–833.

Muhlestein D, et al. Recent progress in the value journey: growth of ACOs and value-based payment in 2018. *HealthAffairs* blog. August 14, 2018.

National Association of Community Health Centers. America's health centers, August 2018.

Rittenhouse DR, et al. Physician organization and care management in California: from cottage to Kaiser. *Health Aff (Millwood)*. 2004;23(6):51–62.

Rittenhouse DR, et al. Primary care and accountable care—two essential elements of delivery-system reform. *N Engl J Med*. 2009;361:2301–2303.

Robinson JC, Casalino LP. Vertical integration and organizational networks in health care. *Health Aff (Millwood)*. 1996;15:7–22.

Rothman SM. *Woman's Proper Place: A History of Changing Ideals and Practices*. New York, NY: Basic Books; 1978.

Rubin HR, et al. Patients' ratings of outpatient visits in different practice settings. *JAMA*. 1993;270:835–840.

Safford BH. How service agreements can improve referrals and shrink the medical neighborhood. *Fam Pract Manage*. 2018;25(5):18–22.

Song Z, Fisher ES. The ACO experiment in infancy—looking back and looking forward. *JAMA*. 2016;316:705–706.

Starr P. *The Social Transformation of American Medicine*. New York, NY: Basic Books; 1982.

Stevens R. *In Sickness and in Wealth: American Hospitals in the Twentieth Century*. New York, NY: Basic Books; 1989.

Stoeckle JD, Candib LM. The neighborhood health center: reform ideas of yesterday and today. *N Engl J Med*. 1969;280:1385–1391.

The Health Care Workforce and the Education of Health Professionals

A health care system is only as good as the people working in it. The most valuable resource in health care is not the latest technology or the most state-of-the-art facility, but the health care professionals and other workers who are the human resources of the health care system.

In this chapter, we discuss the nation's three largest health professions—nurses, physicians, and pharmacists, as well as physician assistants (PAs) and social workers (Table 7–1). What are the educational pathways and licensing processes that produce the nation's practicing physicians, nurses (including nurse practitioners), pharmacists, PAs, and social workers? How many of these health care professionals are working in the United States, and where do they practice? Do we have the right number? Too many? Too few? How would we know if we had too many or too few? Are more women becoming physicians? Are more men becoming nurses? Is the growing racial and ethnic diversity of the nation's population mirrored in the racial and ethnic composition of the health professions? To answer these questions, we begin by providing an overview of each of these professions, describing the overall supply and educational pathways. We then discuss several cross-cutting issues pertinent to all these professions.

PHYSICIANS

As a fourth year medical student preparing to apply for residency training, Susan Unshur needed to make a decision about her choice of a specialty.

She had particularly enjoyed her medical school experiences in pediatrics, and was fascinated by the elective she took in pediatric surgery. But training in pediatric surgery would require at least 6 years of residency and fellowship, and once she completed training, she would face long work hours including being on call for emergency cases. She could complete a pediatrics residency in 3 years to become a general pediatrician, but that was one of the lowest paying specialties and Susan worried about being able to pay off the $175,000 in educational debt she had accumulated in medical school. Dermatology, emergency medicine, and ophthalmology residencies required only one more year of training relative to pediatrics, and those specialties paid very well and allowed for a more controllable lifestyle. The good news was that no matter what specialty Susan chose, there seemed to be plenty of practice opportunities in the region.

Approximately 960,000 physicians are professionally active in the United States (National Center for Health Workforce Analysis, 2018). One-third are in primary care fields and two-thirds in nonprimary care fields. Of physicians who have completed residency training, the great majority have patient care as their principal activity, with the remainder primarily active in teaching, research, or administration. Licensing of all types of health care professionals, including physicians, is a state jurisdiction. State medical boards require that physicians applying for licensure document a passing grade on national licensing examinations, certification

Table 7–1. Number of active practitioners in selected health professions in the United States, 2016–2017

Registered nurses	3,067,256
Nurse practitioners	166,280
Physicians	961,098
Pharmacists	312,500
Dentists	153,500
Physical therapists	239,800
Psychologists	166,600
Social workers	682,100
Chiropractors	47,400
Physician assistants	125,771
Optometrists	40,200

Source: Bureau of Labor Statistics, Department of Labor, Occupational Outlook Handbook, 2018. https://www.bls.gov/ooh/.

of graduation from medical school, and completion of at least 1 year of residency training after medical school.

▶ Medical Education

The University of Pennsylvania opened the first medical school in the colonies in 1765, promoting a curriculum that emphasized the therapeutic powers of bloodletting and intestinal purging. Many other medical sects coexisted in this era, including the botanics, "natural bonesetters," midwives, and homeopaths, without any one group winning dominance. Few regulations impeded entry into a medical career; physicians were as likely to have completed informal apprenticeships as to have graduated from medical schools. Most medical schools operated as small, proprietary establishments profiting their physician owner rather than as university-centered academic institutions (Starr, 1982).

The modern era of the US medical profession dates to the 1890–1910 period. Johns Hopkins University implemented many features that remain the standard of medical education in the United States: a 4-year course of graduate study, competitive selection of students, emphasis on the scientific paradigms of clinical and laboratory science, close linkage between a medical school and a medical center hospital, and cultivation of academically renowned faculty.

A key event in the creation of a 20th-century medical profession was the publication of the Flexner Report in 1910. At the behest of the American Medical Association, the Carnegie Foundation for the Advancement in Teaching commissioned Abraham Flexner to perform an evaluation of medical education in the United States. Flexner's report indicted conventional medical education as conducted by most proprietary, nonuniversity medical schools. Flexner held up the example of Johns Hopkins as the standard by which the nation's institutions of medical education should be judged. Flexner's report was extremely influential. More than 30 medical schools closed in the decades following the Flexner Report, and academic standards at the surviving schools became much more stringent (Starr, 1982). More vigorous regulatory activities in respect to credentialing of medical schools and licensure for medical practice soon enforced the standards promoted in the Flexner Report, and only schools meeting the standards of the Licensing Council on Medical Education (LCME) were allowed to award MD degrees. LCME-accredited schools became known as "allopathic" medical schools to distinguish themselves from homeopathic schools and practitioners. Although homeopaths still practice in the United States (there is now a resurgence of homeopathic practitioners), homeopaths are not officially sanctioned as "physicians" by licensing agencies in the United States. However, one alternative medical tradition has survived in the United States that carries the official imprimatur of the physician rank—osteopathy. Osteopathy originated as a medical practice developed by a Missouri physician, Andrew Still, in the 1890s, emphasizing mechanical manipulation of the body as a therapeutic maneuver (Starr, 1982). Colleges of osteopathy award DO degrees and have their own accrediting organization. Much of the educational content of modern-day osteopathic medical schools has converged with that of allopathic schools. State licensing boards grant physicians with MD and DO degrees equivalent scopes of practice, such as prescriptive authority. By the middle of the 20th century, regulatory restrictions on practice entry, institutionalization of a rigorous standard of academic training, and the rapid growth of medical science and technology solidified the prestige and authority of licensed physicians in the United States.

In 2018, allopathic schools produced 19,553 graduates, and osteopathic colleges (2017) 6,015. The annual number of allopathic school graduates changed little between 1980 and 2008, and only started to increase in 2009 with a surge of medical school expansion. In contrast, the annual number of osteopathic graduates has grown steadily over past decades, increasing sixfold between 1977 and 2017 (AACOM, 2018; AAMC, 2018).

▶ Postdoctoral Education

At least 1 year of formal education after medical school is required for licensure in all states, and most physicians complete additional training to become certified in a particular specialty. Traditionally, the first year of postdoctoral training was referred to as an "internship," with subsequent years referred to as "residency." Now, almost all physicians in the United States complete a full residency training experience of at least 3 years.

Although some residency training programs are integrated into the same large academic medical centers that are home to the nation's allopathic medical schools, many smaller community hospitals sponsor residency-training programs, often in only one or two specialties. The Accreditation Council for Graduate Medical Education (ACGME), a private agency, accredits allopathic residency training programs. Residency training ranges from 3 years for generalist fields, such as family medicine and pediatrics, through 4 to 5 years for specialty training in fields such as surgery and obstetrics–gynecology, to 6 years or longer for physicians pursuing highly subspecialized training. Beginning in 2015, the ACGME also became the accrediting organization for osteopathic residency programs.

Once physicians have completed residency training, the American Board of Medical Specialties certifies physicians for board certification in their particular specialty field. Criteria for board certification usually consist of completion of training in an ACGME-accredited program and passing of an examination administered by the specific specialty board (e.g., the American Board of Pediatrics). Board certification

is not required for state licensure. Physicians may advertise to patients their status as specialty board-certified to promote their expertise and qualifications, and board certification may be a factor considered by hospitals when deciding whether to allow a physician to have "privileges" to care for patients in the hospital or for managed care organizations deciding whether to include a physician in the organization's physician network. Many specialty boards now require periodic reexamination to maintain certification, with some also requiring physicians to perform and document a quality improvement project in their practice.

In 2017, graduates of US allopathic medical schools constituted 63% of the physicians entering ACGME residency programs. The remainder were graduates of schools of osteopathy and physicians graduating from medical schools outside the United States. A complex regulatory structure exists to govern which international medical graduates are eligible to enter US residency training, involving state licensing board sanctioning of the graduate's foreign medical school and graduates completing US medical licensing examinations. There is almost no opportunity for international graduates to become licensed to practice in the United States without first undergoing residency training in the United States, even if the physician has been fully trained abroad and has years of practice experience. About half of international medical graduates are US citizens who decided to train abroad, often because they were not admitted to a US medical school. Many who are residents of other countries come from India, Pakistan, and Canada. International medical graduates who are not US citizens receive only a temporary educational visa while in residency training, and it is expected that these individuals will return to their nations of origin once they have completed training. However, various visa-waiver programs exist to allow these physicians to remain in the United States, usually linked to a period of service in a US community with a physician shortage. Controversy exists about this reliance on international medical graduates to meet US physician workforce needs. Critics argue that the United States fosters a "brain drain," depleting developing nations of vital human resources (Karan et al., 2016), with others responding that emigration to seek better life opportunities is a human right.

▶ Financing Medical Education

Who pays the cost of medical education in the United States? Unlike the case in most developed nations, where medical schools are government-supported and charge no or only nominal tuition, students pay high tuition and fees to attend US medical schools. Approximately half of US medical schools are public state institutions, with state tax revenues helping to subsidize medical school education. The Federal Government plays a minor role in financing medical student education, but pays more than $10 billion per year in Medicare funds to hospitals that sponsor residency programs, including "direct" education payments for resident stipends and faculty salaries plus indirect education payments to defray other costs associated with being a teaching hospital. $4 billion more in federal-state Medicaid funds also support residency training. Although in 1997, Medicare capped the number of residency program slots it would pay for, Medicare gives hospitals considerable latitude in how to spend their Medicare medical education dollars. Hospitals can decide which specialties, and how many slots in each specialty, they wish to sponsor for residency training. As a result, the imbalance between the inadequate number of primary care physicians and the number of specialists is reinforced by the graduate medical education system (Iglehart, 2015). Hospitals have tended to add new residency positions in nonprimary care fields, guided more by the value of residents as low-cost labor to staff hospital-based specialty services than by an assessment of regional physician workforce needs and priorities. Between 2002 and 2019, the number of first-year residency positions increased by 11,600 despite the cap on Medicare-funded positions, with many of the positions funded from hospital clinical revenues and virtually all the gains occurring in specialist, rather than primary care, positions (Chen, 2013; The Match, 2019).

PHYSICIAN ASSISTANTS

Jillian Boca was a speech therapist at a community hospital. She liked her work but wanted to advance in her career. She was talking to some of her colleagues who were physical therapists and x-ray technicians; they were thinking of going back to school to become physician assistants. One of the registered nurses at the hospital was also planning to go back to school to become a nurse practitioner. A local medical school sponsored a program with physician assistant and nurse practitioner students receiving their training together. Jillian and two of her colleagues were admitted to the program.

As the name suggests, PAs are closely linked with physicians. The profession of PA originated in the United States in 1965 with the establishment of the first PA training program at Duke University School of Medicine. The PA profession developed to fill the niche of a broadly skilled clinician who could be trained without the many years of medical school and residency education required to produce a physician, and who would work in close collaboration with physicians to augment the medical workforce. The first wave of PAs trained in the United States included many veterans who had acquired clinical skills working as medical corpsmen in the Vietnam War. PA training programs served as an efficient means to allow these veterans to "retool" their skills for civilian practice.

The American Academy of Physician Assistants defines PAs as "health professionals licensed to practice medicine with physician supervision" (Jones, 2007). PAs are usually licensed by the same state boards that license physicians, with the requirement that PAs work under the delegated authority of a physician. In practical terms, "delegated authority" means that PAs are permitted to perform many of the tasks performed by physicians as long as the tasks are completed under physician supervision. To be eligible for licensure in most states, PAs must have graduated from an accredited training program and pass the Physician Assistant National Certifying Examination, administered by the National Commission on Certification of Physician Assistants. An estimated 125,000 PAs are professionally active in the United States (National Center for Health Workforce Analysis, 2018). Traditionally, the majority of PAs worked in primary care fields. However, only 27% of PAs now practice in primary care, with many finding employment opportunities in emergency departments and surgical specialties (National Commission on Certification of Physician Assistants, 2018). PAs work in diverse settings, including private physician offices, community clinics, HMOs, and hospitals.

Physician Assistant Education

PA training has been described as a "condensed version of medical school" (Jones, 2007), lasting 2 to 3 years. Many of the initial training programs did not award degrees and accepted applicants with varying levels of prior formal education. Currently, the 238 accredited PA training programs in the United States award a master's degree and require applicants to have attained a baccalaureate degree. Approximately half of PA training programs are based at academic health centers and are directly affiliated with medical schools. Several PA programs have established postgraduate training programs, typically 1 year in duration and focused on subspecialty training.

PA programs produce over 8,000 graduates annually, compared with the approximately 25,000 graduates of allopathic and osteopathic medical schools. Enrollment in PA programs has grown steadily over the past decades, with the number of PA graduates more than doubling between 2000 and 2016.

REGISTERED NURSES

Felicia Comfort has worked for 20 years as a registered nurse on hospital medical–surgical wards. Although the work has always been hard, Felicia has found it gratifying to care for patients when they are acutely ill and need the clinical skills and compassion of a good nurse. But lately the work seems even more difficult. The pressure to get patients in and out of the hospital as soon as possible has meant that the only patients occupying hospital beds are those who are severely ill and require a tremendous amount of nursing care. At age 45, Felicia finds that her back has problems tolerating the physical labor of moving patients around in bed. Making matters worse, the hospital recently decided to "re-engineer" its staffing as a cost containment strategy and has hired more nursing aides and fewer registered nurses, adding to Felicia's work responsibilities. Felicia decides that it is time for a change. She takes a job as a visiting nurse with a home health care agency, providing services to patients after their discharge from a hospital. She likes the pace of her new job and finds the greater clinical independence refreshing after her years of dealing with rigid hospital regimentation of nurses and physicians.

Registered nurses represent the single largest health profession in the United States. In 2016, 3,000,000 registered nurses were licensed in the United States, with hospitals the primary employment setting for 61% of nurses. 18% work in ambulatory care or other community-based settings and 7% in long-term care (US Bureau of Labor Statistics, 2018a). The national licensing examination for registered nurses is administered by the National Council of State Boards of Nursing, a nonprofit organization comprising representatives of each of the state boards of nursing.

Registered Nurse Education

Historically, many nurses received their education in vocational programs administered by hospitals not integrated into colleges and universities. These programs awarded diplomas of nursing rather than college degrees and tended to have the least demanding curricula. Over time, nursing education shifted into academic institutions. Most nurses are now educated either in 2- to 3-year associate degree programs administered by community colleges, or in baccalaureate programs administered by 4-year colleges. Of registered nurses active in 2017, 7% were trained in diploma programs, 28% in associate degree programs, 45% in baccalaureate degree programs, and 17% in master's degree programs (National Council of State Boards of Nursing, 2017). Many nursing leaders have called for nursing education to move completely to baccalaureate-level programs. Patient outcomes are better when hospitals are staffed with baccalaureate trained nurses (Yakusheva, 2014). However, associate degree programs have remained a more affordable and accessible option than baccalaureate programs for many students.

Enrollment in registered nurse training programs has had a cyclical pattern over recent decades (US Health Services and Resources Administration, 2017), with periods of RN shortage during which growing numbers of foreign-educated nurses, particularly from the Philippines, entered the US health workforce. Unlike the situation for physicians, international nursing school graduates do not have to undergo training in the United States to become eligible for taking the

US registered nurse licensing examination. Since 2007, as the number of US-trained nurses grew, the volume of nurses from other nations fell rapidly.

NURSE PRACTITIONERS

Felicia Comfort has been working as a home care nurse for 2 years. She has taken on growing responsibility as a case manager for many home care patients with chronic, debilitating illnesses, coordinating services among the physicians, physical therapists, social workers, and other personnel involved in caring for each patient. She decides that she would like to become the primary caregiver for these types of patients, and applies to a nurse practitioner training program in her area. After completing her 2 years of nurse practitioner education, she finds a job as a primary care clinician at a geriatric clinic.

A growing number of registered nurses in the United States have obtained advanced practice degrees in addition to their basic nursing training. Advanced practice nurses include clinical nurse specialists, nurse anesthetists, clinical nurse midwives, and nurse practitioners. The approximately 160,000 professionally active nurse practitioners represent the largest single group of advanced practice nurses (US Bureau of Labor Statistics, 2018b).

Nurse practitioner education typically involves a 2-year master's degree program for individuals who previously attained a baccalaureate degree in nursing. A minority of programs have special tracks for students with baccalaureate degrees in fields other than nursing. Education emphasizes primary care, prevention, and health promotion, preparing nurse practitioners for a broad scope of clinical practice, although some training programs also prepare nurse practitioners for work in nonprimary care fields. Half of nurse practitioners work in primary care settings.

Many nurse practitioner programs were established in the 1970s with federal funding as part of the same national effort to boost the number of primary care clinicians that gave rise to PA training programs. Enrollment in nurse practitioner programs grew slowly in the 1980s and exploded in the 21st century, as the number of nurse practitioner training programs grew from 282 to 424 between 2000 and 2016 (Auerbach

et al., 2018). From 2003 to 2014, the number of annual nurse practitioner graduates rose from 6,600 to 18,000 (Bodenheimer & Bauer, 2016).

Licensing and related regulations for nurse practitioners are less uniform across states than those for physicians, PAs, and registered nurses. State boards of nursing vary in the scope of practice they allow nurse practitioners. Twenty-three states allow nurse practitioners to practice with complete independence from physicians while other states require physician supervision (American Association of Nurse Practitioners, 2018).

Similar to PAs, nurse practitioners working in primary care settings typically perform approximately 80% of the types of tasks performed by physicians. Decades of research provide evidence that nurse practitioners can deliver care of equivalent quality to that delivered by primary care physicians (Stanik-Hutt et al., 2013).

Nurse practitioners both substitute for physicians in an era of primary care physician shortage and complement physicians in health care teams, often playing a leading role in chronic care management, health promotion, and instruction in patient self-care. The boldest effort to promote advance practice nurses as substitutes for physicians comes from proponents of doctoral-level professional degrees for nurses, known as doctor of nursing practice (DNP) degrees. In 2017, over 300 programs were producing 6,000 DNP graduates. The programs, which require a baccalaureate nursing degree for admission, take 3 to 4 years. Leaders of these programs wish to create nursing graduates carrying the title of "doctor," who will be able to practice autonomously with a scope equivalent to that of physicians, including independent practice in acute care hospital settings.

PHARMACISTS

Rex Hall has worked for 5 years as a pharmacist at a chain drug store. He is not sure that his extensive professional education and skills as a pharmacist are being fully utilized in his current job. Some of his time is spent in discussing possible drug interactions with physicians and suggesting alternative drug regimens, as well as counseling patients about side effects and proper use of their medications.

But too much of his time is taken up answering calls from physicians and patients who are ordering prescription refills, counting out pills, filling pill bottles, and figuring out which medications are covered by which health plan. He sees a job posting for a new pharmacist position at a local hospital. The job description states that the pharmacist will review drug use in the hospital and develop strategies to work with physicians, nurses, and other staff to minimize drug errors and inappropriate prescribing practices. Rex decides to apply for the job.

More than 310,000 pharmacists were actively practicing in 2017, 43% in community pharmacies, 25% in hospitals, and the remainder in grocery or department stores with pharmacies (US Bureau of Labor Statistics, 2018c). Although historically most pharmacists were educated in baccalaureate degree programs, in 2004 all programs were required to extend the training period by 1 to 2 years and award Doctorate of Pharmacy degrees. The number of accredited schools increased from 82 in 2000 to 142 in 2018, with the number of graduates growing from 7,300 in 2000 to 14,500 in 2017. Over the past decades, drug store chains such as Walgreens and CVS have largely displaced the independently owned pharmacy. Hospitals are the second largest employer of pharmacists, with managed care organizations, long-term care facilities, and clinics also offering practice settings for pharmacists. The content of pharmacists' work is changing, as noted in the vignette above and in a further discussion later in this chapter.

SOCIAL WORKERS

Social work is a growing profession, with the number of social workers topping 680,000 in 2017. Forty-four percent of social workers are dedicated to health care, with about 40% of these in the fields of mental health and substance abuse. Social workers are trained in assessment skills, diagnostic impressions, psychosocial support to patients and families; and assistance with navigation of the health and social service systems including transitions between hospital, extended care facilities, and home. Some specific tasks carried out by social workers include assessing patients' personal, behavioral, and family/home/job situation for the health care team, connecting patients to durable medical equipment and in-home services, finding

placements for hospital in-patients unable to go home, helping patients to get health insurance and other community services, investigating possible neglect or abuse, and counseling patients on healthy behavior change (US Bureau of Labor Statistics, 2018d).

The minimum educational requirement is a bachelor's degree, but most social work positions in the health care field require a master's degree in social work plus state licensure. Licensed clinical social workers (LCSWs) must have at least a master's degree plus 2 years of academic and practical experience in the field, during which they serve as members of care teams in hospital, primary care, and behavioral health settings. LCSWs may be generalists or be specialized in the management of geriatric patients, children, or persons with developmental disabilities, mental health, and substance abuse diagnoses.

LCSWs have gained greater prominence in primary care as a result of the national movement toward behavioral health integrated into primary care (Block, 2018). Behavioral health professionals, generally LCSWs or psychologists, are colocated within primary care teams, and primary care clinicians seeing a patient with behavioral health problems, such as depression, can introduce the patient to the LCSW in a "warm hand-off." The LCSW would then take over the care of the depression in consultation with the clinician. This model has become part of the patient-centered medical home described in Chapter 5.

SUPPLY, DEMAND, AND NEED

Teresa was working as a per diem hospital registered nurse when she became pregnant with her first child in 1993. Because of ample availability of nurses, she wasn't always able to get scheduled for the shifts she preferred, and wages hadn't increased in several years. She decided to take time off from nursing when her daughter Amanda was born. When Amanda started kindergarten, Teresa went back to school to get her NP degree. She received many job offers when she completed her training and went to work for a community health center. In 2011, when Amanda started college with an interest in following her mother into the nursing profession, the college career counselor explained that registered nurses were in great demand and local hospitals were paying salaries almost as high as those for nurse practitioners. Amanda decided to enter the RN baccalaureate program and become a hospital nurse.

The supply of health workers in all the professions discussed in this chapter has been growing over past decades (Figs. 7–1 to 7–3). Between 1975 and 2005, the number of active registered nurses per capita in the United States nearly doubled, the number of physicians per capita grew by approximately 75%, and the number of pharmacists per capita increased by approximately 50%. Increases in the supply of PAs and nurse practitioners have been even more dramatic (Auerbach et al., 2018). For physicians, virtually all the growth in supply is accounted for by increasing numbers of nonprimary care specialists. Interestingly, although supply has steadily increased during these years, health workforce analysts have alternated between sounding alarms about shortages and surpluses of physicians and nurses. For example, in the 1980s and 1990s, several commissions warned of a surplus of physicians in the United States (Graduate Medical Education National Advisory Committee, 1981; Pew Health Professions Commission, 1995; Council on Graduate Medical Education, 1996). By the early years of the 21st century, some policy analysts were declaring a physician shortage (Council on Graduate Medical Education, 2005). Similarly, concerns about an oversupply of nurses in the mid-1990s were supplanted in 1998 by declarations of a nursing shortage (Buerhaus et al., 2000), with many analysts concluding the shortage had ended by 2010 (Staiger et al., 2012).

What explains why perceptions turned from surplus to shortage when supply was continuing to steadily increase over these decades? The supply of health care professionals is only one part of the equation for determining the adequacy of the workforce. The other part of the equation is a judgment about how many physicians, nurses, or pharmacists are actually required. Even when the supply of health

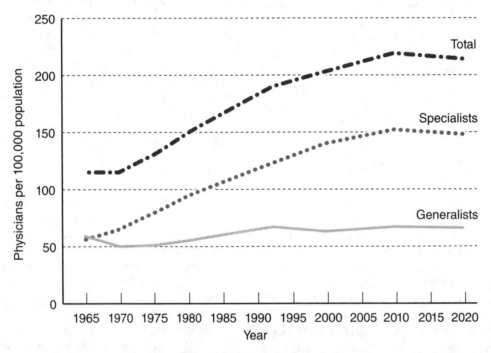

▲ **Figure 7–1.** Supply of practicing physicians in the United States. Note: Includes patient care physicians who have completed training and excludes physicians employed by the federal government. (From Council on Graduate Medical Education [COGME]. Patient Care Physician Supply and Requirements: Testing COGME Recommendations. US Department of Health and Human Services; 1996 [HRSA-P-DM 95–3].)

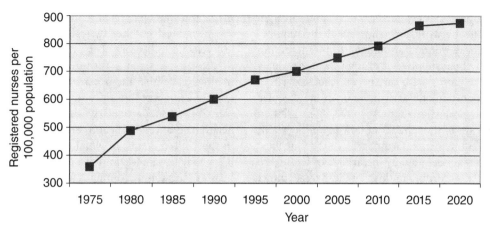

▲ **Figure 7–2.** Supply of active registered nurses per 100,000 population in the United States. (From Auerbach DI, et al. Will the RN workforce weather the retirement of the baby boomers? *Medical Care* 2015;53:850−856.)

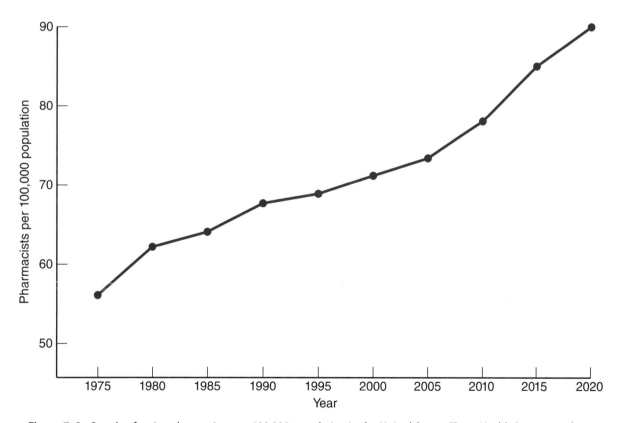

▲ **Figure 7–3.** Supply of active pharmacists per 100,000 population in the United States. (From Health Services and Resources Administration. The Adequacy of Pharmacist Supply: 2004 to 2030. December 2008.)

care professionals per capita is growing, there may be a perception of a workforce shortage if the requirements for these workers are judged to be increasing more rapidly than supply. For example, as individuals age they have more health care needs; a society with a growing proportion of elderly individuals may require more health professionals per capita. There are two general schools of thought about how to define health workforce requirements (Grumbach, 2002). One view considers market demand as the arbiter of workforce requirements. According to this view, if there is unmet market demand for, let us say, nurses, as indicated by many vacant nursing positions at hospitals, then a shortage exists. Or, to the contrary, if many nurses are unemployed or underemployed, a surplus exists. An alternative approach defines workforce requirements on the basis of population need rather than market demand. For example, a need-based approach for nursing would attempt to evaluate whether a certain level of nursing supply optimizes patient outcomes, such as by determining whether higher registered nurse staffing levels for a given volume and acuity of hospital inpatients result in fewer medication errors and hospital-acquired infections and better overall patient outcomes.

In the case of registered nursing, both demand and need perspectives converged to conclude that a shortage existed in the late 1990s (Bureau of Health Professions, 2002). As the intensity of hospital care increased and hospitals sought more highly trained registered nurses to staff their facilities, vacancy rates increased for hospital nurses. In response, hospitals began to increase wages to attract nurses into the workforce. Researchers around this time also began to produce evidence that lower levels of registered nurse staffing in hospitals were associated with worse clinical outcomes for hospitalized patients (Needleman et al., 2011), suggesting a true medical need for more registered nurses in hospitals. One state, California, proceeded to codify a need-based approach to nurse supply by enacting legislation requiring a minimum nurse staffing level per occupied hospital bed (Spetz, 2004).

The case of the physician workforce has been less straightforward. While most nurses work as employees of hospitals or other employers, until recently most physicians were self-employed or part-owners of a medical group that acted as their employer, making vacancy rates or other typical labor market metrics less reliable indicators of the demand for physicians. Moreover, physicians' authority and influence over medical care give them considerable market power and create opportunities for supplier-induced demand (see Chapter 9), particularly when costs are covered by health insurance. In a health care environment like that in the United States, in which demand for physician labor may be almost limitless, physicians tend to keep busy even as supply continues to rise.

Groups such as the Association of American Medical Colleges have been strong proponents in recent years of the view that the supply of physicians in the United States is not keeping up with rising demand driven by advances in medical care and an aging population (AAMC, 2019). Tempering the enthusiasm for this policy direction is research that raises questions about whether the health of the public benefits from more physicians. For example, mortality rates for high-risk newborns are worse in regions with a very low supply of neonatologists than in regions with a somewhat greater supply, but above that level, further increases in the supply of neonatologists are not associated with better clinical outcomes for newborns (Goodman et al., 2002). At the other age extreme, Medicare beneficiaries residing in areas with high physician supply do not report better access to physicians or higher satisfaction with care and do not receive better quality of care (Goodman & Grumbach, 2008). A recent study suggests that an increase in physician supply may result in better health, but that the effect is much greater from increasing primary care physician supply than from increasing the supply of specialists. This study examining changes in physician supply and life expectancy in US counties between 2005 and 2015 found that every 10 additional primary care physicians per 100,000 population was associated with a 51.5-day increase in life expectancy, while an increase in 10 specialist physicians per 100,000 population corresponded to a 19.2-day increase (Basu et al., 2019). The authors expressed concern that the average supply of primary care physicians per capita in US counties decreased during this time while the per capita supply of specialists increased. In assessing the adequacy of health care professional supply, it is important not just to count the number of workers, but to examine how these workers are deployed. The quest for effective deployment of the workforce has been characterized using the following analogy: "Before adding another spoonful of sugar to your tea, first stir up the sugar already in your tea cup." In other words, does the health system make the most of its existing supply of highly trained health care professionals? The case of the pharmacist workforce highlights this issue. Many pharmacists spend a great deal of time performing the basic "pill counting" tasks of drug dispensing. Should pharmacists continue to perform most dispensing functions, or would their extensive training be better utilized in more clinically challenging activities—especially now that all newly graduated pharmacists in the United States are required to have doctoral-level training? The occupation of pharmacy technician has been developed in the United States to assist pharmacists with drug dispensing (Cooksey et al., 2002). An estimated 69% of pharmacists' time is spent on activities that properly trained technicians could perform—counting, packaging, and labeling prescriptions, and resolving insurance formulary issues. Greater use of properly supervised pharmacy technicians might increase the productivity of the existing pharmacists. In addition, innovations in automation of pill dispensing could reduce pharmacist workload. Delegating more tasks to pharmacy assistants and automated systems would allow pharmacists to optimize their clinical training and skills for patient counseling about medications, collaborating on patient safety programs to reduce the epidemic of medication errors, monitoring drug use for chronic disease management programs, and participating in multidisciplinary clinical teams in both hospitals and ambulatory settings (Smith et al., 2013).

These same types of concerns have been raised about whether other health care professionals are being deployed with maximum efficiency and productivity and working at their highest level of skill. For example, new models of primary care are emphasizing that many preventive and chronic care tasks traditionally performed by physicians could be reallocated to medical assistants, nurses, and pharmacists, allowing more productive use of the work effort of primary care clinicians (Bodenheimer & Smith, 2013). Within a profession, the relative mix of specialties may also influence the health outcomes produced by the total supply. As the study on physician supply and life expectancy mentioned above suggests, redistributing physician supply from specialists to primary care physicians might yield greater benefit for the health of a population (Basu et al., 2019).

WOMEN IN THE HEALTH PROFESSIONS

Dr. Jenny Wong works as a general internist for the Suburbia Medical Group. She never has to check her schedule in advance, because she knows that every appointment is always booked, not to mention the last minute add-ons. As one of only two women in a group of 11 primary care physicians, she is in demand. In particular, female patients in the practice have sought her out to become their primary care physician. While gratified to be responding to this demand, Dr. Wong also finds it a bit daunting. She senses that her patients expect her to spend more time with them to explain diagnoses and treatments and discuss their overall well-being. But Dr. Wong has the same 15-minute appointment times as every other physician in the practice and continually finds herself falling behind in her schedule. Today Dr. Wong is feeling especially stressed. She is scheduled to meet at lunchtime with the director of Suburbia Medical Group to discuss plans for her impending maternity leave. She knows he will not take kindly to her intention of taking 4 months off after the birth of her child.

Historically, most physicians and pharmacists in the United States have been men, and most nurses women. For physicians and pharmacists, this demographic pattern is in the midst of a dramatic change (Fig. 7–4). In 1970, 13% of pharmacists were women, but by 2012, more than half of pharmacists were women. The proportion of women among physicians increased from 8% in 1970 to 35% in 2015. The figures are even more dramatic when examining the makeup of current students: women constituted 53% of entering medical students in 2018 and 63% of pharmacy students in 2017. In contrast, nursing has long been a profession mainly comprising women, and this is changing very slowly. In 2015, only 10% of registered nurses were men, up slightly from 5% in 1996 (US Department of Health and Human Services, 2017).

Female health care professionals on average work fewer hours per week than men and are more likely

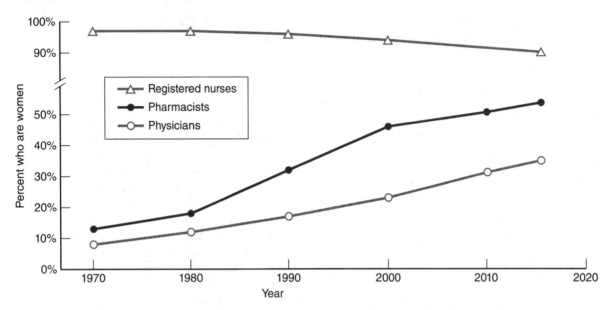

▲ **Figure 7–4.** Women as a percentage of physicians, nurses, and pharmacists in the United States, 2011–2015. (From US Bureau of Health Workforce. Sex, Race and Ethnic Diversity of U.S. Health Occupations (2011–2015). August 2017. https://bhw.hrsa.gov/sites/default/files/bhw/nchwa/diversityushealthoccupations.pdf.)

to work on a part-time basis. However, the practices of male and female health care professionals differ in ways other than simply the number of hours worked. Female physicians attract more female patients and tend to spend more time with their patients than do male physicians. Studies have shown that female physicians deliver more preventive services than male physicians, especially for their female patients (Lurie et al., 1993). Female physicians appear to communicate differently with their patients, with both adults and children, being more likely to discuss lifestyle and social concerns, and to give more information and explanations during a visit (Elderkin-Thompson & Waitzkin, 1999; Roter et al., 2002). Female physicians are more likely to involve patients in medical decision-making than male physicians (Cooper-Patrick et al., 1999).

A gender gap exists in health professional pay. Female physicians and nurses earn less than their male counterparts, even after adjusting for specialty, hours worked, and other factors (Muench et al., 2015; Ly et al., 2016).

UNDERREPRESENTED MINORITIES IN THE HEALTH PROFESSIONS

Cynthia Cuidado is the first person in her family to go to college, much less the first to become a health professional. A large contingent of her extended family celebrates her graduation from her master's degree family nurse practitioner training program. Although hospitals in the city where Cynthia trained had several open positions for nurse practitioners, she has decided to take a job at a migrant farm worker clinic in a rural community near where she grew up.

The United States is a nation of growing racial and ethnic diversity. African Americans, Latinos, and American Indians account for nearly one-third of the population, yet the health professions fail to reflect this rich racial and ethnic diversity. Only about 10% of pharmacists, 11% of physicians, 18% of PAs, 17% of nurses, and 9% of dentists are from these three underrepresented racial and ethnic groups (Fig. 7–5) (US Department of Health and Human Services, 2017).

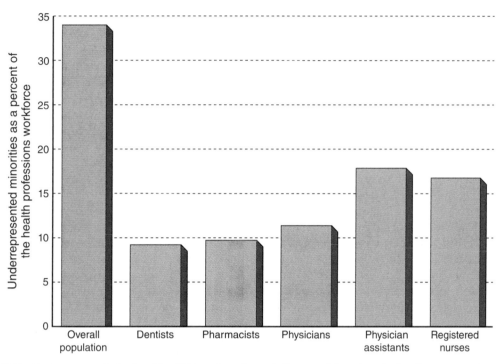

▲ **Figure 7–5.** Underrepresented minorities (African Americans, Latinos, and American Indians) as a percent of the health professions workforce, 2011–2015. (From US Department of Health and Human Services, Health Resources and Services Administration, National Center for Health Workforce Analysis. Sex, Race, and Ethnic Diversity of U.S. Health Occupations (2011–2015), August 2017. https://bhw.hrsa.gov/sites/default/files/bhw/nchwa/diversityushealthoccupations.pdf.)

Health professions have made efforts to increase the number of underrepresented minorities enrolling in their training programs. In nursing, these efforts appear to be paying dividends. Underrepresented minorities as a proportion of students in baccalaureate nursing programs increased from 12% in 1991 to 22% in 2017 (American Association of Colleges of Nursing, 2018). Medical schools have experienced a different trend. Underrepresented minorities as a percentage of medical students increased in the early 1990s, from 12.2% in 1991 to 15.5% in 1997. However, the percentage of underrepresented minority medical students dropped after 1997, falling to 13.9% in 2005. The decrease in underrepresented minority student enrollment in medical schools beginning in the mid-1990s coincided with the onset of a wave of anti-affirmative action policies, such as Proposition 209 in California and the Hopwood versus Texas federal court ruling that curtailed the ability of university admissions committees to give special consideration to applicants' race and ethnicity (Grumbach & Mendoza, 2008). By 2016, the percentage of underrepresented minority students in US medical schools remained only 13.2% (Association of American Medical Colleges, 2016). Pharmacy schools have had a modest increase in underrepresented minority enrollment in recent decades, from 11% of pharmacy students in 1990 to 15% in 2017 (American Association of Colleges of Pharmacy, 2017).

The lack of greater racial and ethnic diversity in the health professions is a compelling policy concern. As discussed in Chapter 3, minority communities experience poorer health and access to health care compared with communities populated primarily by non-Latino whites. Minority health care professionals are more likely to practice in underserved minority communities and serve disadvantaged patients, such as the uninsured and those covered by Medicaid (Komaromy et al., 1996; Mertz & Grumbach, 2001; Walker et al., 2012; Tweedy, 2015). Research has also found salutary effects of ethnically concordant relationships between minority patients and health care professionals on the use of preventive services, patient satisfaction, and ratings of the physician's participatory decision-making style (Saha et al., 2000; Cooper et al., 2003; US Department of Health and Human Services, 2006; Gonzalez et al., 2018; Alsan et al., 2018). Some studies focusing specifically on language concordance when patients have limited English proficiency have also found that access to language concordant clinicians is associated with better patient experiences and outcomes such as reductions in patient reports of medication errors (Wilson et al., 2005; Ortega, 2018). Thus, the underrepresentation of minorities is not just a matter of equality of opportunity; it has profound implications for racial and ethnic disparities in access to care and in health status.

CONCLUSION

An intricate array of educational pathways, accreditation of teaching institutions, and credentialing of individuals to legally practice a healing profession defines the composition of the health workforce. Access, cost, and quality—the three overriding issues in health care—are all inextricably linked to trends in the health care workforce. An inadequate supply of health care professionals may impede patients' access to care or compromise the quality of care. But increases in the supply of health care professionals may fuel escalation of health care costs. It is not surprising, then, to find disagreement about whether a health system has enough, too few, or too many of a particular class of health care professionals. The recent consensus in the United States about a shortage of registered nurses is one of the rare instances in which analyses based on demand models and on need models arrived at similar conclusions. The current debate over the adequacy of the physician workforce in the United States is more typical of the challenges in coming to agreement about the adequacy of supply, revealing how different frames of reference for judging the nation's requirement for health care professionals lead to different

policy conclusions. In addition to the overall supply of health professionals, the demographic composition of the workforce in terms of gender and race–ethnicity also has important policy implications.

Although making definitive determinations about the "right" number of health care professionals often proves elusive, two conclusions may be made with more confidence. First, all health systems should deploy their workers in a manner that makes the best use of their training and skills, creating practice structures that allow each health care professional to operate at his or her highest level of capability and ensuring that those patients most in need benefit from the clinical expertise of the health care professionals working in the system. Most systems fall short of this goal and have not fully "stirred the sugar in the cup of tea," failing to continually reassess and adapt the roles and responsibilities of the members of the health care team to the changing needs of modern-day health systems. Second, all systems need to ensure that their health professionals are highly qualified and embrace a culture of continuous quality improvement (discussed in Chapter 10). To echo the opening of this chapter, a health care system is only as good as the people working in it.

REFERENCES

AAMC (Association of American Medical Colleges). FACTS: applicants, matriculants, enrollment, graduates. 2018. www.aamc.org/data/facts. Accessed September 22, 2019.

AACOM (American Association of Colleges of Osteopathic Medicine). Trends in osteopathic medical school applicants, enrollment, and graduates. 2018. www.aacom.org. Accessed September 22, 2019.

Alsan M, et al. Does diversity matter for health? Experimental evidence from Oakland. NBER Working Paper No. 4787; 2018. https://differencesmatter.ucsf.edu/.../differencesmatter.../oakland_0%20%281%29.pdf. Accessed September 22, 2019.

American Association of Colleges of Nursing. 2018. https://www.aacnnursing.org/Portals/42/News/Surveys-Data/EthnicityTbl.pdf. Accessed September 22, 2019.

American Association of Colleges of Pharmacy. Profile of pharmacy students. Fall 2017. https://www.aacp.org/node/1657. Accessed September 22, 2019.

American Association of Nurse Practitioners. State practice environment. 2018. https://www.aanp.org/advocacy/state. Accessed September 22, 2019.

Association of American Medical Colleges. Current trends in medical education: facts and figures, 2016. https://www.aamcdiversityfactsandfigures2016.org/report-section/section-3/. Accessed September 22, 2019.

Association of American Medical Colleges. The complexities of physician supply and demand: projections from 2017 to 2032. Washington, DC; 2019. Association of American Medical Colleges › workforce-studies › reports. Accessed October 4, 2019.

Auerbach DI, et al. Growing ranks of advanced practice clinicians—implications for the physician workforce. *N Engl J Med.* 2018;378:2358–2360.

Basu S, et al. Association of primary care physician supply with population mortality in the United States, 2005–2015. *JAMA Intern Med.* 2019;179(4):506–514.

Block R. Behavioral health integration and workforce development. Milbank Memorial Fund issue brief, May 2018. https://www.milbank.org/.../behavioral-health-integration-workforce-development/. Accessed September 22, 2019.

Bodenheimer T, Bauer L. Rethinking the primary care workforce: an expanded role for nurses. *N Engl J Med.* 2016:375:1015–1017.

Bodenheimer T, Smith MD. Primary care: proposed solutions to the physician shortage without training more physicians. *Health Aff (Millwood).* 2013;32:1881–1886.

Buerhaus PI, et al. Implications of an aging registered nurse workforce. *JAMA.* 2000;283:2948–2954.

Bureau of Health Professions. *Projected Supply, Demand, and Shortages of Registered Nurses, 2000–2020.* Rockville, MD: Health Resources and Services Administration; 2002. https://www.ahcancal.org/research_data/.../Registered_Nurse_Supply_Demand.pdf. Accessed September 22, 2019.

Chen C. The redistribution of Graduate Medical Education positions in 2005 failed to boost primary care or rural training. *Health Aff (Millwood).* 2013;32:102–110.

Cooksey JA, et al. Challenges to the pharmacist profession from escalating pharmaceutical demand. *Health Aff (Millwood).* 2002;21(5):182–188.

Cooper LA, et al. Patient-centered communication, ratings of care and concordance of patient and physician race. *Ann Intern Med.* 2003;139:907–915.

Cooper-Patrick L, et al. Race, gender and partnership in the patient-physician relationship. *JAMA.* 1999;282:583–589.

Council on Graduate Medical Education (COGME). *Eighth Report: Patient Care Physician Supply and Requirements: Testing COGME Recommendations.* Rockville, MD: Council on Graduate Medical Education; 1996. https://www.hrsa.gov/advisorycommittees/.../cogme/Reports/eighthreportfull.pdf. Accessed September 22, 2019.

Council on Graduate Medical Education (COGME). *Sixteenth Report: Physician Workforce Policy Guidelines for the United States, 2000–2020.* Rockville, MD: Council on Graduate Medical Education; 2005. https://www.hrsa.gov/advisorycommittees/.../cogme/Reports/sixteenthreport.pdf. Accessed September 22, 2019.

Elderkin-Thompson B, Waitzkin H. Differences in clinical communication by gender. *J Gen Intern Med.* 1999;14:112–121.

Gonzalez CM, et al. Patient perspectives on racial and ethnic implicit bias in clinical encounters: Implications for curriculum development. *Patient Educ Couns.* 2018;101:1669–1675.

Goodman D, et al. The relation between the availability of neonatal intensive care and neonatal mortality. *N Engl J Med.* 2002;346:1538–1544.

Goodman D, Grumbach K. Does having more physicians lead to better health system performance? *JAMA.* 2008;299:335–337.

Graduate Medical Education National Advisory Committee. *Summary report.* DHHS Pub. No. (HRA) 81–651. Washington, DC; 1981. https://searchworks.stanford.edu/view/2583545. Accessed September 22, 2019.

Grumbach K. Fighting hand to hand over physician workforce policy. *Health Aff (Millwood).* 2002;21(5):13–17.

Grumbach K, Mendoza R. Disparities in human resources: addressing the lack of diversity in the health professions. *Health Aff (Millwood).* 2008;27(2):413–422.

Iglehart JK. Institute of Medicine report on GME—a call for reform. *N Eng J Med.* 2015;372:376–381.

Jones PE. Physician assistant education in the United States. *Acad Med.* 2007;82:882–887.

Karan A, et al. Medical "brain drain" and health care worker shortages. *AMA J Ethics.* 2016;18:665–675.

Komaromy M, et al. The role of black and Hispanic physicians in providing health care for underserved populations. *N Engl J Med.* 1996;334:1305–1310.

Lurie N, et al. Preventive care for women: Does the sex of the physician matter? *N Engl J Med.* 1993;329:478–482.

Ly DP, Seabury SA, Jena AB. Differences in incomes of physicians in the United States by race and sex: observational study. *BMJ.* 2016;353:i2923.

The Match. National Resident Matching Program. 2019. www.nrmp.org. Accessed September 22, 2019.

Mertz EA, Grumbach K. Identifying communities with low dentist supply in California. *J Public Health Dent.* 2001;61:172–177.

Muench U, et al. Salary differences between male and female registered nurses in the United States. *JAMA.* 2015;313(12):1265–1267.

National Center for Health Workforce Analysis. The U.S. Health Workforce chartbook. US Department of Health and Human Services, September 2018. https://bhw.hrsa.gov/national-center-health-workforce-analysis. Accessed September 22, 2019.

National Commission on Certification of Physician Assistants. May 2018. *2017 statistical profile of certified physician assistants.* http://www.nccpa.net/research. Accessed September 22, 2019.

National Council of State Boards of Nursing. National Nursing Workforce Study, 2017. https://www.ncsbn.org/workforce.htm.

Needleman J, et al. Nurse-staffing levels and inpatient hospital mortality. *N Engl J Med.* 2011;364:1037–1045.

Ortega P. Spanish language concordance in U.S. medical care: a multifaceted challenge and call to action. *Acad Med.* 2018;90:1276–1280.

Pew Health Professions Commission. *Critical Challenges. Revitalizing the Health Professions for the Twenty-First Century.* San Francisco, CA: UCSF Center for the Health Professions; December 1995. https://healthforce.ucsf.edu/publications/critical-challenges-revitalizing-health-professions-twenty-first-century. Accessed September 22, 2019.

Roter D, et al. Physician gender effects in medical communication: a meta-analytic review. *JAMA.* 2002;288:756–764.

Saha S, et al. Do patients choose physicians of their own race? *Health Aff (Millwood).* 2000;19(4):76–83.

Smith M, et al. Pharmacists belong in accountable care organizations and integrated care teams. *Health Aff (Millwood).* 2013;32:1963–1970.

Spetz J. California's minimum nurse-to-patient ratios: the first few months. *J Nurs Adm.* 2004;34:571–578.

Staiger DO, et al. Registered nurse labor supply and the recession—are we in a bubble? *N Engl J Med.* 2012;366:1463–1465.

Stanik-Hutt J, et al. The quality and effectiveness of care provided by nurse practitioners. *J Nurse Pract.* 2013;9:492–500.

Starr P. *The Social Transformation of American Medicine.* New York, NY: Basic Books; 1982.

Tweedy D. The case for black doctors. *New York Times,* May 15, 2015.

US Bureau of Labor Statistics, Occupational outlook handbook. Registered nurses. 2018a. https://www.bls.gov/ooh/healthcare/registered-nurses.htm. Accessed September 22, 2019.

US Bureau of Labor Statistics, Occupational outlook handbook. Nurse practitioners. 2018b. https://www.bls.gov/.../nurse-anesthetists-nurse-midwives-and-nurse-practitioners.htm. Accessed September 22, 2019.

US Bureau of Labor Statistics, Occupational outlook handbook. Pharmacists. 2018c. https://www.bls.gov/ooh/healthcare/pharmacists.htm. Accessed September 22, 2019.

US Bureau of Labor Statistics, Occupational outlook handbook. Social workers. 2018d. https://www.bls.gov/OOH/community-and-social-service/social-workers.htm. Accessed September 22, 2019.

US Department of Health and Human Services, Bureau of Health Workforce. Sex, Race and Ethnic Diversity of U.S. Health Occupations, August 2017. https://bhw.hrsa.gov/national-center-health-workforce-analysis. Accessed November 18, 2019.

US Department of Health and Human Services. The rationale for diversity in the health professions: a review of the evidence. Health resources and services administration; 2006. http://bhpr.hrsa.gov/healthworkforce/reports/diversityreviewevidence.pdf. Accessed September 22, 2019.

US Health Services and Resources Administration. Supply and demand projections of the nursing workforce: 2014–2030. July 21, 2017. https://bhw.hrsa.gov/sites/default/.../projections/NCHWA_HRSA_Nursing_Report.pdf. Accessed September 22, 2019.

Walker KO, et al. The association among specialty, race, ethnicity, and practice location among California physicians in diverse specialties. *J Natl Med Assoc.* 2012;104(1–2):46–52.

Wilson E, et al. Effects of limited English proficiency and physician language on health care comprehension. *J Gen Intern Med.* 2005;20(9):800–806.

Yakusheva OR. Nurse value-added and patient outcomes in acute care. *Health Serv Res.* 2014;49:1767–1786.

Painful Versus Painless Cost Control

Dr. Joshua Worthy is chief of neurology at a large group model health maintenance organization (HMO) and serves as the physician representative to the HMO's executive committee. The federal government has just taken the unprecedented step of imposing mandatory cost controls. The HMO's budget for the coming year will be frozen at the current year's level. In past years, the annual growth in the HMO's budget has averaged 8%.

The HMO's CEO begins the committee meeting by groaning, "These cuts are draconian! To meet these new budget limits we'll have to cut staff and ration life-saving technologies. Patients will suffer." A consumer member responds, "We all know there's fat in the system. Why, in the newspaper just the other day there was an article about how rates of back surgery in our city are twice the national average. And if we're going to talk about cuts, maybe we should start by looking at your salary and the number of administrators working here. I'm not so sure patients have to suffer just because we're adopting the kind of reasonable spending limits that they have in most countries."

Dr. Worthy remains silent for much of the meeting. He wonders to himself, "Is the CEO right? Is cost containment inevitably a painful process that will deprive our patients of valuable health services? Or, could we be doing a better job with the resources we're already spending? Is there a way that our HMO could implement these cost controls in a relatively painless fashion as far as our

patients' health is concerned?" Interpreting Dr. Worthy's silence as an indication of great wisdom and judgment, the committee assigns him to chair the HMO's task force charged with developing a cost-control strategy to meet the new budgetary realities.

With the United States spending $3.5 trillion on health care in 2017, concerns over health care costs dominate the health policy agenda in the United States. The lack of adequate insurance and access to care for millions of people—which spawned the Affordable Care Act—is in part attributable to the problem of rising costs. Health care inflation has made health insurance and health services unaffordable to many families and employers.

Private and public payers in the United States have taken aim at health care cost increases and discharged volleys of innovative strategies attempting to curb expenditure growth, such as creating new approaches to utilization review, encouraging HMO and Accountable Care Organization (ACO) enrollment, making patients pay more out-of-pocket for care, and a multitude of other measures. Yet national health expenditures per capita increased almost tenfold between 1980 and 2017, rising from $1,110 to $10,739 (Fig. 8–1). Viewed as a percentage of gross domestic product (GDP), US health expenditures increased from 9.2% in 1980 to 17.9% in 2017 (Fig. 8–2). While growth slowed from 2009 to 2013 due to the economic recession, it accelerated starting in 2014. By 2026, national health expenditures per capita are projected to increase from $10,739 to $16,167 (Cuckler et al., 2018; Martin et al., 2019).

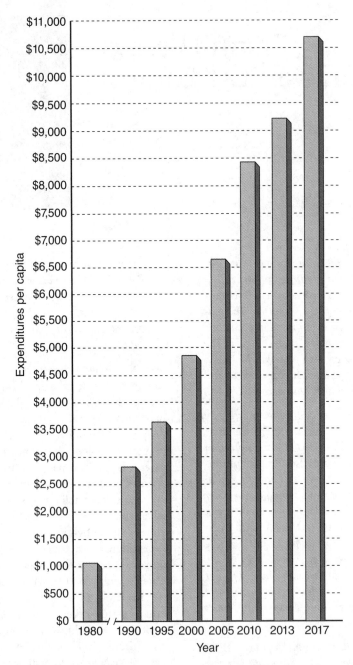

Figure 8–1. US per capita health care expenditures. (From Martin AB et al. National health spending in 2017. *Health Aff (Millwood)*. 2019;38:96–106.)

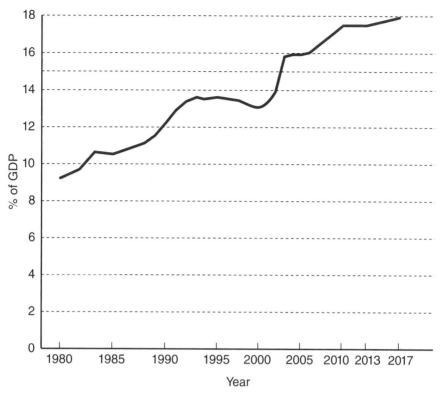

Figure 8–2. US health care expenditures as a percentage of the gross domestic product. (From Martin AB et al. National health spending in 2017. *Health Aff (Millwood)*. 2019;38:96–106.)

Health care providers must consider the prospect of practicing in an era of finite resources. Like Dr. Worthy, physicians and other health caregivers need to deliberate about how constraints on expenditure growth may affect patients' health. Must cost control necessarily be painful, leading to rationing of beneficial services? Or, is there a painless route to containing costs, reached by eliminating unnecessary medical treatments and administrative expenses?

In this chapter, the painful–painless cost-control debate will be explored. First, a model will be constructed describing the relationship between health care costs and benefits in terms of improved health outcomes. Then different general approaches to cost containment and their potential for achieving painless cost control will be discussed. Chapter 9 will describe specific cost-control measures in more detail.

HEALTH CARE COSTS AND HEALTH OUTCOMES

Before entering medical school, Dr. Worthy worked in the Peace Corps in a remote area in Central America. At the time he first arrived in the region, the infant mortality rate was quite high, with many deaths due to infectious gastroenteritis. Dr. Worthy participated in the creation of a sewage treatment system and clean well-water sources for the region, as well as a program for implementing oral rehydration techniques for infants. By the end of Dr. Worthy's 2-year stay, the infant mortality rate had dropped by nearly 25%. The cost for the entire program amounted to 15 cents per capita, paid for by the World Health Organization.

Conditions have been very different for Dr. Worthy as a practicing neurologist in the United States.

Over 25 new magnetic resonance imaging (MRI) scanners have been installed in the city in which his HMO is located, an urban area with a population of 800,000. Dr. Worthy has found that MRI scans provide images that are better than those of computed tomography (CT) scans, allowing him to more accurately diagnose conditions such as multiple sclerosis in earlier stages. But many MRI scans are ordered unnecessarily, and Dr. Worthy wonders if half as many scanners in the city would suffice.

From society's point of view, the value of health care expenditures lies in purchasing better health for the population. The concept of "better health" is a broad one, encompassing improved longevity and quality of life, reduced mortality and morbidity rates from specific diseases, relief of pain and suffering, enhanced ability to function independently for those with chronic illnesses, and reduction in fear of illness and death. It is important to know whether investing more resources in health care buys improved health outcomes for society, and if so, the magnitude of the improvement in outcomes relative to the amount of resources invested.

Figure 8–3, drawn from the work of the health economist Robert Evans (1984), illustrates a theoretic relationship between health care resource input and health care outcomes. Initially, as health care resources increase, these outcomes improve, but above a certain level, the slope of the curve diminishes, signifying that increasing investments in health care yield more marginal benefits. In terms of Dr. Worthy's experiences, the Central American region in which he worked lay on the steep slope of this cost–benefit curve: A small investment of resources to create more sanitary water supplies and to administer inexpensive rehydration therapy yielded dramatic improvements in health. On the other hand, purchasing more MRI scanners represents a health care system operating on the flatter portion of the curve: Large investments of resources in new technologies may produce few or no improvements in the overall health of a population.

Naturally, different medical interventions lie on steeper (e.g., childhood immunizations) or on flatter (e.g., the costly prolongation of life for an anencephalic infant) portions of the curve. The curve in Figure 8–3 may be viewed as an aggregate cost–benefit curve for the functioning of a health care system as a whole. The system may be an entire nation or a smaller entity such as an HMO, with its defined population of enrollees.

Overall, the US health care system currently operates along the flatter portion of the curve. Let us assume that Dr. Worthy's HMO system lies at point A

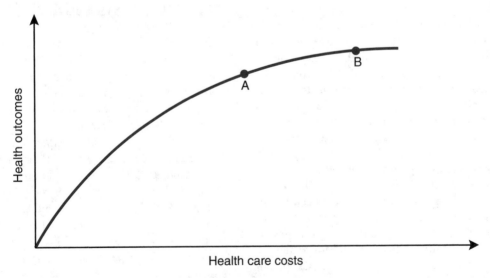

Figure 8–3. A theoretic model of costs and health outcomes. Moving from point A to point B on the curve is associated with both higher costs and better health outcomes.

on the curve in Figure 8–3, with average total health care expenditures per HMO enrollee being the same as the average overall per capita health care cost in the United States ($10,739 in 2017). If stringent new cost containment policies forced the HMO to virtually freeze spending at point A rather than increasing annual expenditures at their usual clip to move to point B, then Figure 8–3 implies that the HMO would sacrifice improving the health of its enrollees by an amount equal to the distance between points A and B on the vertical axis.

Such an analysis would confirm the opinion of those who argue that cost containment requires painful choices that affect the health of the population. Proponents of this view are Aaron and Schwartz (1984 and 1990), who described cost containment as a "painful prescription" requiring rationing of beneficial care. In Figure 8–3, the distance between points A and B on the *y*-axis measures how much health "pain" accompanies the decision to limit spending at point A instead of advancing to point B. Some degree of pain is inherent in the curve. As Evans (1984) observes, "if its slope is everywhere positive, then in a world of finite resources, unmet needs are inevitable." No matter where we sit on the curve, it will always be true that if we spent more we could do a little better.

In Figure 8–3, the distance between points A and B on the *y*-axis is small, given the relatively flat slope of the curve at these points. But reassurances about relatively mild cost containment pain bring to mind the physician, scalpel in hand, hovering over a patient and declaring that "it will only hurt a little bit." A little pain, necessary as it may be, is not the same as no pain; or as Fuchs (1993) puts it, "'low yield' medicine is not 'no yield' medicine."

Before allowing ourselves (and Dr. Worthy) to become overly chagrined at the inevitable painfulness of cost containment, let us add the new dimension of efficiency. We can picture a point C (Fig. 8–4) at which spending is the same as that at point A, but outcomes improve. How does the model account for point C, a point off the curve?

The move to point C requires a shifting of the curve (Fig. 8–5), signifying a new, more efficient (or productive) relationship between costs and health outcomes (Donabedian, 1988). Another way of stating this is that point C represents higher value care. There are numerous possible routes to greater efficiency. For example, diagnostic radiographic imaging services are a rapidly inflating expenditure in the United States. An estimated 30% to 50% of CT scans may be unnecessary and CT radiation exposure is responsible for causing 2% to 5% of all cancers in the United States (Smith-Bindman, 2018). Eliminating unnecessary diagnostic radiographic procedures, such as CT scans for patients with low risk abdominal pain, could simultaneously

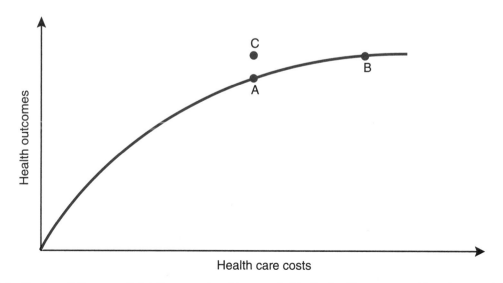

Figure 8–4. Moving off the curve. Point C represents achievement of better health outcome without increased costs.

decrease health care costs and improve health. In the remainder of this chapter, we will examine in greater detail the various possible methods that Dr. Worthy's cost-control task force could consider to achieve more health "bang" for the health care "buck." Before turning to this discussion, however, it is necessary to make explicit three assumptions about this model of costs and outcomes.

1. Implicit in the model is the notion that the relevant outcome of interest is the overall health of a population rather than of any one individual patient. A number of authors have emphasized the need for physicians to broaden their perspective to encompass the health of a general population, as well as their narrower traditional focus on providing the best possible care for each patient (Eddy, 1991; Krieger, 2012). The population-oriented model of costs and outcomes depicted in Figures 8–3 to 8–5 may not fit easily with many physicians' experiences of caring for a particular patient. At the level of the individual patient, the outcome may be all or nothing (e.g., the patient will almost certainly live if he or she receives an operation and die without it) and not easily thought about in terms of curves and slopes. Rather than focusing on any one

particular intervention or patient, the curve attempts to represent the overall functioning of a health care system in the aggregate for the population under its care. (The ethical issues of the population health perspective are discussed in Chapter 13.)

2. The model assumes that it is possible to quantify health at a population level. Traditionally, health status at this level has been measured relatively crudely, using vital statistics such as life expectancy and infant mortality rates. While an index such as infant mortality rates may be a sensitive, meaningful way of evaluating the impact of health care and public health programs in rural Central America, many analysts have questioned whether such crude indicators accurately gauge the impact of health care services in wealthier industrialized nations. In these latter nations, much of health care focuses on "softer" health outcomes such as enhancement of functional status and quality of life in individuals with chronic diseases—aspects more difficult to monitor at the population level than death rates and related vital statistics. In other words, it may be difficult to conceptualize a scale on the y-axis of Figures 8–3 to 8–5 that can register both the effects of managing gastroenteritis in a low-income nation and the addition of MRI scanners in a US city.

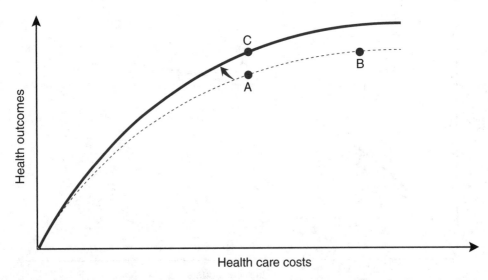

Figure 8–5. Shifting the curve. The shift of the curve represents moving to a more efficient relationship between costs and health outcomes.

3. When evaluating population health, it is difficult to disentangle the effects of health care on health from the effects of such basic social factors as poverty, education, lifestyle, and social cohesiveness (see Chapter 3). For the purpose of our discussion of cost control, we view the curves depicted in Figures 8–3 to 8–5 as representing the workings of the health care system (including public health) per se rather than of the broader economic and social milieu. We therefore use the term *health outcomes* to describe the *y* axis, a term intended to suggest that we are evaluating those aspects of health status directly under the influence of health care. The *x*-axis correspondingly represents expenditures for formal health care services.

Prices and Quantities

We have shown that painless cost control is theoretically possible. But can efficiency be improved in the real world? What strategies could Dr. Worthy's task force propose to move the HMO from point A to point C on the curve? An answer to these questions requires further scrutiny of resource costs in the health care sector.

Costs may be described by the equation

$$\text{Cost} = \text{Price} \times \text{Quantity}$$

Price refers to such items as the hospital daily room charge or the physician fee for a routine office visit. *Quantity* represents the volume and intensity of health service use (e.g., the length of stay in an intensive care unit, or the number of visits to an orthopedic surgeon). Lomas and colleagues (1989), noting this distinction between prices (Ps) and quantities (Qs), refer to cost containment as "minding the Ps and Qs" of health care costs.

Let us look at an example of the $C = P \times Q$ equation:

Blue Shield pays Dr. Morton $750 for 10 office visits at a fee of $75 per visit. The next year, the insurer pays Dr. Morton $900 for 10 visits at $90 per visit.

United Healthcare pays Dr. Norton $750 for 10 office visits, and the next year pays $900 for 12 visits at the same $75 fee. An identical cost increase is a price rise for Dr. Morton but an increase in quantity of care for Dr. Norton.

Changes in prices and quantities have different implications for patients and providers (Reinhardt, 1987). In the preceding example, both physicians increase their income (and both insurance plans increase their expenditures) by $150, though in the case of the price increase, the additional income does not require a higher volume of work. To the patient, however, only the additional $150 spent on a greater number of visits purchases more health care services. (For simplicity's sake, we assume that all visits are identical and that the price rise does not reflect increased quality of service, but simply a higher price for the same product.) A cost increase that merely represents higher prices without additional quantities of health care is an inefficient use of resources from the patient's point of view. Returning to the diagrams in Figures 8–3 and 8–4, if real costs in a health care system were rising only because medical price inflation was exceeding general price inflation while the quantity of care per capita remained static, then increased health costs would not bring about improved health outcomes, and the overall curve would become absolutely flat.

COST-CONTROL STRATEGIES

Controlling Price Inflation

After intense deliberation, Dr. Worthy's task force submits a plan for "painless cost containment" to the HMO executive committee. The first proposal calls for the HMO to aggressively seek discounts on the prices paid for supplies, equipment, and pharmaceuticals by having the HMO selectively contract with suppliers for bulk purchases and stock a more limited variety of product lines and drugs within the same therapeutic class. The proposal also calls for a 10% reduction in salaries for all HMO employees earning over $250,000 per year, as well as a 10% reduction in the capitation fee paid to the HMO's physician group. The executive committee never gets beyond this part of the plan, as furious argument erupts over the proposed income cuts.

Price inflation has been a major contributor to the rise of health care costs in recent decades. The rapid rise of health care prices manifests itself in such ways as prices for prescription drugs in the United States

Table 8–1. Examples of painless cost control

Controlling fees and provider incomes
Cutting the price of pharmaceuticals and other supplies
Reducing administrative waste
Eliminating medical interventions of no benefit
Substituting less costly technologies that are equally effective
Increasing the provision of those preventive services that cost less than the illnesses they prevent

often being more than 50% higher than prices for the same products sold in other nations. Specialist physician incomes are high and continue to rise. Higher prices explain much of the higher costs of health care in the United States compared with the costs in other industrialized nations (Anderson et al., 2019). Limiting price inflation is one way to restrain expenditures without inflicting "pain" on the public's health (Table 8–1).

▶ Eliminating Ineffective and Inappropriate Care

After a brief hiatus to let the furor subside, the HMO executive committee reconvenes. Dr. Worthy introduces his task force's second recommendation—developing appropriateness of care guidelines—by recounting one of his own clinical experiences. When Dr. Worthy first came to the HMO, the neurologists were keeping their stroke patients at bed rest for 1 week before initiating physical therapy. Dr. Worthy, in contrast, began physical therapy and discharge planning for stroke patients the moment their neurologic status was stable. The average length of stay in the acute hospital for his stroke patients was 3 days, compared with 9 days for other neurologists. Dr. Worthy gave a grand rounds presentation demonstrating that 4 days of exercise are required to regain the strength lost from each day of bed rest, meaning that stroke patients would have better outcomes and use fewer resources—shorter acute hospital stays and less rehabilitation—under his care than under the care of his colleagues. Dr. Worthy cites

this as just one example of how the HMO may be devoting resources to ineffective, or even harmful, care.

If controlling prices is one approach to painless cost control, are there also ways to contain the "Q" (quantity) factor in a manner that does not sacrifice beneficial care? Earlier, we cited unnecessary diagnostic imaging studies as an example of inefficient resource use in terms of quantities of services that add to costs and may cause harm. A number of researchers have found convincing evidence of substantial amounts of unnecessary care in the United States (Brownlee, 2007; Kilo & Larsen, 2009; Berwick & Hackbarth, 2012; Lyu et al., 2017). Physicians in the United States perform large numbers of inappropriate procedures (Deyo et al., 2009), and physicians may inappropriately and harmfully accept new technologies as a result of industry influence rather than proven efficacy (Avorn, 2007; Moynihan and Bero, 2017).

Persuasive evidence comes from the work of Fisher, Wennberg, and colleagues, who found that per capita Medicare costs are three times as high in some cities (e.g., Miami) than in others (e.g., Salem OR and Honolulu HI) (Gottlieb et al., 2010). This difference is explained not by prices or degree of illness but is related to the quantity of services provided, which in turn is associated with the predominance of specialists in the higher-cost areas (Fisher et al., 2003). Moreover, residents of areas with a greater per capita supply of hospital beds are up to 30% more likely to be hospitalized than those in areas with fewer beds, after controlling for socioeconomic characteristics and disease burden (Fisher et al., 2000). As for the value of this spending, quality of care and health outcomes are, if anything, worse in the highest spending regions than in areas with less intensive use of services. These findings suggest that a great deal of unnecessary care is taking place in the high-cost areas.

The slope of the cost–benefit curve would become more favorable if a system could eliminate those wasteful components of rising expenditures that have flat slopes (no medical benefit) or negative slopes (harm exceeding benefit, as in the case of inappropriate surgical procedures or prolonged bed rest after strokes). However, inducing physicians and patients to selectively eliminate unnecessary care is no easy matter.

Administrative Waste

The third item on Dr. Worthy's painless cost containment plan targets the HMO's administrative costs. The task force proposes eliminating the HMO's TV and radio advertising budget, laying off 25% of all HMO administrative personnel, and reassigning 25 of the 50 staff members in the department that handles contracts with employers to a new department designed to develop a program to ensure that the HMO provides up-to-date child immunizations and adult preventive care services for 100% of plan enrollees. The HMO's marketing director patiently explains to Dr. Worthy that although he, in principle, agrees with these recommendations, he does not consider it in the HMO's best interest to cut costs in a way that jeopardizes the plan's ability to maintain its market share of enrollees.

Not all quantities in the health care cost equation are clinical in nature. The tremendous administrative overhead of the US health care system has come under increasing scrutiny in recent years as a source of inefficiency in health care expenditures. Woolhandler and colleagues (2003) have estimated that as many as 31 cents of every dollar of US health care spending goes for such quantities of administrative services as insurance marketing, billing and claims processing, and utilization review, rather than for actual clinical services; and that reducing hospital administrative costs to Scottish or Canadian levels would have saved over $150 billion in 2011 (Himmelstein et al., 2014). While some level of administrative service is necessary for health care finance management and related activities such as quality assurance, few argue that the burgeoning administrative and marketing activities translate into meaningful improvement in patient health. Reducing administrative services is another route to painless cost containment.

Eliminating purely wasteful quantities of health care services, be they ineffective clinical services or unnecessary administrative activities, is a relatively straightforward approach to painless cost control. The motto of this approach is: Stop doing things of no clinical benefit. More complicated are approaches to efficiency that involve not simply ceasing completely unproductive activities, but doing things differently. Examples of

this latter approach include innovations that substitute less costly care of equal benefit, preventive care, and redistribution of resources from services with some benefit to services with greater benefit relative to cost. Let us examine each of these examples in turn.

Innovation and Cost Savings

Much of the process of innovation in health care involves the search for less costly ways of producing the same or better health outcomes. A new drug is developed that is less expensive but is equally efficacious and well tolerated as a conventional medication. Services provided by highly paid physicians can often be delivered with the same quality by nurses, nurse practitioners, or physician assistants. Infusion of chemotherapy for many cancer treatments may be done safely on an outpatient basis, averting the expense of hospitalization. Often new technologies are introduced in hopes that they will ultimately prove to be less costly than existing treatment methods.

However, new technologies often fail to live up to cost-saving expectations (Bodenheimer, 2005). A case in point is that of laparoscopic cholecystectomy. Through the use of fiberoptic technology, the gallbladder may be surgically removed using a much smaller abdominal incision than that required for traditional open cholecystectomy, lowering days in the hospital, reducing the cost of each operation, and improving outcomes due to less postoperative pain and disability—seemingly a classic case of "efficient substitution" that lowers costs and improves health outcomes. There's a catch, however. The necessity of gallbladder surgery is not always clear-cut for patients with gallstones. Many patients have only occasional, mild symptoms, and prefer to tolerate these symptoms rather than undergo an operation. Rates of cholecystectomy increased dramatically following the advent of the laparoscopic technique, apparently because more patients with milder symptoms were undergoing gallbladder surgery. In one study, 21% of the surgeries were unnecessary (Pulvirenti et al., 2013). In one HMO, the cholecystectomy rate increased by 59% between 1988 and 1992 after the introduction of the laparoscopic technique. Even though the average cost per cholecystectomy declined by 25%, the total cost for all cholecystectomies in the HMO rose by 11% because of the increased number of procedures done (Legorreta et al., 1993).

Ounces of Prevention

If an ounce of prevention is worth a pound of cure, then replacement of expensive end-stage treatment with low-cost prevention would appear to be an ideal candidate for the "painless cost controller award." Investing in prevention sometimes generates this type of efficiency in health care spending (e.g., many childhood vaccinations cost less than caring for children with infections) (Armstrong, 2007). However, the prevention story is not always so simple. In many cases, the cost of implementing a widespread prevention program may exceed the cost of caring for the illness it aims to prevent (Cohen et al., 2008). For example, screening the general population for elevated blood pressure and providing long-term treatment for those with mild-to-moderate hypertension to prevent strokes and other cardiovascular complications has been found to cost more than the expense of treating the eventual complications themselves (Russell, 2009). For some diseases, this is the case because the complications are rapidly and inexpensively fatal, while successful prevention leads to a long life with high medical costs, perhaps for a different illness, required at some point. Similarly a program of routine mammography screening and biopsy following abnormal test results costs more than it saves by detecting breast cancers at earlier stages. Blood pressure and breast cancer screening programs result in the improved health of the population but require a net investment in additional resources.

Prioritization and Analysis of Cost-Effectiveness

A fourth recommendation of Dr. Worthy's task force involves the diagnosis and treatment of colon cancer. Screening colonoscopy for people over age 50 is associated with a 40% reduction in colon cancer (Nishihara et al., 2013). All the HMO's oncologists strongly recommend chemotherapy for patients who develop widespread metastatic colon cancer. Analysis of cost-effectiveness has demonstrated that screening colonoscopy saves many more years of life per dollar spent than chemotherapy for metastatic colon cancer. Yet chemotherapy allows patients with widespread metastatic disease to enjoy some extra months of life. The task force takes the position that the HMO's physicians should do screening colonoscopies, but that the HMO insurance plan should not cover chemotherapy for widespread metastatic colon cancer.

The most controversial strategy for making health care more efficient is the redistribution of resources from services with some benefit to services with greater benefit relative to cost. This approach is commonly guided by cost-effectiveness analysis, which calculates the net cost of the health care service divided by a defined outcome such as years of life saved (Eisenberg, 1989). For example, a study comparing a comprehensive smoking cessation program with standard tobacco use counseling found that the new program cost $4,137 per additional patient who quit smoking and $7,301 per additional life saved (Levy et al., 2017). Another study of patients with stable coronary artery disease comparing treatment with medication alone versus medication plus coronary artery angioplasty or stenting (procedures to mechanically open the arteries) found that medication plus procedure cost about $150,000 per additional patient relieved of symptoms and more than $200,000 per additional year of life saved (Weintraub et al., 2008). To get the most "bang" for the health care "buck," these studies suggest that a system operating under limited resources would do better by maximizing resources for smoking cessation than by performing invasive procedures on patients with stable coronary artery disease.

Cost-effectiveness analysis must be used with caution. If the data used are inaccurate, the conclusions may be incorrect. Moreover, cost-effectiveness analysis may discriminate against people with disabilities. Researchers are likely to assign less worth to a year of life of a disabled person than does the person himself or herself; thus, analyses using "quality-adjusted life years (QALYs)" may have a built-in bias against persons with less capacity to function independently (Sinclair, 2012). The disability-adjusted life year concept has been proposed to address this bias (Neumann et al., 2018), but QALYs are likely to remain an important metric for cost-effectiveness analysis (Neumann and Cohen, 2018).

Dr. David Eddy (1991, 1992, 1993), in a series of provocative articles in the *Journal of the American Medical Association,* has discussed the practical and ethical challenges of applying cost-effectiveness analysis to medical practice. Two of the essays involve the case of an HMO trying to decide whether to adopt routine use of low-osmolar contrast agents, a type of dye for special x-ray studies that carries a lower risk of provoking allergic reactions than the cheaper conventional dye. With the use of this agent for all x-ray dye studies, 40 nonfatal allergic reactions would be avoided annually and the cost to the HMO would be $3.5 million more per year, compared with costs for use of the older agent in routine cases and use of the low-osmolar dye only for patients at high risk of allergy. The same $3.5 million dollars invested in an expanded cervical cancer screening program in the HMO would prevent approximately 100 deaths from cervical cancer per year.

In discussing how best to deploy these resources, Eddy highlights several points of particular relevance to clinicians:

1. It must be agreed upon that resources are truly limited. Although the cost-effectiveness of low-osmolar contrast dye and cervical cancer screening is quite different, both programs offer some benefit (i.e., they are not flat-of-the-curve medicine). If no constraints on resources existed, the best policy would be to invest in both services.

2. If resources are limited and trade-offs based on cost-effectiveness considerations are to be made, these trade-offs will have professional legitimacy only if it is clear that resources saved from denying services of low cost-effectiveness will be reinvested in services with greater cost-effectiveness, rather than siphoned off for ineffective care or higher profits.

3. Ethical tensions exist between maximizing health outcomes for a group or population as opposed to the individual patient. The radiologist experiences the trauma of patients having severe allergic reactions to the injection of contrast dye. Preventing future deaths from cervical cancer in an unspecified group of patients not directly under the radiologist's care seems an abstract and remote benefit from his or her perspective—one that may be perceived as conflicting with the radiologist's obligation to provide the best care possible to his or her patients.

Many analysts, including those who question the methods of cost-effectiveness analysis, share Eddy's conclusion: Physicians must broaden their perspective to balance the needs of individual patients directly under their care with the overall needs of the population served by the health care system, whether the system is an HMO or the nation's health care system as a whole (see Chapter 13). Professional ethics will have to incorporate social accountability for resource use and population health, as well as clinical responsibility for the care of individual patients (Hiatt, 1975; Greenlick, 1992).

The final recommendation of Dr. Worthy's task force is for the HMO to hire a consultant to advise the HMO on the relative cost-effectiveness of different services offered by the HMO, in order to prioritize the most cost-effective activities. While waiting for the consultant's report, the task force suggests that the HMO begin implementing this strategy by allocating an extra 5 minutes to every routine medical appointment for patients who smoke, so that the physician, nurse practitioner, or physician assistant has time to counsel patients on smoking cessation, as well as by setting up two dozen new community-based group classes in smoking cessation for HMO members. Since only 50.4% of coronary artery stenting for nonacute indications are clearly appropriate (Chan et al., 2011), the smoking cessation costs are to be funded from the HMO's existing budget for coronary artery stenting, and the number of these stent procedures is to be restricted to 30 fewer than the number performed during the current year. The day following the executive committee meeting, the HMO's health education director buys Dr. Worthy lunch and compliments him on his "enlightened" views. On the way back from lunch, the chief of cardiology accosts Dr. Worthy in the corridor and says, "Why don't you just take a few dozen of my patients with severe coronary artery disease out and shoot them? Get it over with quickly, instead of denying them the life-saving stents they need."

CONCLUSION

The relationship between health outcomes and health care costs is not a simple one. The cost–benefit curve has a diminishing slope as increasing investment of resources yields more marginal improvements in the health of the population. The curve itself may shift up or down, depending on the efficiency with which a given level of resources is deployed.

The ideal cost containment method is one that achieves progress in overall health outcomes through the "painless" route of making more efficient use of an existing level of resources. Examples of this approach include restricting price increases, reducing administrative waste, and eliminating inappropriate and ineffective services. "Painful" cost containment represents the other extreme—sacrificing quantities of medically beneficial services. Making trade-offs in services based on relative cost-effectiveness may be felt as painless or painful, depending on one's point of view; some individuals may experience the pain of being denied potentially beneficial services, but at a net gain in health for the overall population through more efficient use of the resources at hand.

Cost containment in the real world tends to fall somewhere between the entirely painless paragon and the completely painful pariah. As the experiences of Dr. Worthy reveal, putting painless cost control into practice may be impeded by political, organizational, and technical obstacles. Price controls may make economic sense but risk intense opposition from providers. Administrative savings may be largely beyond the control of any single HMO or group of providers and require an overhaul of the entire health care system. Identifying and modifying inappropriate clinical practices is a daunting task, as is prioritizing services on the basis of cost effectiveness. But while painless cost control may be difficult to achieve, few would argue that the US health care system currently operates anywhere near a maximum level of efficiency. Regions in the nation with higher health care spending do not have better health outcomes (Fisher et al., 2003). The nation's lackluster performance on indices such as infant mortality and life expectancy rates suggests that the prolific degree of spending on health care in the United States has not been matched by a commensurate level of excellence in the health of the population (Schneider et al., 2017). Making better use of existing resources must be the priority of cost-control strategies in the United States.

REFERENCES

Aaron H, Schwartz WB. *The Painful Prescription: Rationing Hospital Care.* Washington, DC: Brookings Institution; 1984.

Aaron H, Schwartz WB. Rationing health care: the choice before us. *Science.* 1990;247:418–422.

Anderson GF, et al. It's still the prices, stupid: why the US spends so much on health care and a tribute to Uwe Reinhardt. *Health Aff (Millwood).* 2019;38:87–95.

Armstrong EP. Economic benefits and costs associated with target vaccinations. *J Manag Care Pharm.* 2007;13(suppl S-b):S12–S15.

Avorn J. Keeping science on top in drug evaluation. *N Engl J Med.* 2007;357:633–635.

Berwick DM, Hackbarth AD. Eliminating waste in US health care. *JAMA.* 2012;307:1513–1516.

Bodenheimer T. High and rising health care costs. Part 2: Technologic innovation. *Ann Intern Med.* 2005;142:932–937.

Brownlee S. *Overtreated.* New York, NY: Bloomsbury; 2007.

Chan PS, et al. Appropriateness of percutaneous coronary intervention. *JAMA.* 2011;306:53–61.

Cohen JT, et al. Does preventive care save money? *N Engl J Med.* 2008;358:661–663.

Cuckler GA, et al. National health expenditure projections, 2017–26. *Health Aff (Millwood).* 2018;37:482–492.

Deyo RA, et al. Overtreating chronic back pain: time to back off. *J Am Board Fam Med.* 2009;22:62–68.

Donabedian A. Quality and cost: choices and responsibilities. *Inquiry.* 1988;25:90–99.

Eddy DM. The individual vs. society: is there a conflict? *JAMA.* 1991;265:1446–1450.

Eddy DM. Applying cost-effectiveness analysis. *JAMA.* 1992;268:2575–2582.

Eddy DM. Broadening the responsibilities of practitioners. *JAMA.* 1993;269:1849–1855.

Eisenberg JM. Clinical economics. *JAMA.* 1989;262:2879–2886.

Evans RG. *Strained Mercy: The Economics of Canadian Health Care.* Toronto, Ontario, Canada: Butterworths; 1984.

Fisher ES, et al. Associations among hospital capacity, utilization, and mortality of US Medicare beneficiaries, controlling for sociodemographic factors. *Health Serv Res.* 2000;34:1351–1362.

Fisher ES, et al. The implications of regional variation in medicare spending. *Ann Intern Med.* 2003;138:273–287.

Fuchs VR. No pain, no gain: perspectives on cost containment. *JAMA.* 1993;269:631–633.

Gottlieb DJ, et al. Prices don't drive regional Medicare spending variations. *Health Aff (Millwood)*. 2010;29:537–543.

Greenlick MR. Educating physicians for population-based clinical practice. *JAMA*. 1992;267:1645–1648.

Hiatt HH. Protecting the medical commons: who is responsible? *N Engl J Med*. 1975;293:235–241.

Himmelstein DU, et al. A comparison of hospital administrative costs in Eight Nations: US costs exceed all others by far. *Health Aff (Millwood)*. 2014;33:1586–1594.

Kilo CM, Larsen EB. Exploring the harmful effects of health care. *JAMA*. 2009;302:89–91.

Krieger N. Who and what is a "population"? *Milbank Q*. 2012;90:634–681.

Legorreta AP, et al. Increased cholecystectomy rate after the introduction of laparoscopic cholecystectomy. *JAMA*. 1993;270:1429–1432.

Levy DE, et al. Cost-effectiveness of a health system-based smoking cessation program. *Nicotine Tob Res*. 2017;19:1508–1515.

Lomas J, et al. Paying physicians in Canada: minding our Ps and Qs. *Health Aff (Millwood)*. 1989;8(1):80–102.

Lyu H, et al. Overtreatment in the United States. *PLoS One*. 2017;12(9):e0181970.

Martin AB, et al. National health spending in 2017. *Health Aff (Millwood)*. 2019;38:96–106.

Moynihan R, Bero L. Toward a healthier patient voice: more independence, less industry funding. *JAMA Internal Med*. 2017;177:350–351.

Neumann PJ, et al. Comparing cost-per QALYs gained and cost per DALYs averted analysis. *Value in Health*. 2018;21(suppl 1):S118.

Neumann PJ, Cohen JT. QALYs in 2018—advantages and concerns. *JAMA*. 2018;319:2473–2474.

Nishihara, et al. Long-term colorectal-cancer incidence and mortality after lower endoscopy. *N Engl J Med*. 2013;369:1095–1105.

Pulvirenti E, et al. Increased rate of cholecystectomies performed with doubtful or no indications after laparoscopy introduction. *BMC Surgery*. 2013;13:17.

Reinhardt UE. Resource allocation in health care: the allocation of lifestyles to providers. *Milbank Mem Fund Q*. 1987;65:153–176.

Russell LB. Preventing chronic disease: an important investment, but don't count on cost savings. *Health Aff (Millwood)*. 2009;28:42–45.

Schneider EC, et al. Mirror, mirror 2017: international comparison reflects flaws and opportunities for better U.S. health care. The Commonwealth Fund, July 14, 2017. Available at https://www.commonwealthfund.org/publications/fund-reports/2017/jul/mirror-mirror-2017-international-comparison-reflects-flaws-and.

Sinclair S. How to avoid unfair discrimination against disabled patients in healthcare resource allocation. *J Med Ethics*. 2012;38:158–162.

Smith-Bindman R. Use of advanced imaging tests and the not-so-incidental harms of incidental findings. *JAMA Internal Med*. 2018;178:227–228.

Weintraub WS, et al. Cost-effectiveness of percutaneous coronary intervention in optimally treated stable coronary patients. *Circ Cardiovasc Qual Outcomes*. 2008;1:12–20.

Woolhandler S, et al. Costs of health care administration in the United States and Canada. *N Engl J Med*. 2003;349:768–775.

Mechanisms for Controlling Costs

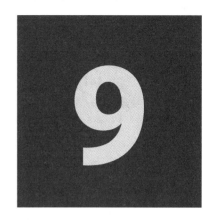

In Chapter 8, we discussed the general relationship between costs and health outcomes and explored the tension between painful and painless approaches to cost containment. In this chapter, we examine specific methods for controlling costs. Our emphasis is on distinguishing among the different types of cost-control mechanisms and understanding their intent and rationale. We briefly cite evidence about how these mechanisms may affect cost and health outcomes.

Financial transactions under private or public health insurance (see Chapter 2, Figs. 2–2, 2–3, and 2–4) may be divided into two components:

1. *Financing*, the flow of dollars (premiums from individuals and employers or taxes) to the health insurance plan (private health insurance or government programs), and
2. *Payment*, the flow of dollars from insurance plans (private or public) to physicians, hospitals, and other providers.

Cost-control strategies can be divided into those that target the financing side versus those that impact the payment side of the funding stream (Fig. 9–1 and Table 9–1).

FINANCING CONTROLS

Cost controls aimed at the financing of health insurance attempt to limit the flow of funds into health insurance plans, with the expectation that the plans will then be forced to modify the outflow of payment. Financing controls come in two basic flavors—regulatory and competitive.

▶ Regulatory Strategies

Dieter Arbeiter, a carpenter in Berlin, Germany, is enrolled in one of his nation's health insurance plans, the "sick fund" operated by the Carpenter's Guild. Each month, Dieter pays 7.5% of his wages to the sick fund and his employer contributes another 7.5%. The German federal government regulates these payroll tax rates. When the government proposes raising the employee rate to 9.2%, Dieter and his coworkers march to the parliament building to protest the increase. The government backs down and as a result, physician fees do not increase that year.

In nations with tax-financed health insurance, government regulation of taxes serves as a control over public expenditures for health care. This regulatory control is most evident when certain tax funds are earmarked for health insurance, as in the case of the German health insurance plans (see Chapter 14) or Medicare Part A in the United States. Under these types of social insurance systems, an increase in expenditures for health care requires explicit legislation to raise the rate of earmarked health insurance taxes. Public antipathy to tax hikes may serve as a political anchor against health care inflation.

A somewhat different model of financing regulation was offered by President Clinton's 1994 health care proposal (which never passed). That proposal called for government regulation of premiums paid to private health insurance plans.

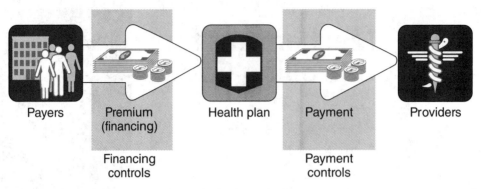

▲ **Figure 9–1.** Cost-control mechanisms may be applied to both the financing and payment components of health care spending under a system of health insurance.

Table 9–1. Categories of cost controls

Financing controls
    Regulatory: limits on taxes or premiums
    Competitive
Payment controls
    Price controls
        Regulatory
        Competitive
    Utilization (quantity) controls
        Aggregate units of payment: capitation, diagnosis-related groups
            (DRGs), global budgets
        Patient cost sharing
        Utilization management
        Supply limits
    Mixed controls

▶ Competitive Strategies

An alternative strategy for containing costs would control the financing flow through competition rather than regulation. The basic premise of competitive financing is to make employers, employees, and individuals more cost-conscious in their health insurance purchasing decisions. Health insurance plans would be encouraged to compete on the basis of price, with lower-cost plans being rewarded with a greater number of enrollees. Instead of having a government agency regulate financing, the competitive market would pressure plans to restrain their premium prices and overall costs.

Giovanni Costa works for General Auto (GA). It is 1995, and he and his family have Blue Cross health insurance that covers most services provided by the health care provider of his choice, with no deductible. Giovanni does not know how much his health plan costs, because GA pays the total premium. Once Giovanni asked his friend in the employee benefits department whether the company was worried about the costs of health insurance. "It's a problem," Giovanni was told, "but it's not too bad because our health insurance premiums are tax deductible for the company. Also, if we gave you higher wages you'd have to pay taxes on those wages, but if we give you better health care coverage, you don't pay taxes on the value of that coverage. So we're both better off by providing generous health care benefits. When it comes right down to it, the government's paying a portion of those premiums."

When considering competitive strategies that attempt to make purchasers more price sensitive, it is important to consider who the purchaser of health insurance really is. For employment-based health insurance, is the purchaser the employer selecting which health plans to offer employees, or is it the individual employee deciding to enroll in a specific plan? As in the case of Giovanni Costa and GA, the answer is often both: GA selects which plans to offer employees and what portion of the premium to subsidize, and Giovanni chooses a particular plan from those offered by GA.

Historically, several factors have blunted both employers' and employees' consideration of price in the purchase of health insurance (Enthoven, 1993; Enthoven and Baker 2018). For employees, the fact that employers who provide health benefits usually pay a large share of the premium for their employees' private health insurance has insulated insured employees from the costs of insurance. Employees view health insurance premiums as an expense to the employer rather than as a cost borne by themselves. In fact, many employees might receive higher wages if the costs of health insurance were lower, but employees do not generally perceive health insurance benefits as foregone wages.

Moreover, the federal policy of treating health care benefits as nontaxable to both employee and employer reduces the employer's burden of paying for such benefits and makes it in the employee's financial interest to receive generous health care benefits. A dollar contributed directly by the employer to a health plan goes farther toward the purchase of health insurance than a dollar in wages that is first taxed as income and then spent by the employee for health insurance. This policy, which cost the federal government about $280 billion in 2018 in employee tax exemptions, has shielded employees from the real price of health insurance and given employees less incentive to be cost-conscious consumers when selecting an insurance plan.

For employers, inflation of health insurance premiums in the 1950s and 1960s was an acceptable part of doing business when the economy was booming and health insurance costs consumed only a small portion of overall business expenses. However, as health insurance costs continued to spiral upward and economic growth slowed, employers became more active in their approach to health insurance costs (see Chapter 16).

It is 2018, and GA now offers Giovanni Costa three choices of health insurance plans: The health maintenance organization (HMO) plan costs $1,600 per month for family coverage, with GA paying 70% and Giovanni paying 30%; the preferred provider organization (PPO) plan is worth $1,800 per month; and the fee-for-service plan runs $2,000 a month. If Giovanni chooses the HMO plan, GA pays $1,120 (70%) and Giovanni pays $480 (30%). If Giovanni signs up for the $1,800 PPO plan, GA still pays $1,120 (70% of

the lowest-cost plan) and Giovanni must pay the rest—$680. If Giovanni wants to choose the fee-for-service plan, GA pays $1,120 and Giovanni pays $880. GA negotiated with all three of its health plans that premium levels would be frozen at their 2018 rates for the next 3 years. A fourth plan previously offered by GA refused to agree to this stipulation, and GA dropped this plan from its portfolio of employee benefits. After 2021, however, the three health plans can demand yearly premium increases, increasing health insurance costs for both GA and Giovanni.

The competitive approach to health insurance financing encourages price-sensitive purchasing by both employer and employee. For employers, the competitive strategy calls for businesses to be more aggressive in their negotiations with health plans over premium rates. Employers bargain actively with health plans and offer employees only plans that keep their rates below a certain level. Moreover, employers make employees more cost aware when selecting a health plan by limiting the amount of the insurance premium that the employer will pay. Rather than paying all or most of the premium, many employers offer a fixed amount of insurance subsidy—often indexed to the cost of the cheapest health plan—and compel employees selecting more costly plans to pay the extra amount. Economist Alain Enthoven, one of the chief proponents of the competitive approach, has called this strategy "managed competition" (Enthoven, 2003). The strategy is also known as the "defined contribution" approach.

Is the evolving competitive approach succeeding at controlling costs? From 2000 to 2010, employer-sponsored health insurance premiums rose by over 10% per year, a major cost-control failure (Claxton et al., 2010). From 2010 to 2018, these premiums grew more slowly, about 5% per year, in part due to the severe economic recession (Claxton et al., 2018). However, competition has never been truly instituted in the United States; 94% of metropolitan markets are controlled by one or two large commercial insurance companies that can extract increasing premiums from employers (Arnst, 2009). Moreover, insurance plans find it easier to compete by "gaming" the market through selection of low-cost enrollees rather than by disciplining providers to deliver a lower-cost, higher-quality product. Studies have shown that competing Medicare HMOs have utilized precisely that strategy (Mehrotra et al., 2006).

If competition could succeed at containing costs, would the outcome be painful or painless cost control? A fundamental concern about market-oriented reforms is that whatever pain may be produced would be experienced most acutely by individuals with lower incomes. Under competition, individuals with higher incomes would be the ones most likely to pay the extra premium costs to enroll in more expensive health plans, while individuals of lesser means could not afford the extra premiums and would be relegated to the lower-cost plans. Enrollees in low-cost plans might experience inferior quality of care and health outcomes.

▶ The Weaknesses of Financing Controls

For cost controls—whether regulatory or competitive—on the financing side of the health care equation to be successful, these strategies ultimately must produce reductions in the flow of funds on the payment side. A government may try to limit the level of taxes earmarked for health care. However, if payments to physicians, hospitals, and other providers continue to grow at a rapid clip, the imbalance between the level of financing and level of payment will produce budget deficits and ultimately force the government to raise taxes. Similarly, under competition, health insurers will attempt to hold down premium increases in order to gain more customers, but if these health plans cannot successfully control what they pay to hospitals, physicians, pharmacies, and other providers, then insurers will be forced to raise their premiums, and competitive relief from health care inflation will prove elusive. It is on the payment side of the equation that the rubber meets the road in health care cost containment. Governments in nations with publicly financed insurance programs do not simply regulate health care financing, but are actively involved in controlling provider payment. Competition places the onus on private health insurance plans—rather than a public agency—to regulate payment costs. We now turn to an examination of the options available to private insurers or government for controlling the flow of funds in the payment transaction.

PAYMENT CONTROLS

In Chapter 8, we distinguished between the "Ps" and "Qs" of health care costs: prices and quantities. Cost equals price multiplied by quantity

$$C = P \times Q$$

Strategies to control costs on the payment side can primarily target either prices or quantities (see Table 9–1).

▶ Price Controls

Under California's fee-for-service Medicaid program, Dr. Vincent Lo's reimbursement for a routine office visit remained below $25 for 8 years.

The Medicare program reduced Dr. Ernesto Ojo's fee for cataract surgery from $900 to $804.

Instead of paying all hospitals in the area the going rate for magnetic resonance imaging (MRI) brain scans ($1,400), Apple a Day HMO contracts only with those hospitals that agree to perform scans for $1,000, and will not allow its patients to receive MRIs at any other hospital.

Metropolitan Hospital wants a contract with Apple a Day HMO at a per diem rate of $2,000. Because Apple a Day can hospitalize its patients at Crosstown Hospital for $1,700 a day, Metropolitan has no choice but to reduce its per diem rate to Apple a Day to $1,700 in order to get the contract. In turn, to make up the $300 per day shortfall, Metropolitan increases its charges to several other private insurers.

Choice Ref PPO asks each hospital in its market region to submit a bid for the total charge for a knee replacement. Most bids are at least $40,000, but High Value Hospital, which has a reputation for good quality care, submits a bid of $33,000. Choice Ref informs the patients enrolled in the plan that they can choose any hospital for a knee replacement, but that Choice Ref will only pay the hospital $35,000 and the patient will be responsible for paying providers any charges above that amount. After this policy is put into effect, 75% of Choice Ref patients needing knee replacement get their operations at High Value Hospital.

In Canada and most European nations, a public or quasipublic agency regulates a uniform fee schedule for physician and hospital payments. Often, negotiations occur between the payers (payer is a general term that includes both purchasers and insurers—see Chapter 16) and professional organizations in establishing these fee schedules. In the United States, as discussed in Chapter 4, Medicare, Medicaid, and many private insurance plans have replaced "usual, customary, and reasonable" physician payment with predetermined prices for particular services. Competitive approaches to controlling prices have also been attempted in the United States. In the 1980s, California initiated competitive bidding among hospitals for Medicaid contracts, with contracts awarded to hospitals offering lower per diem charges. Private insurance plans have also used competitive bidding to bargain for reductions in physician and hospital fees. A recent variation on competitive payment strategies is "reference pricing," such as the approach used by Choice Ref PPO. In theory, public disclosure of prices—price transparency—might deter hospitals and physicians from setting excessively high prices, but such transparency is rarely found in the United States (Mehrotra et al., 2018).

Prices explain much of the difference in health expenditures between the United States and other nations (Anderson et al., 2019). For example, in 2012, the regulated fee for coronary artery bypass surgery in European nations ranged from $14,000 to $23,000; the average fee paid by private insurance plans in the United States was $73,420 (Klein, 2013). A study of reference pricing implemented by one large purchaser in California for joint replacements found that it reduced payments by about 30%, although the purchaser saved only 0.26% in total costs because joint replacements are a relatively small contributor to total costs (Lechner et al., 2013). Two major problems limit the potency of price controls for containing overall costs, particularly when prices are regulated at the fee-for-service level.

1. The first problem occurs when price controls are implemented in a piecemeal fashion by different payers. Providers, like Metropolitan Hospital, often respond to price controls imposed by one payer by increasing charges to other payers with less restrictive policies on fees—a phenomenon known as cost shifting. The cost-shifting problem may be avoided when a uniform fee schedule is used by all payers (as in Germany) or by a single payer (as in Canada).
2. The quantity of services provided often surges when prices are strictly controlled, leading analysts to conclude that providers respond to fee controls by inducing higher use of services in order to maintain earnings (Bodenheimer, 2005).

Price controls have the appeal of being a relatively painless form of cost control insofar as they do not limit the quantity of services provided. However, variations in fee schedules may compromise access to care for certain populations; Medicaid fee-for-service rates to physicians are far below private insurance rates in most states, making it difficult for Medicaid patients to find private physicians who will accept Medicaid payment. In nations with uniform fee schedules, concerns have been voiced that ratcheting down of fees may result in "patient churning" (high volumes of brief visits), with a deterioration in quality of care and patient satisfaction.

▶ Utilization (Quantity) Controls

Because the effectiveness of price controls may be limited by increases in quantity, payers need to consider methods for containing the actual use of services. As indicated in Table 9–1, there are a variety of methods for attempting to control use. We begin by examining one strategy, changing the unit of payment, that we introduced in Chapter 4. We then describe additional mechanisms that attempt to restrain the quantity of services.

Changing the Unit of Payment

Dr. John Wiley is upset when the PPO reduces his fee from $125 to $110 per visit. In order to maintain his income, Dr. Wiley lengthens his day by half an hour so he can schedule more patient visits.

Dr. Jane Stuckey is angry when the HMO reduces her capitation payment from $25 to $20 per patient per month. She is unable to maintain her income by providing more visits because more patient visits do not bring her more money. She hopes that more HMO patients will enroll in her practice so that she can receive more capitation payments.

One simple way to get a handle on the quantity factor is by redefining the unit of payment. In Chapter 4, we discussed how services may be bundled into more aggregate units of payment, such as capitated physician payment, diagnosis-related group (DRG) episode-of-care hospital payment, and bundled payments that combine both physician and hospital payment for an episode of care.

The more aggregated the unit of payment, the more predictable the quantity tends to be. For example, in the case of Dr. Wiley receiving fee-for-service payment, there is a great potential for costs to rise due to increases in the number of physician visits, surgical procedures, and diagnostic tests. When the unit of payment is capitation, as in the case of Dr. Stuckey, the quantity factor is not the number of visits but rather the number of individuals enrolled in a practice or plan. From a health plan's perspective, the $C = P \times Q$ formula still applies when paying physicians by capitation, but now the P is the capitation fee and the Q is the number of individuals covered. Other than by raising birth rates, physicians have little discretion in inducing a higher volume of "quantities" at the capitation level for the health care system as a whole. Similarly, under global budgeting of hospitals, P represents the average global budget per hospital and Q is the number of hospitals.

Shifting payment to a more aggregated unit has obvious appeal as a way for payers to counter cost inflation due to the quantity factor. Life is never so simple, however. In Chapter 4, we discussed how more aggregate units of payment shift financial risk to providers of care. Another way of describing this shifting of risk is that one person's solution to the quantity problem becomes another person's new quantity problem. A hospital paid by global budget instead of by fee-for-service now must monitor its own internal quantities of service lest these quantities drive hospital operating costs over budget. To the extent that providers are unsuccessful in managing resources under more aggregated forms of payment, pressures mount to raise the prices paid at these more aggregated payment units.

Changes in policies for units of payment rarely occur independent of other reforms in cost-control strategies, making it difficult to isolate the specific effects of changing the unit of payment. For example, physician capitation usually occurs in the context of other organizational and cost-control features within a managed care plan. Group model HMOs receiving capitation payments from employers and paying physicians by salary have been shown to reduce costs by reducing the quantity of services provided, in particular by reducing rates of hospitalization (Hellinger, 1996; Bodenheimer, 2005). Compared with group-model HMOs, network model HMOs (see Chapter 6), which often pay physicians fee-for-service, do not significantly control health care costs (Draper et al., 2002).

For hospitals, changing Medicare payments from a fee-for-service to an episode-of-care unit under the DRG-based system in 1983 resulted in a modest slowing of the rate of increase in Medicare Part A expenditures. However, hospitals were able to shift costs to private payers to make up for lower DRG revenues, and national health expenditures as a whole were not affected by Medicare's new payment mechanism (Rice, 1996). Medicare's use of bundled episode-based payments for physicians and hospitals is a more recent development. Bundled Medicare payments for a mixture of cardiovascular and orthopedic inpatient services found no cost reduction (Chen et al., 2018), but payments for hip or knee replacement surgery found modest reductions in cost without an increase in complications (Barnett et al., 2019). Global hospital budgeting in Canada has been a key element of that nation's relative success at containing hospital costs (Commonwealth Fund, 2016).

The health care system in Germany and in some Canadian provinces has countered the open-ended dynamic of fee-for-service payment by introducing global budgeting, called expenditure caps, for physician payment (Bodenheimer, 2005). Under Canadian expenditure caps, a budget is established for all physician services in a province. Although individual physicians continue to bill the provincial health plan on a fee-for-service basis, if increases in the use of services cause overall physician costs to exceed the budget, fees are reduced (or fee increases for the following year are sacrificed) to stay within the expenditure cap. Evidence from Canada suggests that implementation of expenditure caps was associated with stabilization of physician costs in the mid-1990s (Barer et al., 1996). In the United States, Medicare adopted a less-stringent version of an expenditure cap for physician fees, known as the "sustainable growth rate," that was abandoned in 2015 (Aaron, 2015). Expenditure caps for physician payments allow the payer to focus on the aggregate C part of the equation—in this case, the total physician budget. ACO shared savings programs, discussed in Chapters 4 and 6, are a related strategy attempting to provide a global expenditure feedback loop to modulate fee-for-service payments. A 2019 evaluation of the Medicare Shared Savings Program found that through 2014, the ACO program had not reduced costs nor improved quality (Markovitz et al., 2019). A separate review of Medicare, Medicaid, and private insurance ACO contracts found that they were associated with some reduction in in-patient hospital and emergency department use (Kaufman et al., 2019).

Patient Cost Sharing

Randy Payton has an insurance policy with a $2,000 deductible and 20% copayment for all services; if he incurs medical expenses of $6,000, he pays the first $2,000 plus 20% of $4,000, for a total of $2,800.

Joseph Mednick's health plan requires that he pay $20 each time he fills a prescription for a medication, with the health plan paying the cost above $20; because he suffers from diabetes, hypertension, and coronary artery disease, the copayments for his multiple medications cost him $1,200 per year.

Cost sharing refers to making patients pay directly out of pocket for some portion of their health care. In managed competition, cost sharing occurs as part of the financing transaction *at the point of purchasing a health insurance plan*. In this section, we discuss the more traditional notion of cost sharing—using deductibles, copayments, and uncovered services as part of the payment transaction to make patients pay a share of costs *at the point of receiving health care services*.

The primary intent of cost sharing at the point of service is to discourage patient demand for services. (Cost sharing also shifts some of the overall bill for health care from third party payers to individuals in the form of greater out-of-pocket expenses.) As discussed in Chapter 3, when individuals have insurance coverage, they are more likely to use services than when they have no insurance. While protection against individual financial risk is one of the essential benefits of insurance, insurance coverage removes the market restraint

on costs that occurs in a system of out-of-pocket payment.

Cost sharing at the point of service has been one of the few cost-containment devices subjected to the rigorous evaluation of a randomized controlled experiment. In the Rand Health Insurance Experiment conducted in the 1970s, individuals were randomly assigned to health insurance plans with varying degrees of cost sharing. Individuals with cost-sharing plans made about one-third fewer visits and were hospitalized one-third less often than individuals randomized to the plan with no cost sharing (Newhouse et al., 1981).

Although the randomized controlled trial provides an excellent laboratory for scrutinizing the effect of a single cost-containment mechanism, some observers have cautioned that analyses based on controlled research designs may produce results that cannot be generalized to the real world of health policy. For example, the United States has a greater level of cost sharing than many industrialized nations, but also the highest overall costs. Studies have found that when cost sharing begins to produce lower use of services for a large population of patients rather than for a small number of patients in an experiment, physicians may increase the volume of services provided to patients with better insurance coverage. Moreover, 70% of health care expenditures are incurred by 10% of the population—people who are extremely ill and generate huge costs through lengthy ICU stays and other major expenses. Cost sharing has little influence over this component of care. Compared to the micro-world of one not-very-sick patient deciding whether to spend some money on a physician visit, patient cost sharing in the macro-world may remove only a thin slice from a large, expanding pie (Bodenheimer, 2005).

The Rand experiment also evaluated the influence of cost sharing on appropriateness of care and health outcomes. Cost sharing did not reduce medically inappropriate use of services selectively, but equally discouraged use of appropriate and inappropriate services. Study patients (especially those with low incomes) with cost sharing received fewer preventive services and had poorer hypertension control than those without cost sharing (Brook et al., 1983). Patients are less likely to purchase needed medications under cost-sharing policies, for example Medicare Part D's "donut hole" (see Chapter 2), leading to worse control of chronic illnesses and more emergency hospitalizations (Hsu et al., 2006; Goldman et al., 2007; Schneeweiss et al., 2009). Even small copayments are associated with reduced medication adherence in lower income, but not in higher income, populations (Aznar-Lou et al., 2018). These studies suggest that cost sharing is not a painless form of cost control.

Cost sharing for emergency department care may reduce inappropriate use of emergency services without adversely affecting appropriate use or patient health outcomes (Goodell et al., 2009). Cost sharing may be a painless form of cost control when used in modest amounts, not applied to low-income patients, and designed to encourage patients to use lower-cost alternative sources of care (e.g., clinics instead of emergency departments) rather than to discourage use of services altogether.

Utilization Management

Thelma Graves suffers from a severe hyperthyroid condition; she and her physician agree that she will undergo thyroid surgery. Before scheduling the surgery, the physician has to call Ms. Graves' insurance company to obtain preauthorization, without which the insurer will not pay for the surgery.

Fred Brady is hospitalized for an acute myocardial infarction. The hospital contacts the utilization management firm for Mr. Brady's insurer, which authorizes 5 hospital days. On the fourth day, Mr. Brady develops a heart rate of 36 beats/min, requiring the insertion of a temporary pacemaker and prolonging the hospital stay for 10 extra days. After the fifth hospital day, Mr. Brady's physician has to call the utilization management (UM) firm every 2 days to justify why the insurer should continue to pay for the hospitalization.

Derek Jordan has type 1 diabetes and at age 42 becomes eligible for Medicare due to his permanent disability from complications of his diabetes. He is admitted to the hospital for treatment of a gangrenous toe. Under Medicare's DRG method of payment, the hospital receives the same payment for Derek's hospitalization regardless of whether it lasts 2 days or 12 days. Therefore, the hospital wants Derek's physician to discharge Derek as soon

as possible. Each day, a hospital UM nurse reviews Derek's chart and suggests to the physician that Derek no longer requires acute hospitalization.

Utilization management involves the surveillance of and intervention in the clinical activities of physicians for the purpose of controlling costs (Grumbach & Bodenheimer, 1990). In contrast to cost sharing, which attempts to restrict health care use by influencing patient behavior, UM seeks to influence physician behavior. The mechanism of influencing physician decisions is simple and direct: denial of payment for services deemed unnecessary.

UM is related to the unit of payment in the following way: Whoever is at financial risk (see Chapter 4) performs UM. Under fee-for-service reimbursement, insurance companies perform UM to reduce their payments to hospitals and physicians. The DRG system induces hospitals, at risk for losing money if their patients stay too long, to perform UM. Under an HMO capitation contract with a primary physician group, the physician group conducts UM so that it does not pay more to physicians than it receives in capitation payments. If an HMO insurance plan pays a hospital a per diem rate, the insurer may send a UM nurse to the hospital each day to review whether the patient is ready to go home.

Micromanage, Inc., performs UM for several insurance companies. Each day, Rebecca Hasselbach reviews the charts of each patient hospitalized by these insurers to determine whether the patients might be ready for discharge. Usually, if the attending physician wants the patient to remain in the hospital, his or her opinion is honored. By pushing for early discharges, Ms. Hasselbach, her Micromanage colleagues around the country, and the medical director save their insurers about $1,000,000 each year. The annual cost of administering UM is $900,000.

There is little evidence that UM yields substantial savings, particularly when the overhead of administering the UM program itself is taken into account (Wickizer, 1990). UM would appear to be a painless form of cost control because it intends to selectively reduce inappropriate or unnecessary care. However, reviewers often make decisions on a case-by-case basis without explicit guidelines or criteria, with the result that decisions may be inconsistent both between different reviewers for the same case and among the same reviewer for different cases (Light, 1994).

UM has come under fire as a process of micromanagement of clinical decisions that intrudes into the physician–patient relationship and places an unwelcome administrative burden on physicians and other caregivers. Physicians in the United States have been called the most "second-guessed and paperwork-laden physicians in western industrialized democracies" (Lee & Etheredge, 1989). Substantial physician time goes into appealing denials and persuading insurers about the appropriateness of services delivered. A physician and public backlash to UM forced health insurance plans to relax their UM activities in the late 1990s. However, many plans have reintroduced UM and it remains prevalent (Mehrabian, 2018).

Several approaches to UM have been developed that attempt to avoid some of the onerous features of case-by-case utilization review. Practice profiling, rather than focusing on individual cases, uses summary data on practice patterns to identify physicians whose overall use of services significantly deviates from the standards set by other physicians in the community. These outlier physicians can be made subject to strict UM monitoring with denials.

The strategy of "narrow networks" takes UM to its logical conclusion: denying any payments to providers with high-cost profiles by eliminating them from the insurer's provider network. HMOs are the original narrow network, restricting their members to physicians and hospitals within the HMO. Now, many insurers offering policies within the Affordable Care Act's insurance exchanges have narrowed their provider networks by excluding high-price providers. Narrow network plan premiums are 6.7% less than premiums for broad network plans (Polsky et al., 2016). While narrow networks may control costs, a concern has arisen that the networks may lower health care quality by excluding high-quality providers (Corlette et al., 2014).

Supply Limits

Bob is a patient in the Canadian province of Alberta. He develops back pain, and after several visits to his family physician requests an MRI of his spine to rule out disk disease. His physician, who does not suspect a disk herniation, agrees to place him on the waiting list for an MRI, which for nonurgent cases is 5 months long.

Rob lives in Alberta, and after lifting an 80-lb load at work, experiences severe lower back pain radiating down his right leg. Finding a positive straight-leg-raising test on the right with loss of the right ankle reflex, his family physician calls the radiologist and obtains an emergency MRI scan within 3 days.

Supply limits are controls on the number of physicians and other caregivers and on material resources such as the number of hospital beds or MRI scanners. Supply limits can take place within an organized delivery system in the United States, or for an entire geographic region such as a Canadian province.

The number of elective operations and invasive procedures, such as cardiac catheterization, performed per capita increases with the per-capita supply of surgeons and cardiologists, respectively (Bodenheimer, 2005). This phenomenon is sometimes called "supplier-induced demand" (Evans, 1984; Rice & Labelle, 1989; Phelps, 2003). Controlling physician supply may reduce the use of physician services and thereby contribute to cost containment.

Supplier-induced demand pertains to material capacity as well as to physician supply. Per-capita spending for fee-for-service Medicare patients is over twice as high in some regions of the United States than in others (Gawande, 2009, www.dartmouthatlas.org). This remarkable cost variation is not explained by differences in demographic characteristics of the population, prices of services, or levels of illness, but is due to the quantity of services provided. Residents of areas with a greater per-capita supply of hospital beds are up to 30% more likely to be hospitalized than those in areas with fewer beds (Fisher et al., 2000). The maxim that "empty beds tend to become filled" has been known as Roemer's law (Roemer & Shain, 1959). Conversely, strictly regulating the number of centers allowed to perform heart surgery establishes a limit for the total number of cardiac operations that can be performed. In situations of limited supply, physicians must determine which patients are most in need of the limited supply of services. Ideally, those truly in need gain access to appropriate services, with physicians possessing the wisdom to distinguish those patients truly in need (Rob) from those not requiring the service (Bob).

Although there may not always be a directly linear relationship between supply and use of services, there are clear instances in which limitations of capacity restrain use. For example, international comparisons in 2013 demonstrate large variations in use of coronary revascularization procedures (coronary artery bypass surgery and angioplasty), with the United Kingdom's rate of these procedures only 57%, and Canada's 78%, of the US rate (OECD, 2013). These rates correspond to the degree to which these nations regulate (minimally in the case of the United States) the number of centers performing cardiac surgery. In spite of doing more procedures, US coronary heart disease mortality is slightly higher than that of the UK and Canada (OECD, 2013).

A "natural experiment" provides an illustration of how restricting the supply of a high cost resource may be implemented in a relatively painless manner for patients' clinical outcomes. A US hospital experiencing a nursing shortage abruptly reduced the number of staffed intensive care unit beds from 18 to 8 (Singer et al., 1983). For patients admitted to the hospital for chest pain, physicians became more selective in admitting to the intensive care unit only those patients who actually suffered heart attacks. Limiting the use of ICU beds did not result in any adverse health outcomes for patients admitted to nonintensive care unit beds, including those few nonintensive care unit patients who actually sustained heart attacks. This study suggests that when faced with supply limits, physicians may be able to prioritize patients on clinical grounds in a manner that selectively reduces unnecessary services. Establishing supply limits that require physicians to prioritize services based on the appropriateness and urgency of patient need represents a very different (and less intrusive) approach to containing costs than UM, which relies on external parties to authorize or deny individual services in a setting of relatively unconstrained capacity.

Controlling the Type of Supply

A specific form of supply control is regulation of the *types* (rather than the total number) of providers.

Chapter 5 explored the balance between the number of generalist and specialist physicians in a health care system. Increasing the proportion of generalists may yield savings for two reasons. First, generalists earn lower incomes than specialists. Second, and of greater impact for overall costs, generalists appear to practice a less resource-intensive style of medicine and generate lower overall health care expenditures, including less use of hospital and laboratory services (Bodenheimer & Grumbach, 2007).

CONCLUSION

In the real world, cost-containment strategies are applied not as isolated phenomena in a static system, but as an array of policies concerned with modes of financing, organization of health care delivery, and cost control all mixed together. Managed care is a strategy that utilizes a mixture of cost-control mechanisms: changing the unit of payment, utilization management, price discounts, and in some cases supply controls. The Canadian health care system (see Chapter 14) also relies on regulation of prices, global budgets and supply controls.

There is no perfect mechanism for controlling health care costs. Strategies must be judged by their relative success at containing costs and doing so in as painless a manner as possible—without compromising health outcomes. In the view of Dr. John Wennberg, the key to cost control in the United States

> is not in the micromanagement of the doctor–patient relationship but the management of capacity and budgets. The American problem is to find the will to set the supply thermostat somewhere within reason (Wennberg, 1990).

Although US managed care plans and Canadian provincial health plans are often viewed as diametrically opposed paradigms for health care reform, both the Canadian plans and US group model HMOs base their cost-control approaches on what Wennberg terms "the management of capacity and budgets." In Canada, this management is under public control through regulation of physician supply, physician and hospital budgets, and technology. In the United States, private group model HMOs adjust their own "thermostats" by setting their own budgets and numbers of physicians, hospital beds, and high-cost equipment.

If there is a lesson to be learned from attempts to control health care costs in the United States over the past decades, it is that cost-containment policies affecting provider payment need to focus more on macromanagement and less on micromanagement. Trying to manage costs at the level of individual patient encounters (i.e., regulating fees for each service, reviewing daily practice decisions, or imposing cost sharing for every prescription and visit to the physician) is a cumbersome and largely ineffectual strategy for containing overall expenditures. Moreover, one payer lowering its costs by shifting expenses to another payer does not produce systemwide cost savings. Those systems that have been most successful in moderating the inexorable increase in health care costs have tended to emphasize global cost-containment tools, such as paying by capitation or other aggregate units, limiting the size and specialty mix of the physician workforce, and concentrating high-technology services in regional centers. The future debate over cost containment in the United States will center on whether these cost-containment tools are best wielded by private health care plans operating in a price competitive market or by public regulation of health care providers and suppliers.

REFERENCES

Aaron HJ. Three cheers for logrolling–the demise of the SGR. *N Engl J Med*. 2015;372(21):1977–1979.

Anderson GF, et al. It's still the prices, stupid: why the US spends so much on health care and a tribute to Uwe Reinhardt. *Health Aff (Millwood)*. 2019;38:87–95.

Arnst C. In most markets, a few health insurers dominate. *Business Week*. July 23, 2009.

Aznar-Lou I, et al. Effect of copayment policies on initial medication non-adherence according to income: a population-based study. *BMJ Qual Saf*. 2018;27:878–891.

Barer ML, et al. Re-minding our Ps and Qs: cost controls in Canada. *Health Aff (Millwood)*. 1996;15(2):216–234.

Barnett ML, et al. Two-year evaluation of mandatory bundled payments for joint replacement. *N Engl J Med*. 2019;380: 252–262.

Bodenheimer T. High and rising health care costs. *Ann Intern Med*. 2005;142:847–854, 932, 996.

Bodenheimer T, Grumbach K. Improving primary care. *Strategies and Tools for a Better Practice*. New York, NY: McGraw-Hill; 2007.

Brook RH, et al. Does free care improve adults' health? *N Engl J Med*. 1983;309:1426–1434.

Chen LM, et al. Medicare's acute care episode demonstration: effects of bundled payments on costs and quality of surgical care. *Health Serv Res*. 2018;53:632–648.

Claxton G, et al. Health benefits in 2010. *Health Aff (Millwood)*. 2010;29:1942–1950.

Claxton G, et al. Health benefits in 2018: modest growth in premiums, higher worker contributions at firms with more low-wage workers. *Health Aff (Millwood)*. 2018;37: 1892–1900.

Commonwealth Fund. International Profiles of Health Care Systems 2015, January 2016. Available at https://www.commonwealthfund.org/publications/fund-reports/2016/jan/international-profiles-health-care-systems-2015. Accessed October 8, 2019.

Corlette S, et al. Narrow provider networks in new health plans: balancing affordability with access to quality care. Georgetown University Health Policy Institute, 2014. Available at https://www.urban.org/sites/default/files/publication/22601/413135-Narrow-Provider-Networks-in-New-Health-Plans.PDF. Accessed October 8, 2019.

Draper DA, et al. The changing face of managed care. *Health Aff (Millwood)*. 2002;21:11–23.

Enthoven AC. The history and principles of managed competition. *Health Aff (Millwood)*. 1993;12(suppl):24–48.

Enthoven AC. Employment-based health insurance is failing: now what? *Health Aff (Millwood)*. 2003;(suppl web exclusives):W3–W237.

Enthoven AC, Baker LC. With roots in California, managed competition still aims to reform health health care. *Health Affairs*. 2018;37:1425–1430.

Evans RG. *Strained Mercy: The Economics of Canadian Health Care*. Toronto, Ontario, Canada: Butterworths; 1984.

Fisher ES, et al. Associations among hospital capacity, utilization, and mortality of U.S. Medicare beneficiaries, controlling for sociodemographic factors. *Health Serv Res*. 2000;34:1351–1362.

Gawande A. The cost conundrum. *The New Yorker*. June 1, 2009.

Goldman DP, et al. Prescription drug cost sharing: associations with medication and medical utilization and spending and health. *JAMA*. 2007;298:61–69.

Goodell S, et al. *Emergency Department Utilization and Capacity*. Robert Wood Johnson Foundation Policy Brief. No. 17, July 2009. Available at https://www.rwjf.org/en/.../2009/.../emergency-department-utilization-and-capacity0.h. Accessed October 8, 2019.

Grumbach K, Bodenheimer T. Reins or fences: a physician's view of cost containment. *Health Aff (Millwood)*. 1990;9(3):120–126.

Hellinger FJ. The impact of financial incentives on physician behavior in managed care plans: a review of the evidence. *Med Care Res Rev.* 1996;53:294.

Hsu J, et al. Unintended consequences of caps on Medicare drug benefits. *N Engl J Med.* 2006;354:2349.

Kaufman BG, et al. Impact of Accountable Care Organizations on utilization, care and outcomes: a systematic review. *Med Care Research and Review.* 2019;76:255–290.

Klein E. 21 graphs that show America's health-care prices are ludicrous. *Washington Post Blog.* March 26, 2013. Available at http://www.washingtonpost.com/blogs/wonkblog/wp/2013/03/26/21-graphs-that-show-americas-health-care-prices-are-ludicrous/. Accessed October 8, 2019.

Lechner A, et al. The potential of reference pricing to generate health care savings: lessons from a California pioneer. Research Brief No. 30, 2013. Center for Studying Health System Change. Available at http://www.hschange.org/CONTENT/1397/1397.pdf. Accesssed October 8, 2019.

Lee PR, Etheredge L. Clinical freedom: two lessons for the UK from US experience with privatisation of health care. *Lancet.* 1989;1:263–265.

Light DW. Life, death, and the insurance companies. *N Engl J Med.* 1994;330:498–500.

Markovitz AA, et al. Performance in the Medicare Shared Savings Program after accounting for nonrandom exit. *Ann Intern Med.* 2019;171(1):27–36.

Mehrabian N. Reinventing utilization management to bring value to the point of care. 2018. Available at https://www.hcinnovationgroup.com/...value...care/...care.../reinventing-utilization-ma. Accessed October 8, 2019.

Mehrotra A, et al. The relationship between health plan advertising and market incentives: evidence of risk-selective behavior. *Health Aff (Millwood).* 2006;25:759–765.

Mehrotra A, et al. Defining the goals of health care price transparency. *NEJM Catalyst,* June 26, 2018.

Newhouse JP, et al. Some interim results from a controlled trial of cost sharing in health insurance. *N Engl J Med.* 1981;305:1501–1507.

OECD. Health at a glance 2013. Organization for Economic Cooperation and Development, 2013. Available at www.oecd.org/els/health-systems/Health-at-a-Glance-2013.pdf. Accessed October 8, 2019.

Phelps CE. *Health Economics.* Boston, MA: Addison Wesley; 2003.

Polsky D, et al. Marketplace plans with narrow physician networks feature lower monthly premiums than plans with larger networks. *Health Aff (Millwood).* 2016;35:1842–1848.

Rice TH. Containing health care costs. In: Andersen RM, Rice TH, Kominski GF, eds. *Changing the U.S. Health Care System.* San Francisco, CA: Jossey-Bass; 1996.

Rice TH, Labelle RJ. Do physicians induce demand for medical services? *J Health Polit Policy Law.* 1989;14:587–600.

Roemer MI, Shain M. *Hospital Utilization Under Insurance.* Chicago, IL: American Hospital Association; 1959.

Schneeweiss S, et al. The effect of Medicare Part D coverage on drug use and cost sharing among seniors without prior drug benefits. *Health Aff (Millwood).* 2009;28:w305–w316.

Singer DE, et al. Rationing intensive care: physician responses to a resource shortage. *N Engl J Med.* 1983;309:1155–1160.

Wennberg JE. Outcomes research, cost containment, and the fear of health care rationing. *N Engl J Med.* 1990;323:1202–1204.

Wickizer TM. The effect of utilization review on hospital use and expenditures: a review of the literature and an update on recent findings. *Med Care Rev.* 1990;47:327–363.

Quality of Health Care

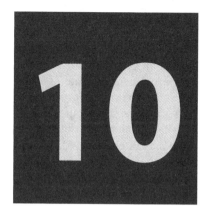

Each year in the United States, millions of people visit hospitals, physicians, and other caregivers and receive medical care of superb quality. But that's not the whole story. Many patients' interactions with the health care system fall short (Institute of Medicine, 1999, 2001). As of 2018, quality was improving slowly overall in the United States but lagging in some regions of the country; moreover, serious disparities exist, harming minority and low-income populations (US Department of Health and Human Services, 2018).

A 2016 study estimated that over 250,000 people each year die as a result of preventable medical errors in hospitals, meaning that medical errors are the third leading cause of death in the United States (Makary & Daniel, 2016). Every year, 1 out of every 25 patients develops an infection while in the hospital—an infection that did not have to happen. A Medicare patient has a 1 in 4 chance of experiencing injury, harm, or death when admitted to a hospital (The Leapfrog Group, 2018).

Hospitals vary greatly in their risk-adjusted mortality rates for Medicare patients; during 2009 to 2012, risk-adjusted deaths from heart failure and pneumonia were three times higher for lower-quality compared with higher-quality hospitals (Medicare Hospital Quality Chartbook, 2013). A previous study showed that if low-quality hospitals reduced mortality rates to the level of high-quality hospitals, 17,000 to 21,000 fewer deaths per year would have occurred (Schoen et al., 2006).

Ambulatory care also has quality problems. A 2003 study found that adults in the United States received just over half of recommended health services (McGlynn et al., 2003). A 2016 follow-up concluded, "Despite more than a decade of efforts, the clinical quality of outpatient care delivered to American adults has not consistently improved" (Levine et al., 2016). Preventable medication errors are estimated to impact more than 7 million patients, contribute to 7,000 deaths, and cost almost $21 billion in direct medical costs (Lahue et al., 2012). In some primary care practices, patients are not informed about abnormal laboratory results more than 20% of the time (Casalino et al., 2009).

Two million lives would have been saved in 2006 if preventive services had been regularly delivered to the entire population (Maciosek et al., 2010). Only 53% of people with hypertension are adequately treated (Yoon et al., 2015) and only 14% of people with diabetes meet their targets for glycemic, blood pressure, and cholesterol control (American Diabetes Association, 2019). Racial and ethnic minority patients experience an inferior quality of care compared with white patients (US Department of Health and Human Services, 2018).

Chassin and Loeb (2011) summarized, "Health care quality and safety today are best characterized as showing pockets of excellence on specific measures or in particular services at individual health care facilities . . . The pockets of excellence mentioned above coexist with enormously variable performance across the delivery system. Along with some progress, we are experiencing an epidemic of serious and preventable adverse events . . . The risk of harmful error in health care may be increasing. As new devices, equipment, procedures, and drugs are added to our therapeutic arsenal, the complexity of delivering effective care increases. Complexity greatly increases the likelihood of error, especially in systems that perform at low levels of reliability."

A prominent Institute of Medicine report (2001) concluded that between what we *know* and what we *do* lies not just a gap, but a chasm. Quality problems have been categorized as overuse, underuse, and misuse (Chassin et al., 1998). We will first examine the factors affecting quality and then explore what can be done to elevate all health care to the highest possible level.

THE COMPONENTS OF HIGH-QUALITY CARE

What is high-quality health care? It is care that assists healthy people to stay healthy, cures acute illnesses, and allows chronically ill people to live as long and fulfilling a life as possible. What are the components of high-quality health care? (Table 10–1)

▶ Adequate Access to Care

Lydia and Laura were friends at a rural high school; both became pregnant. Lydia's middle-class parents took her to a nearby obstetrician, while Laura, from a family on welfare, could not find a physician who would take Medicaid. Lydia became the mother of a healthy infant, but Laura, going without prenatal care, delivered a low–birth-weight baby with severe lung problems.

To receive quality care, people must have access to care. People with reduced access to care suffer worse health outcomes in comparison to those enjoying full access— the quality problem of underuse (see Chapter 3). Quality requires equality (Schiff et al., 1994).

Table 10–1. Components of high-quality health care

Access to care
Adequate scientific knowledge
Competent health care providers
Separation of financial and clinical decisions
Organization of health care institutions to maximize quality

▶ Adequate Scientific Knowledge

Brigitte Levy, a professor of family law, was started on estrogen replacement in 1960 when she reached menopause. Her physician prescribed the hormone pills for 10 years. In 1979, she was diagnosed with invasive cancer of the uterus, which spread to her entire abdominal cavity in spite of surgical treatment and radiation. She died in 1980 at age 68, at the height of her career.

A body of knowledge must exist that informs physicians what to do for the patient's problem. If clear scientific knowledge fails to distinguish between effective and ineffective or harmful care, quality may be compromised. During the 1960s, medical science taught that estrogen replacement, without the administration of progestins, was safe. Sadly, cases of uterine cancer caused by estrogen replacement did not show up until many years later. Brigitte Levy's physician followed the standard of care for his day, but the medical profession as a whole was relying on inadequate scientific knowledge. Treatments of uncertain safety and efficacy may cause harm and cost billions of dollars each year.

▶ Competent Health Care Providers

Ceci Yu, age 77, was waking up at night with shortness of breath and wheezing. Her physician told her she had asthma and prescribed albuterol, a bronchodilator. Two days later, Ms. Yu was admitted to the coronary care unit with a heart attack. Writing to the chief of medicine, the cardiologist charged that Ms. Yu's physician had misdiagnosed the wheezing of congestive heart failure and had treated Ms. Yu incorrectly for asthma. The cardiologist charged that the treatment might have precipitated the heart attack.

The provider must have the skills to diagnose problems and choose appropriate treatments. An inadequate level of competence resulted in poor quality care for Ms. Yu. Medical injuries can be classified as negligent or not negligent.

Jack was given a prescription for a sulfa drug. When he took the first pill, he turned beet red, began to wheeze, and fell to the floor. His friend called 911, and Jack was treated in the emergency department for anaphylactic shock, a potentially fatal allergic reaction. The emergency medicine physician learned that Jack had developed a rash the last time he took sulfa. Jack's physician had never asked him if he was allergic to sulfa, and Jack did not realize that the prescription contained sulfa.

Mack was prescribed a sulfa drug, following which he developed anaphylactic shock. Before writing the prescription, Mack's physician asked whether he had a sulfa allergy. Mack had said "No."

Medical negligence is defined as failure to meet the standard of practice of an average qualified physician practicing in the same specialty. Jack's drug reaction must be considered negligence, while Mack's was not. Of the medical injuries discovered in the 1984 Harvard Malpractice Study, 28% were because of negligence. In those injuries that led to death, 51% involved negligence. The most common injuries were drug reactions (19%) and wound infections (14%). Eight percent of injuries involved failure to diagnose a condition, of which 75% were negligent. Seventy percent of patients suffering all forms of medical injury recovered completely in 6 months or less, but 47% of patients in whom a diagnosis was missed suffered serious disabilities (Brennan et al., 1991; Leape et al., 1991).

Negligence cannot be equated with incompetence. Any good health care professional may have a mental lapse, may be overtired after a long night in the intensive care unit, or may have failed to learn an important new research finding.

▶ Money and Quality of Care

Nina Brown, a 56-year-old woman with diabetes, arrived at her primary care physician's office complaining of chest pain over the past month. Her physician examined Ms. Brown, performed an electrocardiogram (ECG), which showed no abnormalities, diagnosed musculoskeletal pain, and recommended ibuprofen. Five minutes later in the parking lot, Ms. Brown collapsed of a heart attack. The health plan insuring Ms. Brown had an incentive arrangement with primary care physicians whereby the physicians receive a bonus payment if the physicians reduce use of emergency

department and referral services below the community average.

Completely healthy at age 45, Henry Fung reluctantly submitted to a treadmill exercise test at the local YMCA. The study was inconclusive and Mr. Fung, who had fee-for-service insurance, sought the advice of a cardiologist. The cardiologist knew that treadmill tests are sometimes positive in healthy people. Yet he ordered a coronary angiogram, which was perfectly normal. Three hours after the study, a clot formed in the femoral artery at the site of the catheter insertion, and emergency surgery was required to save Mr. Fung's leg.

No one can know what motivated the physician to send Ms. Brown home instead of to an emergency department when unstable coronary heart disease was one possible diagnosis (underuse); nor can one guess what led the fee-for-service cardiologist to perform an invasive coronary angiogram of questionable appropriateness on Mr. Fung (overuse). One factor that bears close attention is the impact of financial considerations on the quantity (and thus the quality) of medical care (Relman, 2007). As noted in Chapter 4, fee-for-service payment encourages physicians to perform more services, whereas capitation payments are sometimes structured to reward those who perform fewer services.

More than 40 years ago, Bunker (1970) found that the United States performed twice the number of surgical procedures per capita than Great Britain. He postulated that this difference could be accounted for by the greater number of surgeons per capita in the United States and concluded that "the method of payment appears to play an important, if unmeasured, part." Most surgeons in the United States are compensated by fee-for-service, whereas most in Great Britain are paid a salary.

An analysis of the National Practitioner Data Base suggests that 10% to 20% of all surgeries in several specialties are unnecessary (Eisler & Hansen, 2013). Surgeons who own and profit from ambulatory surgical centers operate more frequently than those who do not (Morgan et al., 2015). Even though surgery for lumbar spine disc disease often has poorer outcomes than medications and physical therapy, such surgeries more than doubled from 2000 to 2009 in the United States (Yoshihara and Yoneoka, 2015). From 2002 to 2007,

Medicare patients undergoing surgery for lumbar spinal stenosis experienced a doubling of complex rather than simple operations resulting in a major increase in surgical complications, rehospitalizations, and costs. Rates of reoperation (because of worsening pain) are high. Payment for this procedure is greater than that provided for most other procedures performed by orthopedists and neurosurgeons (Deyo et al., 2004, 2010).

> *It was a nice dinner, hosted by the hospital radiologist and paid for by the company manufacturing magnetic resonance imaging (MRI) scanners. After the meal came the pitch: "If you physicians invest money, we can get an MRI scanner near our hospital; if the MRI makes money, you all share in the profits." One internist explained later, "After I put in my $10,000, it was hard to resist ordering MRI scans. With headaches, back pain, and knee problems, the indications for MRIs are kind of fuzzy. You might order one or you might not. Now, I do."*

Relman (2007) writes about the commercialization of medicine: "The introduction of new technology in the hands of specialists, expanded insurance coverage, and unregulated fee-for-service payments all combined to rapidly increase the flow of money into the health care system, and thus sowed the seeds of a new, profit-driven industry."

During the 1980s, many physicians formed partnerships and joint ventures, giving them part ownership in laboratories, MRI scanners, and outpatient surgicenters. By 1990, 93% of diagnostic imaging facilities, 76% of ambulatory surgery centers, and 60% of clinical laboratories in Florida were owned wholly or in part by physicians. In a national study, physicians who received payment for performing x-rays and sonograms within their own offices obtained these examinations four times as often as physicians who referred the examinations to radiologists and received no payment for the studies (Hillman et al., 1990). Physicians who acquire MRI equipment order substantially more scans once they are able to bill for the imaging procedure (Baker, 2010).

Profitable diagnostic, imaging, and surgical procedures have rapidly migrated from the hospital to free-standing physician-owned ambulatory surgery centers, endoscopy centers, and imaging centers, with rapid increases in the number of tests and procedures performed (Berenson et al., 2006). The number of CT scans performed for Medicare patients increased by 300% from 1997 to 2017; 30% to 50% may be unnecessary, increasing patients' risk of radiation-induced cancer (Smith-Bindman, 2018).

Moving to the other side of the overuse–underuse spectrum, payment by capitation, or salaried employment by a for-profit business, may create a climate hostile to the provision of adequate services. In the 1970s, a series of HMOs called prepaid health plans (PHPs) sprang up to provide care to California Medicaid patients. The quality of care in several PHPs became a major scandal in California. At one PHP, administrators wrote a message to health care providers: "Do as little as you possibly can for the PHP patient," and charts audited by the California Health Department revealed many instances of undertreatment. The PHPs received a lump sum for each patient enrolled, meaning that the lower the cost of the services actually provided, the greater the PHP's profits (US Senate, 1975). More recent approaches to capitation payment have attempted to mitigate incentives for undertreatment by requiring providers to achieve quality of care targets and risk-adjusting capitation payments, with payments for patients at greater risk for needing medical services higher than payments for low-risk patients.

The quantity and quality of medical care are inextricably interrelated. Too much or too little can be injurious. The research of Fisher et al. (2003) has shown that similar populations in different geographic areas have widely varying rates of surgeries and days in the hospital, with no consistent difference in clinical outcomes between those in high-use and low-use areas.

▶ Health Care Systems and Quality of Care

> *The personnel cutbacks were terrible; staffing had diminished from four RNs per shift to two, with only two aides to provide assistance. Shelley Rush, RN, was 2 hours behind in administering medications and had five insulin injections to give, with complicated dosing schedules. A family member rushed to the nursing station saying, "The lady in my mother's room looks bad." Shelley ran in and found the patient unconscious. She quickly checked*

the blood sugar, which was disastrously low at 20 mg/dL. Shelley gave 50% glucose, and the patient woke up. Then it hit her—she had injected the insulin into the wrong patient.

Health care institutions must be well organized, with an adequate, competent staff. Shelley Rush was a superb nurse, but understaffing caused her to make a serious error. The book *Curing Health Care* by Berwick et al. (1990) opens with a heartbreaking case:

She died, but she didn't have to. The senior resident was sitting, near tears, in the drab office behind the nurses' station in the intensive care unit. It was 2:00 AM, and he had been battling for 32 hours to save the life of the 23-year-old graduate student who had just suffered her final cardiac arrest.

"Routine screening chest x-ray, taken 10 months ago. The tumor is right there, and it was curable—then. By the time the second film was taken 8 months later, because she was complaining of pain, it was too late. The tumor had spread everywhere, and the odds were hopelessly against her. Everything we've done since then has really just been wishful thinking. We missed our chance. She missed her chance." Exhausted, the resident put his head in his hands and cried.

Two months later, the Quality Assurance Committee completed its investigation . . . . "We find the inpatient care commendable in this tragic case," concluded the brief report, "although the failure to recognize the tumor in a potentially curable stage 10 months earlier was unfortunate . . . . " Nowhere in this report was it written explicitly why the results of the first chest x-ray had not been translated into action. No one knew.

One year later . . . . it was 2:00 AM, and the night custodian was cleaning the radiologist's office. As he moved a filing cabinet aside to sweep behind it, he glimpsed a dusty tan envelope that had been stuck between the cabinet and the wall. The envelope contained a yellow radiology report slip, and the date on the report—nearly 2 years earlier— convinced the custodian that this was, indeed, garbage . . . He tossed it in with the other trash, and 4 hours later it was incinerated along with other useless things.

This patient may have had perfect access to care for an illness whose treatment is scientifically proved; she may have seen a physician who knew how to make the diagnosis and deliver the appropriate treatment; and yet the quality of her care was disastrously deficient. Dozens of people and hundreds of processes influence the care of one person with one illness. In her case, one person—perhaps a file clerk with a near-perfect record in handling thousands of radiology reports—lost control of one report, and the physician's office had no system to monitor whether or not x-ray reports had been received. The result was the most tragic of quality failures—the unnecessary death of a young person.

How health care systems and institutions are organized has a major impact on health care outcomes. For example, large multispecialty group practices in 22 metropolitan areas have better-quality measures at lower cost than dispersed physician practices in those areas (Weeks et al., 2009). Nurse understaffing is associated with higher hospital mortality rates (Needleman et al., 2011). Studies have shown that hospitals with more RN staffing have lower surgical complication rates (Kovner & Gergen, 1998) and lower mortality rates (Aiken et al., 2002).

Oliver Hart lived in a city with a population of 80,000. He was admitted to Neighborhood Hospital with congestive heart failure caused by a defective mitral valve. He was told he needed semi-urgent heart surgery to replace the valve. The cardiologist said "You can go to University Hospital 30 miles away or have the surgery done here." The cardiologist did not say that Neighborhood Hospital performed only seven cardiac surgeries last year. Mr. Hart elected to remain for the procedure. During the surgery, a key piece of equipment failed, and he died on the operating table.

Quality of care must be viewed in the context of regional systems of care (see Chapter 6), not simply within each health care institution. In one study, 27% of deaths related to coronary artery bypass graft (CABG) surgery at low-volume hospitals might have been prevented by referral of those patients to hospitals performing a higher volume of those surgeries (Dudley et al., 2000). Hospitals performing more surgical procedures have lower mortality rates for that surgical procedure (Gonzalez et al., 2014). In addition, surgeons performing more procedures have better outcomes (Morche et al., 2016). Had Mr. Hart been told the relative surgical mortality rates at University Hospital, which performed 500 cardiac surgeries each year, and at Neighborhood Hospital, he would have chosen to be transferred 30 miles down the road. Not only does the volume of surgeries in a hospital matter; equally important is the volume of surgeries performed by the specific surgeon (Birkmeyer et al., 2003).

▶ The Components of Quality: Summary

Good-quality care can be compromised at a number of steps along the way.

Angie Roth has coronary heart disease and may need CABG surgery. (1) If she is uninsured and cannot get to a physician, high-quality care is impossible to obtain. (2) If clear evidence-based guidelines do not exist regarding who benefits from CABG and who does not, Ms. Roth's physician may make the wrong choice. (3) Even if clear guidelines exist, if Angie Roth's physician fails to evaluate her illness correctly or sends her to a surgeon with poor operative skills, quality may suffer. (4) If indications for surgery are not clear in Ms. Roth's case but the surgeon will benefit economically from the procedure, the surgery may be inappropriately performed. (5) Even if the surgery is appropriate and performed by an excellent surgeon, faulty equipment in the operating room or poor teamwork among the operating room surgeons, anesthesiologists, and nurses may lead to a poor outcome.

The Institute of Medicine, in its influential 2001 report *Crossing the Quality Chasm*, conceptualized six core dimensions of quality: safe, effective, patient-centered, timely, efficient, and equitable. These dimensions, defined in greater detail in Table 10–2, are consistent with the components of quality discussed earlier.

PROPOSALS FOR IMPROVING QUALITY

Several infants at a hospital received epinephrine in error and suffered serious medical consequences. An analysis revealed that several pharmacists had made the same mistake; the problem was caused by the identical appearance of vitamin E and epinephrine bottles in the pharmacy. This was a system error.

An epidemic of unexpected deaths on the cardiac ward was investigated. The times of the deaths were correlated with personnel schedules, leading to the conclusion that one nurse was responsible. It turned out that she was administering lethal doses of digoxin to patients. This was not a system error.

Traditionally, quality assurance has focused on individual caregivers and institutions in a "bad apple" approach that relies heavily on sanctions. More recently, quality has been viewed through the lens of the continuous quality improvement (CQI) model that seeks to enhance the clinical performance of all systems of care, not just the outliers with poor quality of care. The move to a CQI model has required development of more formalized standards of care that can be used as benchmarks for measuring quality, and more systematic collection of data to measure overall performance and not just performance in isolated cases (Table 10–2).

▶ Traditional Quality Assurance: Licensure, Accreditation, and Peer Review

Traditionally, the health care system has placed great reliance on educational institutions and licensing and accrediting agencies to ensure the competence

Table 10–2. Quality aims as defined by the Institute of Medicine

- *Safe*—avoiding injuries to patients from the care that is intended to help them
- *Effective*—providing services based on scientific knowledge to all who could benefit and refraining from providing services to those not likely to benefit (avoiding underuse and overuse, respectively)
- *Patient-centered*—providing care that is respectful of and responsive to individual patient preferences, needs, and values and ensuring that patient values guide all clinical decisions
- *Timely*—reducing waits and sometimes harmful delays for both those who receive and those who give care
- *Efficient*—avoiding waste, including waste of equipment, supplies, ideas, and energy
- *Equitable*—providing care that does not vary in quality because of personal characteristics such as gender, ethnicity, geographic location, and socioeconomic status

Source: Institute of Medicine. *Crossing the Quality Chasm: A New Health System for the 21st Century.* Washington, DC: National Academies Press; 2001.

of individuals and institutions in health care. Health care professionals undergo rigorous training and pass special licensing examinations intended to ensure that caregivers have at least a basic level of knowledge and competence. However, clinicians may have been competent practitioners at the time they took their examinations, but their skills lapsed or they developed impairment from alcohol or drug use, depression, or other conditions (Leape & Fromson, 2006).

Many organizations that confer specialty board certification require physicians to pass examinations on a periodic basis and perform systematic quality reviews of their own clinical practices to maintain active specialty certification. However, while some hospitals may require active specialty certification for a physician to be granted privileges to practice in the hospital, certification is not required for medical licensure.

The traditional approach to quality assurance has also relied heavily on physician self-regulation (Madara & Burkhart, 2015). Peer review, which has been part of medicine for decades, is the evaluation by health care practitioners of the appropriateness and quality of services performed by other practitioners, usually in the same specialty (Edwards, 2018). Medicare anointed the Joint Commission on Accreditation of Hospitals (now named the Joint Commission) with the authority to terminate hospitals from the Medicare program if quality of care was found to be deficient. The Joint Commission requires hospital medical staff to set up peer review committees for the purpose of maintaining quality of care.

The Joint Commission uses criteria of structure, process, and outcome to assess quality of care. Structural criteria include such factors as whether the emergency department defibrillator works properly. Process criteria include whether medical records are completed in a timely manner, or if the credentials committee keeps minutes of its meetings. Outcomes include such measures as mortality rates for surgical procedures, proportions of deaths that are preventable, and rates of adverse drug reactions and wound infections. Medicare also contracts with quality improvement organizations (QIOs) to promote better quality of care among physicians caring for Medicare beneficiaries (US Department of Health and Human Services, 2018).

Angela Lopez, age 57, suffered from metastatic ovarian cancer but was feeling well and prayed

she would live 9 months more. It was decided to infuse chemotherapy directly into her peritoneal cavity. As the solution poured into her abdomen, she felt increasing pressure. She asked the nurse to stop the fluid. The nurse called the physician, who said not to worry. Two hours later, Ms. Lopez became short of breath and demanded that the fluid be stopped. The nurse again called the physician, but an hour later Ms. Lopez died. Her abdomen was tense with fluid, which pushed on her lungs and stopped circulation through her inferior vena cava. The quality assurance committee reviewed the case as a preventable death and criticized the physician for giving too much fluid and failing to respond adequately to the nurse's call. The physician replied that he was not at fault; the nurse had not told him how sick the patient was. The case was closed.

The traditional quality assurance strategies of licensing and peer review have not been effective tools for improving quality (Chassin & Baker, 2015). Peer review often adheres to the theory of bad apples, attempting to discipline physicians (to remove them from the apple barrel) for mistakes rather than to improve their practice through education. The physician who caused Ms. Lopez's preventable death responded to peer criticism by blaming the nurse rather than learning from the mistake. With the hundreds of decisions physicians make each day, often in time-constrained situations, serious errors are relatively common in medical practice. One-third of physicians surveyed in 2009 did not agree with disclosing serious errors to patients and 20% had not disclosed errors to their patients (Iezzoni et al., 2012).

Even if sanctions against the truly bad apples had more teeth, these measures would not solve the quality problem. Removing the incontrovertibly bad apples from the barrel does not address all the quality problems that emanate from competent caregivers who are not performing optimally. Health care systems do need to forcefully sanction caregivers who, despite efforts at remediation, cannot operate at a basic standard of acceptable practice. But measures are also needed to "shift the curve" of overall clinical practice to a higher level of quality, not just to trim off the poor-quality outliers.

Peer reviewers frequently disagree as to whether the quality of care in particular cases is adequate or not (Laffel & Berwick, 1993). Because of these limitations, efforts are underway to formalize standards of care using clinical practice guidelines and to move from individual case review to more systematic monitoring of overall practice patterns (Table 10–3).

▶ Clinical Practice Guidelines

Dr. Benjamin Waters was frustrated by patients who came in with urinary incontinence. He never learned about the problem in medical school, so he simply referred these patients to a urologist. In his managed care plan, Dr. Waters was known to overrefer, so he felt stuck. He could not handle the problem, yet he did not want to refer patients elsewhere. He solved his dilemma by prescribing incontinence pads and diapers, but did not feel good about it.

Dr. Denise Drier learned about urinary incontinence in family medicine residency but did not feel secure about caring for the problem. On the web, she found "Urinary Incontinence in Adults: Clinical Practice Guideline Update." She studied the material and applied it to her incontinence patients. After a few successes, she and the patients were feeling better about themselves.

For many conditions, there is a better and a worse way to make a diagnosis and prescribe treatment. Physicians may not be aware of the better way because of gaps in training, limited experience, or insufficient time or motivation to learn new techniques. For these problems, clinical practice guidelines can be helpful in improving quality of care. Practice guidelines make specific recommendations to physicians on how to treat clinical conditions such as diabetes, osteoporosis, urinary incontinence, or cataracts.

In 2014, 2,619 guidelines existed, written by dozens of organizations including specialty societies and commercial companies. The US Preventive Services Task Force and other respected professional organizations issue widely accepted guidelines based on a rigorous and objective review of scientific evidence. However, many guidelines are unreliable and tainted by monetary interests (Graham et al., 2011). Nearly 90% of clinical practice guideline authors in one survey had ties to the pharmaceutical industry, a bias often not disclosed (Shaneyfelt & Centor, 2009). For example, 8 of the 15 members of the panel recommending new cholesterol guidelines in 2013—which increased the number of people who would be taking statin drugs—had industry ties (Ioannidis, 2014). Moreover, clinical practice guidelines developed based on research on a narrowly defined population, such as nonelderly patients with a single chronic condition, may not be applicable to different patient populations, such as elderly patients with multiple diseases (Boyd et al., 2005). To address the pervasive conflicts of interest in many guidelines, the number of guidelines was reduced to 1,402 by 2018, but many are still unreliable (Shekelle, 2018).

In 2012, the American Board of Internal Medicine Foundation and Consumer Reports launched the Choosing Wisely campaign, which called on professional societies and health care providers to reduce the unnecessary and potentially harmful health services that cost about $200 billion in wasteful spending in the United States in 2011. By the end of 2016, over 70 medical societies had joined the campaign and 500 recommendations had been issued, for example avoiding routine cholecystectomy for patients with asymptomatic gallstones and reducing the number of CT scans for several clinical conditions (www.choosingwisely.org). Nearly 40% of physicians surveyed had heard about Choosing Wisely. Consumer Reports developed patient-oriented materials describing the recommendations. A number of health systems began

Table 10–3. Proposals for improving quality

Licensure, accreditation, peer review
Clinical practice guidelines
Measuring practice patterns
Continuous quality improvement
Computerized information systems
Public reporting of quality
Pay for performance
Financially neutral clinical decision making

to implement the recommendations. During the first 5 years of the campaign, actual reductions in unnecessary services have been slow in coming, but the momentum is gathering (Kerr et al., 2017).

Practice guidelines are not appropriate for many clinical situations. Uncertainty pervades clinical medicine, and practice guidelines are applicable only for those cases in which we enjoy "islands of knowledge in our seas of ignorance." Practice guidelines can assist but not replace clinical judgment in the quest for high-quality care.

Pedro Urrutia, age 59, noticed mild nocturia and urinary frequency. His friend had prostate cancer, and he became concerned. The urologist said that his prostate was only slightly enlarged, his prostate-specific antigen (blood test) was normal, and surgery was not needed. Mr. Urrutia wanted surgery and found another urologist to do it.

At age 82, James Chin noted nocturia and urinary hesitancy. He had two glasses of wine on his wife's birthday and later that night was unable to urinate. He went to the emergency department, was found to have a large prostate without nodules, and was catheterized. The urologist strongly recommended a transurethral resection of the prostate. Mr. Chin refused, thinking that the urinary retention was caused by the alcohol. Five years later, he was in good health with his prostate intact.

Even when guidelines have been defined, patient preferences vary markedly. Some, like Mr. Urrutia, want prostate surgery, even though it is not needed; others, like Mr. Chin, have strong indications for surgery but do not want it. Practice guidelines must take into account not only scientific data, but also patient preferences (Montori et al., 2013).

Do practice guidelines in themselves improve quality of care? The evidence is murky (Djulbegovic & Guyatt, 2014). However, guidelines can be an important foundation for more comprehensive quality improvement strategies, such as computer systems to remind physicians when patients are in need of certain services according to a guideline (e.g., a reminder system about women due for a mammogram) (Chen & Bodenheimer, 2011) or having trusted colleagues ("opinion leaders") or visiting experts ("academic detailing") conduct small group sessions with clinicians to review and reinforce practice guidelines (Avorn, 2017).

▶ Measuring Practice Patterns

A central tenet of the CQI approach is the need to systematically monitor how well individual caregivers, institutions, and organizations are performing. Two types of indicators used to evaluate clinical performance are process measures and outcome measures. *Process* of care refers to the types of services delivered by caregivers. Examples are prescribing aspirin to patients with coronary heart disease, or turning immobile patients in hospital beds on a regular schedule to prevent bed sores. *Outcomes*—e.g., death, symptoms, mental health, physical functioning, laboratory studies, and health status—are the gold standard for measuring quality. However, outcomes (particularly those dealing with quality of life) may be difficult to measure. More easily counted outcomes such as mortality may be rare events, and therefore uninformative for evaluating quality of care for many conditions that are not immediately life-threatening. Also, outcomes may be heavily influenced by the underlying severity of illness and related patient characteristics, and not just by the quality of health care that patients received (King, 2016). When measuring patient outcomes, it is necessary to "risk adjust" these outcome measurements for differences in the underlying characteristics of different groups of patients. Because of these challenges in using outcomes as measures to monitor quality of care, process measures are commonly used. For process measures to be valid indicators of quality, there must be solid research demonstrating that the processes do in fact influence patient outcomes.

Dr. Susan Cutter felt horrible. It was supposed to have been a routine hysterectomy. Somehow she had inadvertently lacerated the large intestine of the patient, a 45-year-old woman with symptomatic fibroids of the uterus but otherwise in good health prior to surgery. Bacteria from the intestine had leaked into the abdomen, and after a protracted battle in the ICU the patient died of septic shock.

Dr. Cutter met with the Chief of Surgery at her hospital. The Chief reviewed the case with

Dr. Cutter, but also pulled out a report showing the statistics on all of Dr. Cutter's surgical cases over the previous 5 years. The report showed that Dr. Cutter's mortality and complication rates were among the lowest of surgeons on the hospital's staff. However, the Chief did note that another surgeon, Dr. Dehisce, had a complication rate that was much higher than that of all the other staff surgeons. The Chief of Surgery asked Dr. Cutter to serve on a departmental committee to review Dr. Dehisce's cases and to meet with Dr. Dehisce to consider ways to address his poor performance.

The contemporary approach to quality monitoring moves beyond examining a few isolated cases toward measuring processes or outcomes for a large population of patients. A traditional peer review approach is to review every case of a patient who dies during surgery. Reviewing an individual case may help a surgeon and the operating team understand where errors may have occurred—a process known as "root cause" analysis. However, it does not indicate whether the case represented an aberrant bad outcome for a surgeon or team that usually has good surgical outcomes, or whether the case is indicative of more widespread problems. To answer these questions requires examining data on all the patients operated on by the surgeon and the operating team to measure the overall rate of surgical complications, and having some benchmark data that indicate whether this rate is higher than expected for similar types of patients.

Many practice organizations, from small groups of office-based physicians to vertically integrated health systems are starting to monitor patterns of care and provide feedback on this care to physicians and other staff. A typical example of this practice profiling is measuring the rate at which diabetic patients receive recommended services, such as annual eye examinations, periodic testing of HbA1c levels, and evaluation of kidney function. Diabetes process of care profiles demonstrate which clinicians are providing high quality care and which would benefit from improvement advice; and indicate what systematic reforms would improve care, such as health coaching for diabetic patients in poor control (Bodenheimer & Grumbach, 2007).

▶ Continuous Quality Improvement

Maximizing excellence for individual health care professionals is only one ingredient in the recipe for high-quality health care. Improving institutions is the other, through CQI techniques. CQI involves the identification of concrete problems and the formation of interdisciplinary teams to gather data and propose and implement solutions to the problems.

In LDS Hospital in Salt Lake City, variation in wound infection rates by different surgeons was related to the timing of the administration of prophylactic antibiotics. Patients who received antibiotics 2 hours before surgery had the lowest infection rates. The surgery department adopted a policy that all patients receive antibiotics precisely 2 hours before surgery; the rate of postoperative wound infections dropped from 1.8% to 0.9%. (Burke, 2001)

Such successes only dot, but do not yet dominate, the health care quality landscape (Solberg, 2007). The Institute for Healthcare Improvement (IHI) has led efforts to spread CQI efforts by sponsoring "collaboratives" to assist institutions and groups of institutions to improve health care outcomes and access while ideally reducing costs. Hundreds of health care organizations have participated in collaboratives concerned with such topics as improving the care of chronic illness, reducing waiting times, improving care at the end of life, and reducing adverse drug events. Collaboratives involve learning sessions during which teams from various institutions meet and discuss the application of a rapid change methodology within institutions. Some of IHI's successes have taken place in the area of chronic disease, with a variety of institutions—from large integrated delivery systems to tiny rural community health centers—implementing the chronic care model to improve outcomes for conditions such as diabetes, asthma, and congestive heart failure. Collaboratives have shown modest improvement in patient outcomes (Burton et al., 2018). In the area of patient safety, in 2004, IHI launched the 100,000 Lives Campaign (www.ihi.org) to reduce mortality rates in hospitals; more than 4,000 hospitals in the United States participated. There is evidence that the campaign contributed to reductions in hospital mortality (Berwick et al., 2006; Wachter & Pronovost, 2006).

Related to CQI is the Lean improvement method. Lean principles were developed by Toyota as a structured process for eliminating waste and improving value in automobile manufacturing. Lean includes elements such as identifying all the steps in the production process and analyzing potential sources of inefficiency and quality defects, and engaging front-line workers in the improvement process (NEJM Catalyst, 2018a). Many prominent health care organizations have adopted Lean as their model for value improvement. Although many case studies attest to improvements in health care quality after implementing Lean methods, only a few rigorous evaluations of Lean have been conducted, demonstrating improvements in some process measures such as handwashing by hospital staff but no consistent benefit on clinical outcomes such as hospital mortality and rates of readmission (Moraros et al., 2016).

Computerized Information Systems

The advent of computerized information systems has created opportunities to improve care and to monitor the process and outcomes of care for entire populations. Electronic medical records can create lists of patients who are overdue for services needed for preventive care or the management of chronic illness and can generate reminder prompts for physicians and patients. Computerized physician order entry systems can alert the physician about inappropriate medication doses or medications to which the patient is known to be allergic. Development of protocols for sharing electronic medical record data across practices and health systems allows key clinical information to flow with patients across the care continuum, improving care coordination and potentially enhancing patient safety and reducing duplication of services. However, studies on the impact of electronic medical records on quality are mixed (McCullough et al., 2013). Electronic medical records are a tool that can improve care, but transformation of practice organization is required to take full advantage of this tool (Wachter, 2015).

The digital revolution in health care is opening up vistas for the application of artificial intelligence

to mine the massive amounts of data in electronic medical records, digital radiographic images, genomic assays, and other health data repositories. "Machine learning" synthesizes these data for computer-assisted enhancement of diagnosis, prognosis, and treatment (Rajkomar et al., 2019). Although there have been a few emerging successful applications of artificial intelligence to improve the accuracy and efficiency of interpretation of diagnostic studies such as CT scans and retinal imaging, many questions remain about the broader application of artificial intelligence to the very human work of care and healing.

Public Reporting of Quality

The CQI approach emphasizes systematic monitoring of care to provide internal feedback to clinicians and health organizations to spur improved processes of care. A different approach to monitoring quality of care is to direct this information to the public. This approach views public release of systematic measurements of quality of care—commonly referred to as health care "report cards"—as a tool to empower health care consumers to select higher-quality caregivers and institutions. In 2003, Medicare initiated public reporting for hospitals, called Hospital Compare, focusing on risk-adjusted quality of care for heart attacks, heart failure, and pneumonia. In 2010, Medicare added a Physician Compare website. It is uncertain whether these public reports have significantly improved quality (Ryan et al., 2012; Findlay, 2015). The Healthcare Effectiveness Data and Information Set (HEDIS), developed by the National Committee for Quality Assurance (NCQA, 2019), a private organization controlled by insurers and large employers, tracks many performance indicators at the level of health insurance plans, making it less useful to consumers, physicians, and hospitals. Some states and health systems issue report cards on hospital and physician quality.

An important experiment in physician report cards was initiated by the New York State Department of Health in 1990. The department released data on risk-adjusted mortality rates for coronary bypass surgery performed at each hospital in the state, and in 1992, mortality rates were also published for each cardiac surgeon. Each year's list was big news and highly controversial. However, difficulties in measurement were highlighted by the fact that within 1 year, 46% of the surgeons had moved from one-half of the ranked list to the other half.

Several fascinating results came of this project: (1) Patients did not switch from hospitals with high mortality rates to those with lower mortality rates. (2) With the release of each report, one in five bottom quartile surgeons relocated or ceased practicing. (3) In 4 years, overall risk-adjusted coronary artery bypass mortality dropped by 41% in New York State. Mortality for this operation also dropped in states without report cards, but not as much. (4) Some surgeons, worried about the report cards, may have elected not to operate on the most risky patients in order to improve their report card ranking. It is possible that the reduction in surgical mortality in part resulted from withholding surgery for the sickest patients. The New York State experiment had less effect on changing the market decisions of patients and purchasers than on motivating quality improvements in hospitals that had poor surgical outcomes (Marshall et al., 2000; Jha & Epstein, 2006). Similarly, public reporting of diabetes measures can stimulate physicians to improve their care (Smith et al., 2012). Despite resources such as HEDIS report cards on health plan quality, few employers use quality data when selecting health plans for their employees; cost is the driving factor in most employer decisions (Galvin & Delbanco, 2005).

Report cards are based on a philosophy that says "if you can't count it, you can't improve it." Albert Einstein expressed an alternative philosophy that might illuminate the report card enterprise: "Not everything that can be counted counts, and not everything that counts can be counted." Increasingly, the focus on quality is switching to a focus on value, with value referring to quality divided by cost. Thus, an increase in a quality measure associated with a growth in cost may not improve value, where improved quality with a stable or reduced cost increases value (Owens et al., 2011).

▶ Pay for Performance

Pay-for-performance (P4P) programs provide financial rewards or penalties to individual health care providers, groups of providers, or institutions according to their performance on measures of quality. If properly targeted and designed, P4P programs would help drive the behavior of providers and health care systems to improve the quality of care delivered (Mendelson et al., 2017). One of the oldest P4P programs is the Integrated Healthcare Association (IHA) program in California which began in 2002 with performance measures including clinical care, patient satisfaction, use of information technology, and health care costs. In 2017, 9 health plans and 200 physician organizations—impacting 9.6 million patients—participated in the IHA program. From 2001 to 2015, physician organizations received over $500 million in performance-based payments (Integrated Healthcare Association, 2016). Overall performance improved an average of 3% annually but varied substantially among physician organizations (Chee et al., 2016).

The IHA program is unique in that all major health plans collaborate in choosing the measures upon which performance bonuses are based. If only one health plan sets up a P4P program with physicians, there may not be enough patients from that health plan to accurately measure the physician's quality; with all health plans participating, a substantial portion of a physician's patient panel is included in the measures. In addition, IHA targets large physician organizations with many patients; if measures are linked to individual physicians, the small numbers of patients may distort the results. The ability of the California experience to aggregate a large number of patients allows for more accurate performance evaluation.

Medicare has initiated three hospital P4P programs. The Value-Based Purchasing Program reduces Medicare hospital payments by 1.75% and uses that "value pool" to award high quality hospitals who achieve high quality scores compared with their own past scores and with the scores of other hospitals. The Hospital Acquired Condition Reduction Program reduces Medicare payments by 1% for hospitals with higher rates of patient injuries from such events as surgical site infections or hip fractures from falls (NEJM Catalyst, 2018b). The Hospital Readmissions Reduction Program penalizes hospitals up to 3% of their Medicare payments if they have high rates of readmissions for such diagnoses as heart attacks, heart failure, pneumonia, or hip/knee replacement. This program has not achieved significant readmission reduction (Joshi et al., 2019).

The 2015 Medicare Access and CHIP Reauthorization Act (MACRA) established a new P4P program for physicians who care for a substantial number of Medicare patients. Under MACRA, Medicare payments to physicians are adjusted up or down based on the quality and efficiency of their care starting in 2019. Physicians whose practice participates in an alternative payment system with upside and downside financial risk (see Chapter 4) would receive a 5% bonus and not be subjected to the quality-adjusted Medicare payments (Spivack et al., 2018; Wilensky, 2018).

A P4P program described as "the world's largest pay-for-performance healthcare scheme" was launched in the United Kingdom in 2004 (Minchin et al., 2018). This program is described in Chapter 14.

Some authors urge caution, pointing out that P4P programs could encourage physicians and hospitals to avoid high-risk patients in order to keep their performance scores up (McMahon et al., 2007). Another difficulty is that many patients see a large number of physicians in a given year, making it impossible to determine which physician should receive a performance bonus (Pham et al., 2007). Moreover, P4P programs could increase disparities in quality by preferentially rewarding physicians and hospitals caring for higher-income patients and having greater resources available to invest in quality improvement, and penalizing those institutions and physicians attending to more vulnerable populations in resource-poor environments (Casalino et al., 2007).

► Financially Neutral Clinical Decision Making

The quest for quality care encompasses a search for a financial structure that does not reward over- or undertreatment and that separates physicians' personal incomes from their clinical decisions. Balanced incentives (see Chapter 4), combining elements of capitation or salary and fee-for-service, may have the best chance of minimizing the payment–treatment nexus (Robinson, 1999), encouraging physicians to do more of what is truly beneficial for patients while not inducing inappropriate and harmful services. Completely financially neutral decision making will always be an ideal and not a reality.

WHERE DOES MALPRACTICE REFORM FIT IN?

During a coronary angiogram, emboli traveled to the brain of Ivan Romanov, resulting in a serious stroke, with loss of use of his left arm and leg. The angiogram was appropriate and performed without technical errors. Mr. Romanov had suffered a medical injury (an injury caused by his medical treatment), but the event was not because of negligence.

During a dilation and curettage (D&C), Judy Morrison's physician unknowingly perforated her uterus and lacerated her colon. Ms. Morrison reported severe pain but was sent home without further evaluation. She returned 1 hour later to the emergency department with persistent pain and internal bleeding. She required extensive surgical repair over the following 4 months. This medical injury was found by the legal system to have been caused by negligence.

A peculiar set of institutions called the malpractice liability system forms an important part of US health care (Mello et al., 2014). The goals of the malpractice system are twofold: To financially compensate people who in the course of seeking medical care have suffered medical injuries and to prevent physicians and other health care personnel from negligently causing harm to their patients.

The malpractice system has scored miserably on both counts. According to the Harvard Medical Practice Study, only 2% of patients who suffer from medical negligence file malpractice claims that would allow them to receive compensation, meaning that the malpractice system fails in its first goal. Thus the system does not deal with 98% of negligent acts performed by physicians, making it difficult to attain its second goal. More recent research has confirmed the findings of the Harvard study (Localio et al., 1991; Sage & Kersh, 2006).

On the other hand, as many as 40% of malpractice claims do not involve true medical errors (Studdert et al., 2006), with an even smaller proportion representing actual negligence. Nonetheless, one-quarter of these inappropriate claims result in the patient receiving monetary compensation. Overall, for every dollar in compensation received by patients in malpractice awards, legal costs and fees consume 40 to 60 cents (Shepherd, 2013).

The malpractice system has serious negative side effects on medical practice (Localio et al., 1991).

1. The system assumes that punishment, which usually involves physicians paying large amounts of money to a malpractice insurer plus enduring the overwhelming stress of a malpractice jury trial, is a reasonable method for improving the quality of medical care. In fact, fear of a lawsuit closes physicians' minds to improvement and leads to unnecessary and costly diagnostic testing (Carrier et al., 2013). The atmosphere created by malpractice litigation clouds a clear analytic assessment of quality.

2. The system is wasteful, with a huge portion of malpractice insurance premiums spent on lawyers, court costs, and insurance overhead rather than payments to patients (Mello et al., 2010). Many claims have no merit but wreak unnecessary stress upon physicians (Seabury et al., 2013). Between 2005 and 2014, only 6% of physicians had a paid malpractice claim and 1% of physicians accounted for 32% of paid claims (Studdert et al., 2016). Patients granted malpractice award payments sometimes experienced no negligent care, and patients subjected to negligent care often receive no malpractice payments (Brennan et al., 1996).

3. The system is based on the belief that trial by jury is the best method of determining whether there has been negligence, a questionable assumption.

4. People with lower incomes generally receive smaller awards (because wages lost from a medical injury are lower) and are therefore less attractive to lawyers, who are paid as a percentage of the award. Accordingly, low-income patients, who suffer more medical injury, are less likely than wealthier people to file malpractice claims (McClellan et al., 2012).

In summary, the malpractice system is burdened with expensive, unfounded litigation that harasses physicians who have done nothing wrong, fails to discipline or educate most physicians committing actual medical negligence and does not compensate most true victims of negligence.

A number of proposals have been made for malpractice reform (Mello et al., 2017).

▶ Tort Reform

Medical malpractice fits into the larger legal field of torts (wrongful acts or injuries done willfully or negligently). Tort reforms limit the amount of compensation that plaintiffs may recover and place caps on attorneys' fees. Thirty states have enacted tort reforms, which have reduced claims payments by 20% to 30% and may have contributed to slowing the growth of malpractice insurance premiums. However, caps on awards can be unfair to patients, limiting payments to those with the worst injuries (Localio, 2010; Mello et al., 2014).

▶ Communication-and-Resolution Programs

Several medical centers have initiated dispute resolution programs in which hospitals disclose adverse events to patients, apologize, and in some cases offer compensation. Interviews with patients found that 60% had a positive experience with the process and over half who received compensation were satisfied with it (Moore et al., 2017). Such alternatives to the jury trial could bring more compensation to injured parties by reducing legal costs and shift the dispute settlement to a more scientific, less emotional theater.

CONCLUSION

Each year people in the United States make over 1 billion ambulatory care visits and have more than 36 million hospital admissions. While quality of care provided during most of these encounters is excellent, the goal of the health care system should be to deliver high-quality care every day to every patient. This goal presents an unending challenge to each health caregiver and health care institution. Health professionals make hundreds of decisions each day, including which questions to ask in the patient history, which parts of the body to examine in the physical examination, which laboratory tests and x-rays to order and how urgently, which diagnoses to entertain, which treatments to offer, when to have the patient return for follow-up, and whether other clinicians need to be consulted. It is humanly impossible to make all of these decisions correctly every day. For health care to be of high quality, mistakes should be minimized, mistakes with serious consequences should be avoided, and systems should be in place that reduce, detect, and correct errors to the greatest extent possible. Even when all decisions are technically accurate, if caregivers are insensitive or fail to provide the patient with a full range of informed choices, quality is impaired.

For the clinician, each decision that influences quality of care may be simple, but the sum total of all decisions of all caregivers impacting on a patient's illness makes the achievement of high-quality care elusive. To safeguard quality of care, laws and regulations are needed, including standards for health professional education, rules for licensure, boards with the authority to discipline violators, and measurement to inform institutions, practitioners, and patients about the quality of their care. Improvement of health care quality cannot solely rely on regulators in Washington, DC, in state capitals, or across town; it must come from within each institution, whether a huge academic center, a community hospital, or a small medical office.

REFERENCES

Aiken LH, et al. Hospital nurse staffing and patient mortality, nurse burnout, and job dissatisfaction. *JAMA*. 2002;288:1987.

American Diabetes Association. Standards of medical care in diabetes—2019 abridged for primary care providers. *Clinical Diabetes*. 2019;37:11–34.

Avorn J. Academic detailing. *JAMA*. 2017;317:361–362.

Baker LC. Acquisition of MRI equipment by doctors drives up imaging use and spending. *Health Aff (Millwood)*. 2010;29:2252–2259.

Berenson RA, et al. Hospital–physician relations: cooperation, competition, or separation? *Health Aff (Millwood)*. 2006;26:w31–W43.

Berwick DM, et al. *Curing Health Care*. San Francisco, CA: Jossey-Bass; 1990.

Berwick DM, et al. IHI replies to "The 100,000 Lives Campaign: a scientific and policy review." *Jt Comm J Qual Patient Saf*. 2006;32:628–630.

Birkmeyer JD, et al. Surgeon volume and operative mortality in the United States. *N Engl J Med*. 2003;349:2117–2127.

Bodenheimer T, Grumbach K. *Improving Primary Care: Strategies and Tools for a Better Practice*. New York, NY: McGraw-Hill; 2007.

Boyd CM, et al. Clinical practice guidelines and quality of care for older patients with multiple comorbid diseases. *JAMA*. 2005;294:716–724.

Brennan TA, et al. Incidence of adverse events and negligence in hospitalized patients. *N Engl J Med*. 1991;324:370–376.

Brennan TA, et al. Relation between negligent adverse events and the outcomes of medical-malpractice litigation. *N Engl J Med*. 1996;335:1963–1967.

Bunker J. Surgical manpower. *N Engl J Med*. 1970;282:135–144.

Burke JP. Maximizing appropriate antibiotic prophylaxis for surgical patients. *Clin Infect Dis*. 2001;33(suppl 2): S78–S83.

Burton RA, et al. Perspectives on implementing quality improvement collaboratives effectively. *Joint Commission J Qual Safety*. 2018;44:12–22.

Carrier ER, et al. High physician concern about malpractice risk predicts more aggressive diagnostic testing in office-based practice. *Health Aff (Millwood)*. 2013;32:1383–1391.

Casalino LP, et al. Will pay-for-performance and quality reporting affect health care disparities? *Health Aff (Millwood)*. 2007;26:w405–w414.

Casalino LP, et al. Frequency of failure to inform patients of clinically significant outpatient test results. *Arch Intern Med*. 2009;169:1123–1129.

Chassin MR, Baker DW. Aiming higher to enhance professionalism. *JAMA*. 2015;313:1795–1796.

Chassin MR, Loeb J. The ongoing quality improvement journey: next stop, high reliability. *Health Aff (Millwood)*. 2011;30:559–568.

Chassin MR, et al. The urgent need to improve health care quality. *JAMA*. 1998;280:1000–1005.

Chee TT, et al. Current state of value-based purchasing programs. *Circulation*. 2016;133:2197–2205.

Chen E, Bodenheimer T. Improving population health through team-based panel management. *Arch Intern Med*. 2011;171:1558–1559.

Deyo RA, et al. Spinal fusion surgery—the case for restraint. *N Engl J Med*. 2004;350:722–726.

Deyo RA, et al. Trends, major medical complications, and charges associated with surgery for lumbar spinal stenosis in older adults. *JAMA*. 2010;303:1259–1265.

Djulbegovic B, Guyatt GH. Evidence-based practice is not synonymous with delivery of uniform health care. *JAMA*. 2014;312:1293–1294.

Dudley RA, et al. Selective referral to high-volume hospitals: estimating potentially avoidable deaths. *JAMA*. 2000;283:1159–1166.

Edwards MT. In pursuit of quality and safety: an 8-year study of clinical peer review best practices in US hospitals. *Intern J Qual in Health Care*. 2018;30:602–607.

Eisler P, Hansen B. Doctors perform thousands of unnecessary surgeries. *USA Today*, June 20, 2013.

Findlay S. Physician compare. Health Affairs Health Policy Brief. October 29, 2015.

Fisher ES, et al. The implications of regional variations in Medicare spending. Part 1: the content, quality, and accessibility of care. *Ann Intern Med.* 2003;138:273–287.

Galvin RS, Delbanco S. Why employers need to rethink how they buy health care. *Health Aff (Millwood).* 2005;24:1549–1553.

Gonzalez AA, et al. Understanding the volume-outcome effect in cardiovascular surgery: the role of failure to rescue. *JAMA Surg.* 2014;149:119–123.

Graham R, et al. *Clinical Practice Guidelines We Can Trust.* Washington, DC: National Academies Press; 2011. https://www.ncbi.nlm.nih.gov/books/NBK209539/. Accessed October 18, 2019.

Hillman BJ, et al. Frequency and costs of diagnostic imaging in office patients: a comparison of self-referring and radiologist-referring physicians. *N Engl J Med.* 1990;323:1604–1608.

Iezzoni LI, et al. Survey shows that at least some physicians are not always open or honest with patients. *Health Aff (Millwood).* 2012;31:383–391.

Institute of Medicine. *To Err Is Human: Building a Safer Health System.* Washington, DC: National Academies Press; 1999. http://www.nationalacademies.org/hmd/~/media/Files/Report%20Files/1999/To-Err-is-Human/To%20Err%20is%20Human%201999%20%20report%20brief.pdf. Accessed October 18, 2019.

Institute of Medicine. *Crossing the Quality Chasm: A New Health System for the 21st Century.* Washington, DC: National Academies Press; 2001. http://www.nationalacademies.org/hmd/~/media/Files/Report%20Files/2001/Crossing-the-Quality-Chasm/Quality%20Chasm%202001%20%20report%20brief.pdf. Accessed October 18, 2019.

Integrated Healthcare Organization. Value Based Pay for Performance in California. September 2016. Integrated Healthcare Association › files › vbp4p-fact-sheet-final-2016. Accessed October 18, 2019.

Ioannidis JP. More than a billion people taking statins?: Potential implications of the new cardiovascular guidelines. *JAMA.* 2014;311:463–464.

Jha AK, Epstein AM. The predictive accuracy of the New York State coronary artery bypass surgery report-card system. *Health Aff (Millwood).* 2006;25:844–855.

Joshi S, et al. Regression to the mean in the Medicare Hospital Readmissions Reduction Program. *JAMA Intern Med.* 2019. [Epub ahead of print]

Kerr EA, et al. Choosing wisely: how to fulfill the promise in the next 5 years. *Health Aff (Millwood).* 2017;36:2012–2018.

King T. *The Medical Management of the Vulnerable and Underserved Patient.* New York, NY: McGraw-Hill; 2016.

Kovner C, Gergen PJ. Nurse staffing levels and adverse events following surgery in U.S. hospitals. *Image J Nurs Sch.* 1998;30:315.

Laffel GL, Berwick DM. Quality health care. *JAMA.* 1993;270:254–255.

Lahue BJ, et al. National burden of preventable adverse drug events associated with inpatient injectable medications. *Am Health Drug Benefits.* 2012;5:1–10.

Leape LL, et al. The nature of adverse events in hospitalized patients. *N Engl J Med.* 1991;324:377–384.

Leape LL, Fromson JA. Problem doctors: is there a system-level solution? *Ann Intern Med.* 2006;144:107–115.

The Leapfrog Group. Leapfrog hospital safety grade. 2018. https://www.hospitalsafetygrade.org/. Accessed October 18, 2019.

Levine DM, et al. The quality of outpatient care delivered to adults in the United States, 2002 – 2013. *JAMA Intern Med.* 2016;176:1778–1790.

Localio AR. Patient compensation without litigation: a promising development. *Ann Intern Med.* 2010;153:266–267.

Localio AR, et al. Relation between malpractice claims and adverse events due to negligence. *N Engl J Med.* 1991;325:245–251.

Madara JL, Burkhart J. Professionalism, self-regulation, and motivation. How did health care get this so wrong? *JAMA.* 2015;313:1793–1794.

Maciosek MV, et al. Greater use of preventive services in U.S. health care could save lives at little or no cost. *Health Aff (Millwood).* 2010;29:1656–1660.

Makary M, Daniel M. Medical error—the third leading cause of death in the US. *BMJ.* 2016;353:i2139.

Marshall MN, et al. The public release of performance data. *JAMA.* 2000;283:1866–1874.

McClellan FM, et al. Do poor people sue doctors more frequently? *Clin Orthop Relat Res.* 2012;470:1393–1397.

McCullough JS, et al. Do electronic medical records improve diabetes quality in physician practices? *Am J Manag Care.* 2013;19:144–149.

McGlynn EA, et al. The quality of health care delivered to adults in the United States. *N Engl J Med.* 2003;348:2635–2645.

McMahon LF, et al. Physician-level P4P—DOA? *Am J Manag Care.* 2007;13:233–236.

Medicare Hospital Quality Chartbook. U.S. Center for Medicare and Medicaid Services. September, 2013. https://www.cms.gov/Medicare/Quality-Initiatives-Patient-Assessment-Instruments/HospitalQualityInits/Downloads/-Medicare-Hospital-Quality-Chartbook-2013.pdf. Accessed October 18, 2019.

Mello MM, et al. National costs of the medical liability system. *Health Aff (Millwood).* 2010;29:1569–1577.

Mello MM, et al. The medical liability climate and prospects for reform. *JAMA*. 2014;312:2146–2155.

Mello MM, et al. Medical liability—prospects for federal reform. *N Engl J Med*. 2017;376:1806–1808.

Mendelson A, et al. The effects of pay-for-performance programs on health, health care use, and processes of care: a systematic review. *Ann Intern Med*. 2017;166:341–353.

Minchin M, et al. Quality of care in the United Kingdom after removal of financial incentives. *N Engl J Med*. 2018;379:948–957.

Montori VM, et al. The optimal practice of evidence-based medicine. *JAMA*. 2013;310:2503–2504.

Moore J, et al. Patients' experiences with communication-and-resolution programs after medical injury. *JAMA Intern Med*. 2017;177:1595–1603.

Moraros J, et al. Lean interventions in healthcare: do they actually work? A systematic literature review. *Int J Qual Health Care*. 2016;28:150–165.

Morche J, et al. Relationship between surgeon volume and outcomes. *Syst Rev*. 2016;5:204.

Morgan DJ, et al. Update on medical overuse. *JAMA Intern Med*. 2015;175:120–124.

National Committee for Quality Assurance. The state of health care quality, 2018. NCQA. 2019. https://www.ncqa.org/report-cards/health-plans/state-of-health-care-quality-report/. Accessed October 18, 2019.

Needleman J, et al. Nurse staffing and inpatient hospital mortality. *N Engl J Med*. 2011;364:1037.

NEJM Catalyst. What is lean healthcare? April 27, 2018a.

NEJM Catalyst. What is pay for performance in healthcare? March 1, 2018b.

Owens DK, et al. High-value, cost-conscious health care. *Ann Intern Med*. 2011;154:174–180.

Pham HH, et al. Care patterns in Medicare and their implications for pay for performance. *N Engl J Med*. 2007;356:1130–1139.

Rajkomar A, et al. Machine learning in medicine. *N Engl J Med*. 2019; 380:1347–1358.

Relman AS. *A Second Opinion: Rescuing America's Health Care*. New York, NY: Public Affairs; 2007.

Robinson JC. Blended payment methods in physician organizations under managed care. *JAMA*. 1999;282:1258–1263.

Ryan AM, et al. Medicare's public reporting initiative on hospital quality had modest or no impact on mortality from three key conditions. *Health Aff (Millwood)*. 2012;31:585–592.

Sage WM, Kersh R. *Medical Malpractice and the US Health Care System*. New York, NY: Cambridge University Press; 2006.

Schiff GD, et al. A better-quality alternative. Single-payer national health system reform. *JAMA*. 1994;272:803–808.

Schoen C, et al. US health system performance: a national scorecard. *Health Aff Web Exclusive*. 2006:w457.

Seabury SA, et al. On average, physicians spend nearly 11 percent of their 40-year careers with an open, unresolved malpractice claim. *Health Aff (Millwood)*. 2013;32:111–119.

Shaneyfelt TM, Centor RM. Reassessment of clinical practice guidelines. *JAMA*. 2009;301:868–869.

Shekelle P. Clinical practice guidelines. What's next? *JAMA*. 2018;320:757–758.

Shepherd J. Uncovering the silent victims of the American medical liability system. *Vanderbilt Law Review*. 2013;67:1.

Smith MA, et al. Public reporting helped drive quality improvement in outpatient diabetes care among Wisconsin physician groups. *Health Aff (Millwood)*. 2012;3:570–577.

Smith-Bindman R. Use of advanced imaging tests and the not-so-incidental harms of incidental findings. *JAMA Intern Med*. 2018;178:227–228.

Solberg LI. Improving medical practice: a conceptual framework. *Ann Fam Med*. 2007;5:251–261.

Spivack SB, et al. No permanent fix: MACRA, MIPS, and the politics of physician payment reform. *J Health Politics, Policy and Law*. 2018;43:1025–1040.

Studdert DM, et al. Claims, errors, and compensation payments in medical malpractice litigation. *N Engl J Med*. 2006;354:2024–2033.

Studdert DM, et al. Prevalence and characteristics of physicians prone to malpractice claims. *N Engl J Med*. 2016;374:354–362.

US Department of Health and Human Services. 2017 National Healthcare Quality and Disparities Report. Agency for Healthcare Research and Quality; September 2018. AHRQ Pub. No. 18-0033-EF. https://www.ahrq.gov/research/findings/nhqrdr/nhqdr17/index.html. Accessed October 18, 2019.

US Department of Health and Human Services. The Administration, Cost, and Impact of the Quality Improvement Organization Program for Medicare Beneficiaries for Fiscal Year 2017. 2018. https://www.cms.gov/medicare/quality...patient.../qualityimprovementorgs/index.html. Accessed October 18, 2019.

US Senate. Hearings Bbfore the permanent subcommittee on investigations, Committee on Government Operations, March 13 and 14, 1975. Prepaid health plans. US Government Printing Office; 1975.

Yoon SS, et al. Hypertension prevalence and control among adults: United States, 2011–2014. NCHS Data Brief, no. 220. Hyattsville, MD: National Center for Health Statistics.

2015. https://www.ncbi.nlm.nih.gov/pubmed/26633197. Accessed October 18, 2019.

Yoshihara H, Yoneoka D. National trends in the surgical treatment for lumbar degenerative disc disease. *Spine J.* 2015;15:265–271.

Wachter R. *The Digital Doctor: Hope, Hype, and Harm at the Dawn of Medicine's Digital Age.* New York: McGraw Hill; 2015.

Wachter RM, Pronovost PJ. The 100,000 Lives Campaign: a scientific and policy review. *Jt Comm J Qual Patient Saf.* 2006;32:621–627.

Weeks WB, et al. Higher health care quality and bigger savings found at large multispecialty medical groups. *Health Aff (Millwood).* 2009;29:991–997.

Wilensky GR. Will MACRA improve physician reimbursement? *N Engl J Med.* 2018;378:1269–1271.

Prevention of Illness

WHAT IS PREVENTION?

In 2017, the United States spent $3.5 trillion on health care. Only 2.5% of this total was dedicated to government public health activities designed to prevent illness.

The renowned medical historian Henry Sigerist, writing in 1941, listed the main items that must be included in a national health program. The first three items were free education, including health education, for all; the best possible working and living conditions; and the best possible means of rest and recreation. Medical care rated only fourth on his list (Terris, 1992a). For Sigerist (1941), medical care was this:

A system of health institutions and medical personnel, available to all, responsible for the people's health, ready and able to advise and help them in the maintenance of health and in its restoration when prevention has broken down.

Many people working in the fields of medical care and public health believe that "prevention has broken down" too often because society has dedicated insufficient resources and commitment to prevention. A serious trend has emerged in the United States: after decades of gains, the average life expectancy has been declining since 2015, driven by increases in midlife mortality rates related to such preventable conditions as drug overdose, alcohol-related diseases, suicide, homicide, hypertensive disease, and chronic respiratory illness (Woolf et al., 2018).

Primary prevention seeks to avert the occurrence of a disease or injury (e.g., immunization against polio; taxes on the sale of cigarettes to reduce their affordability, and thereby their use). *Secondary prevention* refers to early detection of a disease process and intervention to reverse or retard the condition from progressing (e.g., Pap smears to screen for premalignant and malignant lesions of the cervix, and mammograms for early detection of breast cancer).

The promotion of good health and the prevention of illness encompass three distinct levels or strategies (Terris, 1986; Table 11–1):

1. The first and broadest level includes measures to address the fundamental social determinants of illness; as evidence presented in Chapter 3 shows, lower income is associated with higher morbidity and mortality rates. Improvement in the standard of living and social equity (e.g., through job creation programs to reduce or eliminate unemployment) may have a greater impact on preventing disease than specific public health programs or medical care services.

2. The second level of prevention involves public health interventions to reduce the incidence of illness in the population as a whole. Examples are water purification systems, the banning of cigarette smoking in the workplace, and public health education on human immunodeficiency virus (HIV) prevention in the schools. These strategies generally consist of primary prevention. The 2.5% figure cited

Table 11–1. Strategies of prevention

Strategy	Examples
1. Improvement in the standard of living	Job creation Increase in minimum wage
2. Public health interventions to reduce the incidence of illness in the population	Water purification systems in underdeveloped nations Increased tobacco taxes to reduce the purchase of cigarettes Mass education on the dangers of high-fat diets
3. Preventive medical care, performed by health care providers	Screening and treatment of hypertension Periodic breast examinations and mammograms Prenatal care

in the opening paragraph represents these public health activities.

3. The third level of prevention involves individual health care providers performing preventive interventions for individual patients; these activities can be either primary or secondary prevention. The US Preventive Services Task Force and other organizations have established regular schedules for preventive medical care services (US Preventive Services Task Force, 2019).

THE FIRST EPIDEMIOLOGIC REVOLUTION

Until modern times, the conditions that produced the greatest amount of illness and death in the population were infectious diseases. The initial decline of infectious disease mortality rates took place even before the cause of these illnesses was understood. In the 18th and 19th centuries, food production increased markedly throughout the Western world. By the early 19th century, infectious disease mortality rates were dropping in England, Wales, and Scandinavia, probably as a result of improved nutrition that allowed individuals, particularly children, to resist infectious agents. Thus, the initial success of illness prevention took place through the improvement of overall living conditions rather than from specific public health or medical interventions (McKeown, 1990).

In the 19th century, scientists and public health practitioners discovered many of the agents causing infectious diseases. By comprehending the causes (such as bacteria and viruses) and the risk factors (e.g., poverty, overcrowding, poor nutrition, and contaminated water) associated with these illnesses, public health measures (such as water purification, sewage disposal, and pasteurization of milk) were implemented that drastically reduced their incidence. This was the first epidemiologic revolution (Terris, 1985).

From 1870 to 1930, the death rate from infectious diseases fell rapidly. Medical interventions, whether immunizations or treatment with antibiotics, were introduced only after much of the decline in infectious disease mortality had taken place. The first effective treatment against tuberculosis, the antibiotic streptomycin, was developed in 1947, but its contribution to the decrease in the tuberculosis death rate since the early 19th century has been estimated to be a mere 3%. For whooping cough, measles, scarlet fever, bronchitis, and pneumonia, mortality rates had fallen to similarly low levels before immunization or antibiotic therapy became available. Pasteurization and water purification were probably the main reason for the decline in infant mortality rates (McKeown, 1990).

Some illnesses are exceptions to the rule that infectious disease mortality is influenced more by improved living standards and public health measures than by medical interventions. Immunization for smallpox, polio, and tetanus and antimicrobial therapy for syphilis had a substantial impact on mortality rates from those illnesses. Considering infectious diseases as a group, however, medical measures probably account for less than 5% of the decrease in mortality rates for these conditions over the past century (McKinlay et al., 1989; McKeown, 1990).

As infectious diseases waned in importance during the first half of the 20th century and as life expectancy increased, rates of noninfectious chronic illness grew rapidly. Eleven infectious diseases accounted for 40% of total deaths in the United States in 1900, but less than 10% in 1980. In contrast, heart disease, cancer, and stroke (cerebrovascular disease) caused 16% of total deaths in 1900 but 64% by 1980 (McKinlay et al., 1989).

THE SECOND EPIDEMIOLOGIC REVOLUTION

Beginning in 1950, epidemiologists began to understand the causes of noninfectious diseases and initiated a second epidemiologic revolution (Terris, 1992b).

Table 11–2. Causes of death in the United States, 2016[a]

Total	2,744,000
Top 10 causes	
Heart disease	635,000
Cancer	598,000
Unintentional injuries (accidents)	161,000
Chronic lower respiratory diseases	155,000
Cerebrovascular disease	142,000
Alzheimer's disease	116,000
Diabetes	80,000
Pneumonia and influenza	52,000
Kidney disease	50,000
Suicide	45,000
Top 3 contributors to mortality (2006)	
Tobacco	480,000
Diet and inactivity	460,000
Alcohol	88,000

[a]Xu J et al. Deaths: Final Data for 2016. National Vital Statistics Reports, July 26, 2018; Centers for Disease Control and Prevention. CDC fast stats. 2014. www.cdc.gov/nchs/fastats.

It was learned that the major illnesses in the United States have a few central causes and are in large part preventable. In 2016, 2.7 million people died in the United States (Table 11–2). A surprisingly small number of risk factors are implicated in 40% of these deaths. It has been estimated that use of tobacco causes 480,000 fatalities, an unhealthful diet and inactivity contributes to 460,000 more, and alcohol is responsible for 88,000 deaths annually in the United States (Centers for Disease Control and Prevention, 2014). By discovering and educating the population about the risk factors of smoking, unhealthful diet, and lack of exercise, the second epidemiologic revolution has already shown success. From 1980 to 2016, age-adjusted mortality rates for coronary heart disease (CHD) declined by an astonishing 73% (Health United States, 2017) (Fig. 11–2). This decline was associated with reduced rates of tobacco use and lowered mean serum cholesterol levels in the population. As with infectious diseases a century earlier, this decline was mostly related to public health interventions regarding smoking and diet. The unfortunate side of this success story is that those in the poorest socioeconomic position and the least education have considerably higher mortality rates than those with higher socioeconomic status (Zheng, 2012).

INDIVIDUAL OR POPULATION?

Chronic disease prevention may be viewed from two distinct perspectives: that of the individual and that of the population (Rose, 1985). The medical model seeks to identify high-risk individuals and offer them individual protection, often by counseling on such topics as smoking cessation and low-fat diet. The public health approach seeks to reduce disease in the population as a whole, using such methods as mass education campaigns to counter drinking and driving, the taxation of tobacco to drive up its price, and the labeling of foods to indicate fat and cholesterol content. Both approaches have merit but the medical model suffers from important drawbacks.

The individual-centered approach of the medical model may target its interventions to the wrong individuals. In the United States, most people with high cholesterol levels remain healthy for years, and some people with low levels have heart attacks at an early age. Why is this so? Because the risk of CHD for persons with high cholesterol levels or low cholesterol levels is not so different. A "low" cholesterol level of 180 mg/dL is low by US standards, but high when compared with levels in poor nations. A large number of people at small risk for a disease may give rise to more cases of the disease than the smaller number of people who are at high risk (Brown et al., 1992). This fact limits the utility of the medical model's "high-risk" approach to prevention. A public health approach (e.g., mass educational campaigns on the health effects of unhealthful diets and the labeling of foods) strives to reduce the mean population cholesterol level. A 10% reduction in the serum cholesterol distribution of the entire population would do more to reduce the incidence of heart disease than a 30% reduction in the cholesterol levels of those relatively few individuals with counts greater than 300 mg/dL.

A coherent ideology underlies the medical model of chronic disease prevention—the concept that in the arena of noninfectious chronic disease, individuals play a major role in causing their own illnesses by such behaviors as smoking, drinking alcohol, and eating high-fat foods. The corollary to this view is that chronic disease mortality rates can be reduced by persuading individuals to change their lifestyles. These statements are true, but they do not tell the whole story.

An alternative ideology, which fits more closely with the public health approach to chronic disease prevention, argues that modern industrial society creates the conditions leading to heart disease, cancer, stroke, and other major chronic diseases of the developed world. Tobacco advertising; processed high-salt foods in "supersized" portions; easy availability of alcoholic beverages; societal stress; an urbanized and suburbanized existence that substitutes automobile travel for exercise; and a markedly unequal distribution of wealth are the substrates upon which the modern epidemic of chronic disease has flourished. Such a worldview leads to an emphasis on societal rather than individual strategies for chronic disease prevention (Fee & Krieger, 1993).

Both the medical and public health models (seeing responsibility as both individual and societal) must be joined to further implement the second epidemiologic revolution; medical caregivers attempt to change high-risk lifestyles of their individual patients, and society searches for ways to reduce the consumption of tobacco, alcohol, and unhealthful foods. One model that bridges the medical and public health approaches is Community-Oriented Primary Care. In this model, primary care clinicians systematically define a target population, determine its health needs, and develop community-based interventions to address these needs (Nutting, 1990). The target population could be the patients enrolled in a primary care practice or an entire neighborhood. For example, a pediatrician might review data on her enrolled patients and find that many children are obese. In addition to counseling individual families in her practice, in the Community Oriented Primary Care model the pediatrician would work with community members and agencies on broader public health interventions, such as advocating for improved school lunch programs and more time for physical education classes in the local schools, or encouraging the local health department to launch a media campaign promoting consumption of water instead of sweetened beverages.

In 2009, Thomas Frieden, then Director of the US Centers for Disease Control and Prevention, proposed a prevention pyramid uniting the public health and medical models (Fig. 11–1). The pyramid emphasizes that improving the population's socioeconomic status and implementing public health measures have the greatest impact on health (Frieden, 2010a).

MODELS OF PREVENTION

To provide examples of different approaches to preventing illness, we have chosen to discuss two serious health problems in the United States: CHD and breast cancer.

▶ Coronary Heart Disease

CHD is associated with several major risk factors including: unhealthy foods, cigarette smoking, and hypertension. Primary prevention strategies are available for CHD because the causes of the disease are well understood. Primary CHD prevention involves risk factor reduction, including cessation of tobacco use; replacement of unhealthy foods with fruits, vegetables, and whole foods; and control of hypertension. These strategies have been largely responsible for the decrease in CHD death rates (Fig. 11–2).

Tobacco Use

Tobacco has been called the smallpox virus of chronic disease—a harmful agent, elimination of which from the planet would benefit humankind (Fee & Krieger, 1993). Since the 1964 release of the first Surgeon General's Report on the Health Consequences of Smoking, the smoking behavior of the US population has changed dramatically. Between 1965 and 2016, the percentage of adult men who were current smokers dropped from 51% to 18%; for adult women, the decline was from 34% to 14 % (Fig. 11–3). These reductions in smoking prevalence avoided an estimated 3 million deaths between 1964 and 2000—a major public health achievement (Warner, 1989). However, rates of smoking are far higher among people with low educational levels and low income, harmful e-cigarette use is increasing (Glantz & Bareham, 2018), and smoking continues to be the leading cause of death in the United States (Health United States, 2017).

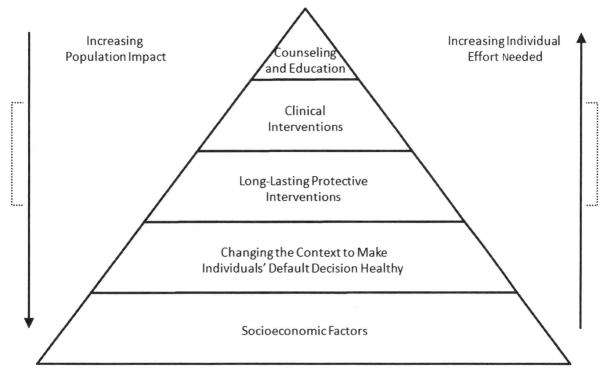

▲ Figure 11–1. The health impact pyramid. (From Frieden TR. A framework for public health action: the health impact pyramid. *Am J Public Health.* 2010;100:590.)

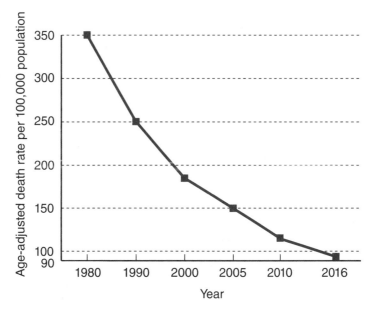

▲ Figure 11–2. Trends in age-adjusted mortality from coronary heart disease in the United States, 1980–2016. (From US Department of Health and Human Services. Health United States, 2017. https://www.cdc.gov/nchs/data/hus/hus17.pdf.)

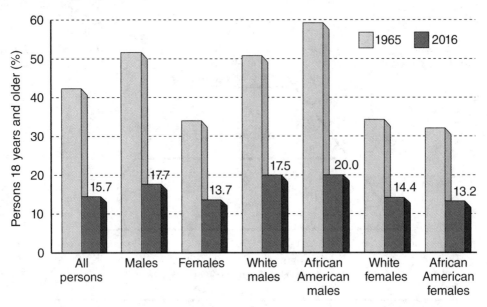

▲ **Figure 11–3.** Cigarette smoking by persons 18 years and older in the United States in 1965 (light red bars) and 2016 (dark red bars). Percentages are age adjusted. (Health United States, 2017.)

Antismoking campaigns have been relatively successful for well-educated people, but less so for people with less education, who also tend to be poorer. Between 1974 and 2012, cigarette smoking declined 40% among the least educated persons, while it dropped 71% among the most educated. In 2016, 26% of the least educated persons smoked cigarettes, compared with only 7% of the most educated (Health United States, 2017).

Since the 1969 ban on radio and television cigarette advertising, the tobacco industry has increased its advertising expenditures dramatically in the print media and through sponsorship of community events. In 2016, tobacco advertising expenditures exceeded $9 billion, with the principal target group young adults (Centers for Disease Control, 2018). The antismoking campaign of the past 30 years has merged the medical and public health models of prevention. Physician counseling can influence smokers to quit. In 2006, however, only 34% of low-income smokers had smoking cessation discussions with their health care provider (Cokkinides et al., 2009). Public health measures are more effective, including public education, cigarette taxes, and restriction of smoking in public places. A 10% increase in the price of cigarettes reduces cigarette

consumption by 3% to 5%. Yet compared with other developed nations, the United States has relatively low taxes on tobacco (Cokkinides et al., 2009; Schroeder & Warner, 2010).

Unhealthy Eating

Dietary patterns in the United States are too low in vegetables, fruit, whole grains, and low-fat dairy, and too high in refined grains, saturated fat, sugars, and sodium. This diet produces CHD in part by causing an increase in low-density lipoprotein cholesterol. Lowering cholesterol levels reduces the risk of heart attacks caused by CHD.

In the late 1980s, a major national campaign was launched by the National Institutes of Health (NIH) to reduce serum cholesterol levels. This National Cholesterol Education Program is based on the medical model, with health care providers screening individuals for elevated cholesterol and aggressively treating hyperlipidemic patients with diet, cholesterol-lowering medications, or both (Grundy et al., 2004).

Public health analysts have criticized the NIH strategy as relying too heavily on a medical model of prevention that is expensive and of potentially limited effectiveness. The NIH approach targeted more than 100 million people who need dietary changes and recommended drug treatment for many of these individuals. The use of statin drugs to treat hyperlipidemia in people with known CHD (secondary prevention) and in some people without CHD (primary prevention) has been shown to reduce deaths from CHD, but the effectiveness of drug treatment is much greater if it is used in secondary rather than primary prevention (Hayward et al., 2010). The traditional orientation of physicians toward individual patients (the medical model) has led the medical profession and the NIH to emphasize identification and treatment of high-risk individuals with elevated cholesterol levels. Pharmaceutical manufacturers also have an interest in promoting a medical model that relies on prescribing medications.

Currently, public health efforts to curb the consumption of unhealthy foods have not had the success of anti-tobacco policy. Sixty-nine percent of adults in the United States were classified as overweight or obese during 2013–2016, compared with 56% in 1988 (Health United States, 2017). The food industry spends billions of dollars on advertising, a substantial portion of which promotes fast foods and sugary drinks. Sugary beverage consumption is associated with increased all-cause mortality (Collin et al., 2019). Proposals have been made to copy the strategy used by tobacco prevention campaigns in reducing the availability of unhealthy foods; for example, taxing sugary drinks, changing school lunch and food stamp programs to increase their healthy content, restricting food advertising directed at children, and eliminating school-based candy and soft-drink vending machines are primary preventive measures that are slowly gaining public acceptance (Frieden et al., 2010b; Basu et al., 2014). The imposition of taxes on sugar-sweetened beverages has been shown to reduce the purchase and consumption of these beverages (Backholer & Baker, 2018). Attention is also being paid to the billions of dollars annually in federal subsidies to agribusinesses for growing corn, which contributes to the flooding of the nation with low-cost, high-fructose corn sweeteners and other high-calorie processed foods. Public health advocates have called for reforms to the federal farm bill to reduce subsidies for obesogenic foods and to provide more support for sustainable farming of healthful fruits and vegetables (Pollan, 2007; Wallinga, 2010).

Hypertension

Nearly half of deaths from cardiovascular disease (heart attacks and strokes) are attributable to high blood pressure (hypertension), which affects one-third of the US adult population. High sodium intake is a major risk factor for developing hypertension and reducing salt intake is effective in reducing blood pressure (Bibbins-Domingo et al., 2010; Coxson et al., 2013).

Most efforts at hypertension control are based on the medical model, treating individuals with medications. Yet, similar to the cholesterol situation, the greatest impact in reducing hypertension-related mortality rates will come from a reduction in the blood pressure of the large number of borderline hypertensives rather than from focusing solely on people with very high blood pressure (Stamler, 1992).

There has been a long-held belief that primary prevention of high blood pressure can be accomplished by a reduction in the daily intake of sodium from the 2015 average level of 3,400 mg per day to the recommended level of 1,500 mg per day. In 2018, this sodium intake goal is being questioned, and salt as a contributor to hypertension may be true only at higher levels of sodium intake. The sodium intake recommendations are likely to change (DiNicolantonio and O'Keefe, 2018).

▶ Breast Cancer

Whereas mortality rates for cardiovascular disease declined since the late 1960s, cancer mortality rates peaked in 1990 before decreasing by 24% between 1990 and 2016, in part due to reductions in cigarette smoking. Breast cancer mortality rates have also decreased during those years, but are 40% higher for African American women than for white women (Health United States, 2017).

The designing of effective primary prevention for a disease generally depends on an understanding of the epidemiology of that disease. In the case of lung cancer, the discovery of the link with cigarette smoking allowed a widespread primary prevention program to be developed. But the causes of many cancers are still unclear, meaning that preventive strategies must use secondary rather than primary prevention. Pap smears for early detection of cervical cancer, fecal occult blood testing and colonoscopy for early detection of colorectal cancer, and mammography for early detection of breast cancer are examples of secondary prevention.

Multiple risk factors for breast cancer have been uncovered, including age greater than 65 years, family history of breast cancer, overweight after menopause, more years of ovulatory menstrual cycles, and taking hormone replacement therapy after menopause (Centers for Disease Control and Prevention, 2018).

However, only one-third of breast cancer cases can be accounted for by known risk factors. The differences between high and low age-adjusted breast cancer risks in the United States are small compared with the huge differences between such high-incidence nations as the United States and low-incidence (generally underdeveloped) nations. Perhaps unknown agents related to modern industrialization are the primary causes of breast cancer, while such influences as female hormones are secondary promoters of the disease.

From the 1940s to the 1980s, industrial production of synthetic organic chemicals rose from 1 billion to 400 billion pounds annually, and the volume of hazardous wastes also increased 400-fold during that period (Epstein, 1990, 1994). In 2010, the President's Cancer Panel reported that "the true burden of environmentally induced cancer has been grossly underestimated." Studies have linked breast cancer risk to organochlorine insecticides, polycyclic aromatic hydrocarbons, and organic solvents, but research on these environmental causes of breast cancer has been inadequate and inconsistent (Rodgers et al., 2018). Until the main causes of breast cancer are known, public health has been forced to retreat to secondary prevention to reduce mortality rates in women with the disease. Periodic mammograms can reduce breast cancer mortality rates in women above 50 years of age. Yet many breast cancer activists decry the paltry sums going for basic epidemiologic research to determine the causes of breast cancer.

▶ Summary

The examples of CHD and breast cancer illustrate different aspects of illness prevention. Primary prevention,

using both public health and medical approaches, has been successful in reducing mortality rates for CHD and lung cancer. Secondary prevention has had some success in reducing breast cancer mortality rates, but the incidence of the disease remains high and primary prevention is badly needed.

DOES PREVENTION REDUCE MEDICAL CARE COSTS?

The influence of prevention on medical care costs is a complex one. As a rule, primary prevention using public health measures is far more cost-effective than prevention through medical care; public health measures do not require millions of expensive one-to-one interactions with medical care providers.

In the arena of individual medical care prevention, some measures save money and some do not. Every dollar invested in measles, mumps, and rubella immunizations saves many more dollars in averted medical care costs. Physician counseling on smoking cessation is a low-cost activity that can reduce the multibillion dollar cost of caring for people with tobacco-related illness. These preventive care activities do reduce health care spending in the long run (Maciosek et al., 2017). In contrast, medical care to reduce cholesterol and high blood pressure are unlikely to result in significant savings to the health care system (US Government Accountability Office, 2014).

Primary prevention through public health action can be enormously effective in reducing the burden of human suffering and the cost of treating disease. From 1900 to 1940, the nation's public health efforts achieved a 97% reduction in the death rate for typhoid fever; 97% for diphtheria; 92% for infectious diarrhea; 91% for measles, scarlet fever, and whooping cough; and 77% for tuberculosis (Winslow, 1944). Higher cigarette taxes reduce the annual cost of tobacco-related disease and premature death, while at the same time yielding billions of dollars per year in tax revenues—an ideal preventive measure that actually earns money (Chaloupka et al., 2019). If the three primary preventive methods known to reduce the incidence of CHD, cancer, and stroke (i.e., reduction in smoking, cholesterol levels, and blood pressure) were intensified, the medical care costs of these illnesses could be dramatically reduced. However, these savings are overstated because money saved by preventing disease X will ultimately be spent on the treatment of disease Y or Z, which will strike those people spared from disease X.

CONCLUSION

The goals of disease prevention are to delay disability and death and to maximize illness-free years of life. Improvements in living standards, public health measures, and preventive medical care have made enormous contributions toward the achievement of these goals. Producing further improvements in the overall health of society will likely require focusing on fundamental social and environmental determinants of health, reducing the growing gap between rich and poor, and shifting a greater proportion of the health dollar to disease prevention.

REFERENCES

Backholer K, Baker P. Sugar-sweetened beverage taxes: the potential for cardiovascular health. *Current Cardiovascular Risk Reports.* 2018;12:28.

Basu S, et al. Ending SNAP subsidies for sugar-sweetened beverages could reduce obesity and type 2 diabetes. *Health Aff (Millwood).* 2014;33:1032–1039.

Bibbins-Domingo K, et al. Projected effect of dietary salt reductions on future cardiovascular disease. *N Engl J Med.* 2010;362:590–599.

Brown EY, et al. Preventive health strategies and the policy makers' paradox. *Ann Intern Med.* 1992;116:593–597.

Centers for Disease Control and Prevention. CDC fast stats. 2014. www.cdc.gov/nchs/fastats. Accessed October 18, 2019.

Centers for Disease Control and Prevention. Tobacco related spending. 2018. https://www.cdc.gov/tobacco/data_statistics/fact_sheets/economics/econ.../index.htm. Accessed October 18, 2019.

Centers for Disease Control and Prevention, 2018. What are the risk factors for breast cancer? September 2018. https://www.cdc.gov/cancer/breast/basic_info/risk_factors.htm. Accessed October 18, 2019.

Chaloupka, et al. The use of excise taxes to reduce tobacco, alcohol, and sugary beverage consumption. *Annu Rev Public Health.* 2019;40:10.1–10.15.

Cokkinides V, et al. Tobacco control in the United States: recent progress and opportunities. *CA Cancer J Clin.* 2009;59:352–365.

Collin LJ, et al. Association of sugary beverage consumption with mortality risk in US adults. *JAMA Network Open.* 2019; May 17.

Coxson PG, et al. Mortality benefits from US population-wide reduction in sodium consumption. *Hypertension.* 2013;61:564–570.

DiNicolantonio JJ, O'Keefe JH. Salt and hypertension: what do we know? *Curr Opin Cardiol.* 2018;33:377–381.

Epstein SS. Losing the war against cancer: who's to blame and what to do about it. *Int J Health Serv.* 1990;20:53–71.

Epstein SS. Environmental and occupational pollutants are avoidable causes of breast cancer. *Int J Health Serv.* 1994;24:145–150.

Fee E, Krieger N. Thinking and rethinking AIDS: implications for health policy. *Int J Health Serv.* 1993;23:323–346.

Frieden TR. A framework for public health action: the health impact pyramid. *Am J Public Health.* 2010a;100:590–595.

Frieden TR, et al. Reducing childhood obesity through policy change. *Health Aff (Millwood).* 2010b;29:357–363.

Glantz SA, Bareham DW. E-cigarettes: use, effects on smoking, risks, and policy implications. *Ann Rev Public Health.* 2018;39:215–235.

Grundy SM, et al. Implications of recent clinical trials for the national cholesterol education program adult treatment panel III guidelines. *Circulation.* 2004;110:227–239.

Health United States, 2017. US Department of Health and Human Services. https://www.cdc.gov/nchs/data/hus/hus17.pdf. Accessed October 18, 2019.

Hayward RA, et al. Optimizing statin treatment for primary prevention of coronary artery disease. *Ann Intern Med.* 2010;152:69–77.

Maciosek MV, et al. Updated priorities among effective clinical preventive services. *Ann Fam Med.* 2017;15:14–22.

McKeown T. Determinants of health. In: Lee PR, Estes CL, eds. *The Nation's Health.* Boston, MA: Jones & Bartlett; 1990.

McKinlay JB, et al. A review of the evidence concerning the impact of medical measures on recent mortality and morbidity in the United States. *Int J Health Serv.* 1989;19:181–208.

Nutting PA, ed. *Community Oriented Primary Care: From Principle to Practice.* Albuquerque, NM: University New Mexico Press; 1990.

Pollan M. You are what you grow. *N Y Times Mag.* April 22, 2007.

President's Cancer Panel. Reducing environmental cancer risk. National Cancer Institute. 2010. https://deainfo.nci.nih.gov/advisory/pcp/annualreports/.../pcp_report_08-09_508.pdf. Accessed October 18, 2019.

Rodgers KM, et al. Environmental chemicals and breast cancer: an updated review of epidemiological literature informed by biologic mechanisms. *Environ Res.* 2018;160:152–182.

Rose G. Sick individuals and sick populations. *Int J Epidemiol*. 1985;14:32–38.

Schroeder SA, Warner KE. Don't forget tobacco. *N Engl J Med*. 2010;363:201–204.

Sigerist HE. *Medicine and Human Welfare*. New Haven, CT: Yale University Press; 1941.

Stamler R. The primary prevention of hypertension and the population blood pressure problem. In: Marmot M, Elliott P, eds. *Coronary Heart Disease Epidemiology*. New York, NY: Oxford University Press; 1992.

Terris M. The changing relationships of epidemiology and society: the Robert Cruikshank lecture. *J Public Health Policy*. 1985;6:15–36.

Terris M. What is health promotion? *J Public Health Policy*. 1986;7:147–151.

Terris M. Concepts of health promotion: dualities in public health theory. *J Public Health Policy*. 1992a;13:267–276.

Terris M. Healthy lifestyles: the perspective of epidemiology. *J Public Health Policy*. 1992b;13:186–194.

US Government Accountability Office, Health Prevention. Cost-effective services in recent peer-reviewed health care literature. 2014. www.gao.gov/products/GAO-14–789R. Accessed October 18, 2019.

US Preventive Services Task Force. *Published Recommentations, March* 2019. www.uspreventiveservicestaskforce.org. Accessed October 18, 2019.

Wallinga D. Agricultural policy and childhood obesity. *Health Aff (Millwood)*. 2010;29:405–410.

Warner KE. Smoking and health: a 25-year perspective. *Am J Public Health*. 1989;79:141–143.

Winslow CEA. Who killed Cock Robin? *Am J Public Health*. 1944;34:658–659.

Woolf SH, et al. Changes in midlife death rates across racial and ethnic groups in the United States: systematic analysis of vital statistics. *BMJ*. 2018;362:k3096.

Zheng H. Do people die from income inequality of a decade ago? *Soc Sci Med*. 2012;75:36–45.

Long-Term Care

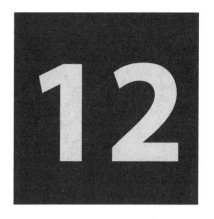

Eddie Taylor awoke one morning at his home in California unable to speak or to move the right side of his body, but able to understand other people around him. After 3 terrifying days in a hospital and 3 frustrating weeks in a stroke rehabilitation center, Eddie failed to improve. Because he no longer required hospital-level care, he became ineligible for Medicare hospital coverage. Since his spouse, James, was wheelchair-bound with crippling rheumatoid arthritis and unable to care for him, Eddie was transferred to a nursing home. Medicare did not cover the $245 per day cost. After 2 years, Medicaid began to pick up the nursing home bills. Much of the couple's life savings—earned during the 50 years Eddie worked in a men's clothing store—had been spent down to allow Medicaid eligibility. Because Medicaid paid only $130 per day, few recreational activities were offered, and Eddie spent each day lying in bed next to a demented patient, who screamed for hours at a time. Unable to voice his complaints at the inhuman conditions of his life, he became severely depressed, stopped eating, and within 3 months was dead.

On high school graduation night, Lyle celebrated with a few drinks and drove to his girlfriend's house. He lost control of the car, hit a tree, and suffered a fractured cervical spine, unable to move his arms or legs. After 9 months in a rehabilitation unit, Lyle remained quadriplegic. He returned home, with a home care agency providing total

24-hour-a-day care at a cost of $300 per day, not covered by insurance. Lyle's father, a businessman, became increasingly angry at his wife, the principal flutist in the city's professional orchestra, because she refused to leave the orchestra to care for Lyle. After 1 year and $110,000 in long-term care expenses, Lyle's parents were close to divorce. One night Lyle's father awoke in a cold sweat; in his dream, he had placed a plastic bag over Lyle's head and suffocated him.

Time and again physicians and other caregivers witness the tragedy of chronic illness compounded by the failure of the nation's health care system to meet the social needs created by the illness. The crisis of long-term care is twofold: Thousands of families each year lose their savings to pay for the chronic illness of a family member, and long-term care often takes place in dehumanizing institutions that rob their occupants of their last remaining vestiges of independence.

Long-term care includes those health, social, housing, transportation, and other supportive services needed by persons with physical, mental, or cognitive limitations sufficient to compromise independent living. The need for long-term care services is usually determined by evaluating a person's impairment of activities of daily living (ADLs; e.g., eating, dressing, bathing, toileting, and getting in or out of bed or a chair) and in instrumental activities of daily living (IADLs; e.g., laundry, housework, meal preparation, grocery shopping, transportation, financial management, taking medications, and telephoning) (Table 12–1).

Table 12–1. Activities requiring assistance in long-term care

Activities of daily living (ADLs) (basic human functions)
Feeding
Dressing
Bathing or showering
Getting to and from the toilet and caring for incontinence
Getting in and out of a bed or chair
Instrumental activities of daily living (IADLs) (activities necessary to remain independent)
Doing housework and laundry
Preparing meals
Shopping for groceries
Using transportation
Managing finances
Making and keeping appointments
Taking medications
Telephoning

Thirteen million people in the United States require assistance with one or more ADLs or IADLs, and can therefore be considered as needing long-term care services (Nguyen, 2017).

Projections of growth for the elderly population in the United States are startling. In 2000, the population 65 years of age and older numbered 35 million; this figure is expected to reach 72 million by the year 2030. The number of people 85 years and older will more than double from 4.2 million in 2000 to 8.7 million in 2030. Those 75 years and older are most likely to need long-term care because 54% have severe disability (U.S. Census Bureau, 2018). As more and more people need long-term care, the answers to two questions become increasingly urgent: How shall the nation finance long-term care? Should most long-term care be delivered through institutions or in people's homes and communities?

WHO PAYS FOR LONG-TERM CARE?

Phoebe McKinnon was in good health until she fell, broke her hip, and suffered a postoperative joint infection. She was placed on complete bed rest with oral antibiotics for 3 months, after which time she would have another surgery. Widowed, Ms. McKinnon lived alone; her only daughter lived 1,500 miles away. Because Ms. McKinnon

required 24-hour-a-day help, the social worker, after carefully researching the financial options, reluctantly suggested that Ms. McKinnon spend the 3 months in a nursing home. Ms. McKinnon and her daughter agreed but were shocked when the social worker explained that the cost would be $220 a day, for a total bill of $19,800.

The United States spent $263.3 billion on long-term care in 2017, including $166.3 billion on nursing home care (Martin et al., 2019). In 2017, the median cost of a 1-year nursing home stay was over $97,000.

In 2014, direct out-of-pocket payments by patients and their families financed 17% of long-term care services in the United States. A common scenario is that of Eddie Taylor: After a portion of their life savings are spent for long-term care, families finally become eligible for Medicaid long-term care coverage. Medicaid paid for 52% of US long-term care expenditures and private insurance paid for 10%. Many people expect the Medicare program to pay for nursing home stays, and like Phoebe McKinnon and her daughter, are surprised and shocked when they find that Medicare will barely assist them. Only 20% of long-term care costs are financed by Medicare (Kaiser Family Foundation, 2016).

What are the precise roles of Medicare, Medicaid, and private insurance in the financing of long-term care services?

▶ Medicare Long-Term Coverage

Glenn Whitehorse developed diabetes-related gangrene of his right leg requiring above-the-knee amputation. He was transferred from the acute care hospital to the hospital's skilled nursing facility, where he received physical therapy services. Because he was generally frail, he was unable to move from bed to chair without assistance. Mr. Whitehorse's physical and occupational therapists felt he might do better at home, where he could receive home physical therapy and nursing care. All these services were covered by Medicare.

Mrs. Whitehorse had Parkinson's disease and was unable to assist her husband in bathing, getting out of bed, and going to the bathroom; she was forced to hire someone to assist with these custodial functions, which were not covered by Medicare. When Mr. Whitehorse no longer showed any potential for improvement, Medicare discontinued coverage of his home health services. The situation became too difficult, and he was placed in a nursing home for custodial care. Medicare did not cover the nursing home costs.

Which services provided in a nursing facility or at home are covered by Medicare? The key distinction is between "skilled care," for which Medicare pays, and "custodial care," which is usually not covered. A related issue is that of post-acute versus chronic care. Medicare usually covers services needed for a few weeks or months after an acute hospitalization but often does not pay for care required by a stable chronic condition.

What are some examples of skilled care versus custodial services? Registered nurses in a hospital nursing facility, nursing home, or home care agency provide a wide variety of services, such as changing the dressing on a wound, taking blood pressures, listening to the heart and lungs to detect heart failure or pneumonia, and providing patient education about diabetes, hypertension, heart failure, and other illnesses. Physical and occupational therapists work with stroke, hip fracture, and other patients to help them reach their maximum potential level of functioning. Speech therapists perform the difficult task of teaching stroke patients with speech deficits how to communicate. These are all skilled services, usually covered by Medicare.

Custodial services involve assistance with ADLs and IADLs rather than treatment or rehabilitative care related to a disease process; these are tasks such as cooking, cleaning house, shopping, or helping a patient to the toilet. These services, sometimes provided by home health aides but more commonly by unpaid family members, are considered unskilled and are often not covered by Medicare.

▶ Medicaid Long-Term Coverage

Juan Robles, who lived alone, suffered from deforming degenerative arthritis and was unable to do anything more active than sitting in a chair. Because Mr. Robles had no skilled care medical needs, Medicare would not provide any assistance. Medicaid and the county welfare agency paid for a homemaker to provide 20 hours of help per week,

but that was not sufficient. Mr. Robles had no choice but to enter a nursing home, because that was the only way he could obtain 24-hour-a-day help paid for by Medicaid.

Medicaid differs from Medicare in paying the costs of nursing home care. For home health care, however, Medicaid generally does not cover 24-hour-a-day custodial services for people unable to care for themselves. The completeness of Medicaid's nursing home coverage, in contrast to the limited nature of Medicaid-financed home health care, forces many low-income disabled people like Juan Robles into nursing homes unless they have families capable of providing 24-hour-a-day custodial care. In order to qualify for Medicaid nursing home coverage, families may be forced to spend their savings down to low levels, although in some states, Medicaid allows spouses of nursing home residents to keep some of their assets.

Medicaid's coverage of home health services has increased as a result of home- and community-based care 1915(c) waivers, initially authorized in 1981. This program, which attempts to prevent nursing home admissions, allows Medicaid recipients to receive more home care services than previously. In 2017, 1.7 million Medicaid recipients benefited from the program (Kaiser Family Foundation, 2017).

▶ Private Long-Term Care Insurance

Sue and Lew MacPherson, both aged 72, were worried about their future. They remembered their cousin, who was turned down for private long-term care insurance because of his high blood pressure and later spent his entire savings on nursing home bills. Hoping to protect their $32,000 in savings, they decided to apply for long-term care insurance before an illness would make them uninsurable. Their insurance agent calculated the cost of two policies at $9,000 per year, or 30% of their $30,000 per year income. At that price, Sue and Lew would spend most of their savings on insurance premiums within a few years. They declined the insurance.

Private insurance plays a minor role in long-term care financing; only 11% of the US population over 65 years has private long-term care insurance.

Experience rating (see Chapter 2), with premiums increasing with age, has had a profound effect on the dynamics of private long-term care insurance. Under experience-rated insurance, the elderly are charged high premiums because they are at considerable risk of requiring long-term care services. In 2015, the average premium for a policy with a $180 daily benefit was $2,159 if purchased at age 45 and $4,496 if bought at age 65 (Johnson, 2016). The major attractive market for long-term care insurers is the younger employed population, but only a tiny fraction of this group is interested in long-term care insurance because the prospects of needing such care are so remote.

People purchasing long-term care insurance may find it to be a poor investment. Private policies generally specify that a policyholder must be dependent in two or three ADLs before receiving benefits. Insurers may deny insurance for people with preexisting conditions. Long-term care policies usually have a deductible (measured in days), and most policies pay a fixed daily fee rather than reimbursing actual charges. A typical policy might provide $150 per day after a 60-day deductible. The 2017 average daily nursing home charge was $265, meaning that $115 per day would be the patient's responsibility. Thus, a year's stay would require out-of-pocket expenditures totaling $50,975 (60 days × $265 = $15,900 plus 305 days × $115 = 35,075) over and above payment of the insurance premium. Policies may limit their coverage to a few years, which places a cap on how much the insurance will pay.

WHO PROVIDES LONG-TERM CARE?

▶ Informal Caregivers

Since her husband died, Mrs. Dora Whitney has lived alone. At age 71, she became forgetful and one day left the gas stove on, causing a fire in the kitchen. Two months later, she was unable to find her way home after going to the store and was found by the police wandering in the streets. Her daughter, Kimberly, brought her to the university hospital, where she was diagnosed with Alzheimer's dementia. After a team conference with her mother's physicians, nurses, occupational therapist, and social worker, Kimberly admitted that her only option was to abandon her career as a teacher to care for her mother. Kimberly refused

to place her mother in a nursing home, and funds were not available to hire the needed 24-hour-a-day help.

Most people needing long-term care services receive them from their family and friends. In 2015, about 44 million people served as unpaid family caregivers, of whom 75% of whom are women (Family Caregiver Alliance, 2016). For men, their wives often provide long-term care, and for women, their daughters are frequently caregivers. A growing number of the elderly do not have family living near enough to them to provide informal care; the absence of an informal caregiver is a common reason for nursing home placement. Informal caregivers provide an average of 24 hours per week of care, and the estimated economic value of their unpaid contribution was approximately $470 billion in 2013 (Family Caregiver Alliance, 2016). In 2007, 37% of family caregivers reported quitting their job or reducing their work hours in order to assist their family members, and 40% to 70% suffer from depression (Family Caregiver Alliance, 2012). Caregiver burden can be intense, especially in caring for family members with dementia (Lloyd et al., 2019). Elderly people with caregivers have shorter hospital stays, fewer readmissions, and lower inpatient expenses, demonstrating that unpaid caregivers create a great deal of value for the health care system (AARP, 2015).

▶ Community-Based and Home Health Services

Ana Dominguez insisted that her daughter Juana accept the Yale scholarship. Though at age 49 Ms. Dominguez was bed and wheelchair bound with multiple sclerosis, she would feel too guilty if Juana remained in San Antonio, TX, just to care for her. But Ms. Dominguez needed someone at home 24 hours a day, a service not covered by Medicare. For $15 a day, Juana was able to hire Vilma, an undocumented teenager from El Salvador, to live at home. Adding Vilma's pay and the cost of her food, Juana figured they would spend $35,000 of their $42,000 in savings by the time she graduated from Yale.

Community-based long-term care is delivered through a variety of programs, such as home care, adult day care, assisted living settings, home-delivered meals, board and care homes, hospice care for the terminally ill, mental health programs, and others. During the 1970s, the independent living movement among disabled people created a strong push away from institutional (hospital and nursing home) care toward community-based and home care that fostered the greatest possible independence. During the 1980s, AIDS activists furthered the development of hospice programs that provide intensive home care services for people with terminal cancer and AIDS. The home is a more therapeutic, comforting environment than the hospital or nursing home.

As a product of the intersection of the popular movement toward home care and the DRG-created incentive to reduce Medicare hospital stays, home health services expanded rapidly after 1980. This, in turn, prompted changes in Medicare payment policies to rein in home care expenditures. After concerns were voiced about excessive cuts in Medicare home care payments, in 2000 Medicare instituted a prospective payment system for home care based on the episode-of-illness model (see Chapter 4). Home care agencies are paid a lump sum (which, like DRG hospital payments varies with the severity of the illness) for 60 days of care.

Health caregivers function in teams to perform home care, including nurses, physical, occupational, speech, and respiratory therapists, social workers, home health aides, case managers, and drivers delivering meals-on-wheels. Yet home care, designed to help fill the once low-tech niche in the health care system that assists the disabled with ADLs and IADLs, has become increasingly specialized. Home care agencies now offer intravenous antibiotic infusions, morphine pumps, indwelling central venous lines, and home renal dialysis, administered by skilled intravenous and wound care nurses, respiratory therapists, and other health care professionals. These developments are a major advance in shifting medical care from hospital to home, but they have not been matched by growth in the paid personal custodial care needed to allow disabled people to remain safely in their homes. Similarly, home hospice care, while providing excellent nursing services for patients with terminal illnesses, does not provide 24-hour coverage for ADL support.

Assisted living, which provides housing with a graded intensity of services depending on the functional capabilities of its residents, has been growing rapidly. However, the average annual cost in 2017 was $45,000, most of which comes from out-of-pocket payments, thereby pricing assisting living out of the reach of low- and moderate-income families.

▶ Nursing Homes

According to Vladeck (1980):

Each morning, more than one and a quarter million Americans awaken in nursing homes. Most of them are very old and very feeble. Most will stay in the nursing home for a long time. For most, it will be the last place they ever live . . . . [Nursing home] residents live out the last of their days in an enclosed society without privacy, dignity, or pleasure, subsisting on minimally palatable diets, multiple sedatives, and large doses of television—eventually dying, one suspects at least partially of boredom.

Often, informal help and formal home health services are unable to provide the care required for severely disabled people. Such people may be placed in nursing homes with 24-hour-a-day care provided by health aides and orderlies under the supervision of nurses. In 2014, 1.4 million people resided in US nursing homes. Sixty-six percent of nursing home residents are women, who more often outlive their spouses (Kaiser Family Foundation, 2014). Frequently, after caring for a sick husband at home, women will themselves fall ill and be placed in a nursing home because no one is left to care for them at home. Sixty-one percent of nursing home residents have moderate or severe cognitive impairment, 35% are incontinent, and 47% have four or five ADL impairments (Kaye et al., 2010; CMS, 2015).

The Omnibus Budget Reconciliation Act of 1987 set standards for nursing home quality and mandated surveys to enforce these standards. Quality problems persist. Using the Centers for Medicare and Medicaid Services (CMS) 5-star rating system with one star being the lowest score, 39% of nursing home residents live in facilities with 1 or 2 stars. On average, for-profit nursing homes have lower star ratings than nonprofits (Boccuti et al., 2015). Commonly cited deficiencies are failure to prevent falls, failure to prevent or treat pressure ulcers, and use of restraints (Werner & Konetzka, 2010).

Compared with non-Hispanic whites, Hispanics requiring nursing home are more likely to be placed in low-quality facilities (Fennell et al., 2010).

Lower-income people are housed in close quarters with several other patients and become dependent on an underpaid, inadequately trained staff. Hour after hour may be spent lying in bed or sitting in a chair in front of a TV. While quality of life varies between one nursing home and another, placement in a nursing home almost always thwarts the human yearning for some degree of independence of action and for companionship. A sense of futility overwhelms many nursing home residents, and the desire to live often wanes (Vladeck, 1980).

To keep down costs, most care in nursing homes is provided by nurse's aides, who are paid little, receive minimal training, are inadequately supervised, and are required to care for more residents than they can properly serve. The job of the nursing home aide is difficult, involving bathing, feeding, walking residents, cleaning them when they are incontinent, lifting them, and hearing their complaints. In 2015, 70% of all nursing homes were under for-profit ownership, many operated by large corporate chains. For-profit ownership has been associated with lower staffing levels and poorer quality of care compared with nonprofit ownership (Boccuti et al., 2015).

Offering a humane existence to severely disabled people housed together in close quarters is a nearly impossible task. One view of nursing home reform holds that only the abolition of most nursing homes and the development of adequately financed home and community-based care can solve the nursing home problem.

IMPROVING LONG-TERM CARE

▶ Financing Long-Term Care

Boomer was mad. As a self-employed person, his family's health insurance coverage was costing $800 each month, in addition to his out-of-pocket dental bills. To make matters worse, a big chunk of his social security payments went to Medicare each year, not to mention federal and state income taxes and sales taxes going to finance Medicare and Medicaid, so that other people could get health care. While spending all this money, Boomer was healthy and had not seen a physician for 6 years.

One day Boomer's father, Abraham, suffered a devastating stroke. After weeks in the hospital, largely paid for by Medicare, Abraham was transferred to a nursing home. Because Medicare does not cover most long-term care, Boomer's mother paid the bills out of her savings until most of the money ran out. Abraham then became eligible for Medicaid, which took care of the nursing home bills. After Abraham's illness, Boomer stopped complaining about his social security and tax payments going to medical care. Even though Boomer was paying more than he was receiving, Abraham was receiving far more than he was paying. Boomer was grateful for the care his father received and figured that he might be in Abraham's shoes someday.

In the early 1960s, it was recognized that private insurance was unable to solve the problem of health care financing for people older than 65. The costs of health care for the elderly were too great, making experience-rated health insurance premiums unaffordable for most elderly people. Accordingly, Medicare, a social insurance program, was passed (see Chapter 2). An identical problem confronts long-term care financing: As shown earlier in this chapter, most people who might wish to purchase long-term care insurance are unable to afford an adequate policy. Table 12–2 lists some proposals for improving long-term care.

The Pepper Commission (1990) recommended that the nation institute a social insurance program to finance long-term care. This program, like Medicare Part A, could be financed by an increase in the rate of social security contributions by employers and employees. It would pay for caregivers to provide those services not currently covered by Medicare, especially in-home help in feeding, dressing, bathing, toileting, housework, grocery shopping, transportation, and other assistance with ADLs and IADLs. A similar

Table 12–2. Proposals for improving long-term care

Developing social insurance to finance long-term care
Shifting from nursing home care to home and community-based care
Training and paying for family members as caregivers
Expanding the number of comprehensive long-term care organizations modeled on On Lok Senior Health Services

proposal was offered by Physicians for a National Health Program (Harrington et al., 1991).

▶ Providing Long-Term Care

Mei Soon Wang was desperate to go home. Since a brain tumor had paralyzed her left side and left her incontinent, she had been confined to a nursing home because she had no family in San Francisco to care for her. Her daughter, visiting from Portland, heard of On Lok Senior Health Services, which cared for the frail elderly in their homes. On Lok accepted Ms. Wang, placed her in adult day care, arranged for meals to be delivered to her home, and paid for part-time help on evenings and weekends.

Because a reasonable quality of life and personal independence, within the confines of a patient's illness, are so difficult to achieve in the nursing home environment, long-term care reformers advocate that most long-term care be provided at home. The first step toward deinstitutionalizing long-term care is a financing mechanism that pays for more comprehensive community-based and home long-term care services.

The ideal long-term caregivers are the patient's family and friends; thus, it can be argued that long-term care reform should support, assist, and pay informal caregivers, not replace them. Teams of nurses, physical and occupational therapists, physicians, social workers, and attendants can train and work with informal caregivers, and personnel can be available to provide respite care so informal caregivers can have some relief from the 24-hours-a-day, 7-days-a-week burden. If informal caregivers are not available, all possible efforts can still be made to deliver long-term care in people's homes rather than in nursing homes (Harrington et al., 1991).

An innovative long-term care program that has achieved great success has been the On Lok program in San Francisco. Translated from Chinese, On Lok means peaceful, happy abode. Begun in 1971 in San Francisco's Chinatown, On Lok merges adult day services, in-home care, home-delivered meals, housing assistance, comprehensive medical care, respite care for caregivers, hospital care, and skilled nursing care into one program. Persons eligible for On Lok have chronic illness sufficiently severe to qualify them for nursing home placement, but few spend time in a nursing home. Services for each participant are organized by a multidisciplinary team, including physicians, nurses, social workers, rehabilitation and recreation therapists, and nutritionists.

In 1983, On Lok became the first organization in the United States to assume full financial risk for the care of a frail elderly population, receiving monthly capitation payments from Medicare and Medicaid to cover all services. Whereas 45% of US personal health care expenditures go to hospital and nursing home services, On Lok spent a mere 17% on these items, making 83% of the health care dollar available for ambulatory home- and community-based services (Bodenheimer, 1999). Over 120 On Lok "look alikes" now exist in 31 states under the Program of All-Inclusive Care for the Elderly (PACE). However, PACE sites care for only 49,000 of the 3 million frail elderly and disabled people in the United States. Overall, PACE programs have reduced nursing home use compared to a similar non-PACE population, but Medicare and Medicaid costs appear to be somewhat higher for PACE participants (Ghosh et al., 2015).

The United States has not implemented a social insurance program for long-term care. In contrast, most major industrialized nations have adopted successful long-term care social insurance programs (Gleckman, 2010). A major expansion of the PACE concept combined with comprehensive social insurance for long-term care could provide a badly needed solution to the problems of long-term care in the United States.

REFERENCES

AARP. Valuing the Invaluable: 2015 update. AARP Public Policy Institute. July 2015. https://www.aarp.org/content/dam/aarp/ppi/2015/valuing-the-invaluable-2015-update-new.pdf. Accessed October 19, 2019.

Bodenheimer T. Long-term care for frail elderly people—the On Lok model. *N Engl J Med*. 1999;341:1324–1328.

Boccuti C, et al. Reading the stars: nursing home quality star ratings, nationally and by state. Kaiser Family Foundation Issue Brief, May 14, 2015.

CMS. Nursing Home Data Compendium 2015 Edition. Center for Medicare and Medicaid Services. 2015. https://www.cms.gov/Medicare/Provider.../nursing-homedatacompendium_508-2015.pdf. Accessed October 19, 2019.

Family Caregiver Alliance. Caregiver statistics. 2016. https://www.caregiver.org/caregiver-statistics-demographics. Accessed October 19, 2019.

Fennell ML, et al. Elderly Hispanics more likely to reside in poor quality nursing homes. *Health Aff (Millwood)*. 2010;29:65–73.

Ghosh A, et al. Effect of PACE on costs, nursing home admissions, and mortality 2006–2011). U.S. Department of Health and Human Services, March 2015. https://aspe.hhs.gov/report/effect-pace-costs-nursing-home-admissions-and-mortality-2006-2011. Accessed October 19, 2019.

Gleckman H. Long-term care financing reform: lessons from the US and abroad. The Commonwealth Fund. February 2010. https://www.commonwealthfund.org/publications/fund-reports/2010/feb/long-term-care-financing-reform-lessons-us-and-abroad. Accessed October 19, 2019.

Harrington C, et al. A national long-term care program for the United States: a caring vision. *JAMA*. 1991;266:3023–3029.

Johnson RW. Who is covered by private long-term care insurance? Urban Institute, August 2016. https://www.urban.org/research/.../who-covered-private-long-term-care-insurance. Accessed October 19, 2019.

Kaiser Family Foundation. Distribution of nursing home residents by gender. 2014. www.kff.org/other/state.../distribution-of-nursing-facility-residents-by-gender/. Accessed October 19, 2019.

Kaiser Family Foundation. Streamlining Medicaid Home and Community-Based Services. March 11, 2016. https://www.kff.org/medicaid/issue-brief/streamlining-medicaid-home-and-community-based-services-key-policy-questions/. Accessed October 19, 2019.

Kaiser Family Foundation. Medicaid Section 1915(c) Home and Community-Based Services Waivers Participants, by Type of Waiver. 2017. www.kff.org/health-reform/state-indicator/participants-by-hcbs-waiver-type/. Accessed October 19, 2019.

Kaye HS, et al. Long-term care: who gets it, who provides it, who pays, and how much? *Health Aff (Millwood)*. 2010;29:11–21.

Lloyd J, et al. Self-compassion, coping strategies, and caregiver burden in caregivers of people with dementia. *Clin Gerontol*. 2019;42:47–59.

Martin AB, et al. National health care spending in 2017. *Health Aff (Millwood)*. 2019;38:96–106.

Nguyen V. Long-term support and services. AARP Public Policy Institute, March 2017. https://www.aarp.org/content/dam/aarp/ppi/2017-01/Fact%20Sheet%20Long-Term%20Support%20and%20Services.pdf. Accessed October 19, 2019.

Pepper Commission. *A Call for Action*. Washington, DC: US Government Printing Office; 1990.

U.S. Census Bureau. Americans with disabilities: 2014. November 2018. https://www.census.gov/library/publications/2018/demo/p70-152.html. Accessed October 19, 2019.

Vladeck BC. *Unloving Care: The Nursing Home Tragedy*. New York, NY: Basic Books; 1980.

Werner RM, Konetzka RT. Advancing nursing home quality through quality improvement itself. *Health Aff (Millwood)*. 2010;29:81–86.

Medical Ethics and Rationing of Health Care

For those who work in the healing professions, ethical values play a special role. The specific content of medical ethics was first formulated centuries ago, based on the sayings of Hippocrates and others. The refinement of medical ethics has continued up to the present by practicing health caregivers, health professional and religious organizations, and individual ethicists. As medical technology, health care financing, and the organization of health care transform themselves, so must the content of medical ethics change in order to acknowledge and guide new circumstances.

FOUR PRINCIPLES OF MEDICAL ETHICS

Over the years, participants in and observers of medical care have distilled widely shared human beliefs about healing the sick into four major ethical principles: beneficence, nonmaleficence, autonomy, and justice (Beauchamp & Childress, 2013) (Table 13–1).

Beneficence is the obligation of health care providers to help people in need.

Dr. Rolando Bueno is a hard-working family physician practicing in a low-income neighborhood of a large city. He shows concern for his patients, and his knowledge and judgment are respected by his medical and nursing colleagues. On one occasion, he was called before the hospital quality assurance committee when one of his patients unexpectedly died; he agreed that he had made mistakes in his care and incorporated the lessons of the case into his future practice.

Dr. Bueno tries to live up to the ideal of beneficence. He does not always succeed; like all physicians, he sometimes makes clinical errors. Overall, he treats his patients to the best of his ability. The principle of beneficence in the healing professions is the obligation to care for patients to the best of one's ability.

Nonmaleficence is the duty of health care providers to do no harm.

Mrs. Lucy Knight suffers from insomnia and Parkinson's disease. The insomnia does not bother her, because she likes to read at night, but it irritates her husband. Mr. Knight requests his wife's physician to order strong sleeping pills for her, but the physician declines, saying that the combination of sleeping pills and Parkinson's disease places Mrs. Knight at high risk for a serious fall.

The modern array of medical interventions has the capacity to do good or harm or both, thereby enmeshing the principle of nonmaleficence with the principle of beneficence. In the case of Mrs. Knight, the prescribing of sedatives has more potential for harm than for good, particularly because Mrs. Knight does not see her insomnia as a problem.

Autonomy is the right of a person to choose and follow his or her own plan of life and action.

Mr. Winter is a frail 88-year-old found by Dr. James Choice, his family physician, to have colon cancer, which has spread to the liver. The cancer is causing no symptoms. An oncologist gives Mr. Winter the option of transfusions, parenteral

Table 13–1. The four principles of medical ethics

Beneficence	The obligation of health care providers to help people in need
Nonmaleficence	The duty of health care providers to do no harm
Autonomy	The right of patients to make choices regarding their health care
Justice	The concept of treating everyone in a fair manner

nutrition, and surgery, followed by chemotherapy; or watchful waiting with palliative and hospice care when symptoms appear. Mr. Winter is terrified of hospitals and prefers to remain at home. He feels that he might live a comfortable couple of years before the cancer claims his life. After talking it over with Dr. Choice, he chooses the second option.

The principle of autonomy adds another consideration to the interrelated principles of beneficence and nonmaleficence. Would Mr. Winter enjoy a longer life by submitting himself to aggressive cancer therapy that does harm in order to do good? Or, does he sense that the harm may exceed the good? The balance of risks and benefits confronts each physician on a daily basis (Eddy, 1990). But the decision cannot be made solely by a risk–benefit analysis; the patient's preference is a critical addition to the equation.

Autonomy is founded in the overall desire of most human beings to control their own destiny, to have choices in life, and to live in a society that places value on individual freedom. In medical ethics, autonomy refers to the right of competent adult patients to consent to or refuse treatment. While the physician has an obligation to respect the patient's wishes, he or she also has a duty to fully inform the patient of the probable consequences of those wishes. For children and adults unable to make medical decisions, a parent, guardian, other family member, or surrogate decision maker named in a legal document becomes the autonomous agent on behalf of the patient.

Justice refers to the ethical concept of treating everyone in a fair manner.

Joe, a white businessman in the suburbs, suffers crushing chest pain and within 5 minutes is taken to a nearby private emergency department, where he receives immediate coronary stenting and state-of-the-art treatment for a heart attack. Five miles away, in a poor neighborhood, Josephine, an African-American woman, experiences severe chest pain, calls 911, waits 25 minutes for help to arrive, and is brought to a public hospital whose emergency department staff is attending to five other acutely ill patients. Before receiving appropriate attention, she suffers an arrhythmia and dies.

The principle of justice as applied to medical ethics is newer, more controversial, and harder to define than the principles of beneficence, nonmaleficence, and autonomy. In a general sense, people are treated justly when they receive what they deserve. It is unjust not to grant a medical degree to someone who completes medical school and passes all the necessary examinations. It is unjust to punish a person who did not commit a crime. In another meaning, justice refers to universal rights: to receive enough to eat, to be afforded shelter, to have access to basic medical care and education, and to be able to speak freely. If these rights are denied, justice has been violated. In yet another version, justice connotes equal opportunity: All people should have an equal chance to realize their human potential. Justice might be linked to the golden rule: Treat others as you would want others to treat you. While there is no clear agreement on the precise meaning of justice, most people would agree that the differential treatment of Joe and Josephine is unjust.

▶ Distributive Justice

In exploring the concept of justice, one area of concern is the allocation of benefits and burdens in society. This realm of ethical thinking is called *distributive justice*, involving such questions as: Who receives what amount of wealth, of education, or of medical care? Who pays what amount of taxes?

The principle of justice is linked to the idea of fairness. In the arena of distributive justice, no agreement exists on what formula for allocating benefits and costs is fair. Should each person get an equal share? Should those who work harder receive more? Should the proper formula be "to each according to ability to pay," as determined by a free market? Or "to each according to need?" In allocating costs, should each person pay an equal share or should those with greater wealth pay more? Most societies construct a mixture of these allocation formulas. Unemployment benefits consider effort (having had a job) and need (having lost the job). Welfare benefits are primarily based on need. Job promotions may be based on merit. Many goods are distributed according to ability to pay. Primary education in theory (but not always in practice) is founded on the belief that everyone should receive an equal share (Beauchamp & Childress, 2013; Jonsen et al., 2010).

How is the principle of distributive justice formulated for medical care? The concept that health care is a privilege, allocated according to ability to pay, has long competed with the idea that health care is a right and should be distributed according to need. In most developed nations, the allocation of health care according to need has become the dominant political belief, as demonstrated by the passage of universal or near-universal health insurance laws. In the United States, the failure of the 100-year battle to enact national health insurance, and the widely divergent public opinions on the 2010 Affordable Care Act, attest to the ongoing debate between health care as a privilege and health care as a right (see Chapter 15).

If the overwhelming opinion in the developed world holds that health care should be allocated according to need, then all people should have equal access to a reasonable level of medical care without financial barriers (i.e., people should have a right to health care). In this chapter, we consider that the principle of distributive justice requires all people to equally receive a reasonable level of medical services based on medical need without regard to ability to pay.

ETHICAL DILEMMAS, OLD AND NEW

Ethical dilemmas (Lo, 2013) are situations in which a provider of medical care is forced to make a decision that violates one of the four principles of medical ethics in order to adhere to another of the principles. Financial conflicts of interest on the part of physicians (see Chapters 4 and 10), in contrast, pit ethical behavior against individual gain and are not ethical dilemmas.

Anthony, a 22-year-old Jehovah's Witness, is admitted to the intensive care unit for gastrointestinal

bleeding. His blood pressure is 80/60 mm Hg, and in the past 4 hours, his hematocrit has fallen from 38% to 21%. The medical resident implores Anthony to accept lifesaving transfusions, but he refuses, saying that his religion teaches him that death is preferable to receiving blood products. When the blood pressure reaches 60/20 mm Hg, the desperate resident decides to give the blood while Anthony is unconscious. The attending physician vetoes the plan, saying that the patient has the right to refuse treatment, even if an avoidable death is the outcome.

In Anthony's case, the ethical dilemma is a conflict between beneficence and autonomy. Which principle has priority depends on the particular situation, and in this case, autonomy supersedes beneficence. If the patient were a child without sufficient knowledge or reasoning capability to make an informed choice, the physician would not be obligated to withhold transfusions, even if the family so demanded (Jonsen et al., 2010).

Pedro Navarro has lung cancer that has metastasized to his brain. No effective treatment is available, and Mr. Navarro is confused and unable to understand his medical condition. Ms. Navarro demands that her husband undergo craniotomy to remove the tumor. The neurosurgeon refuses, arguing that the operation will do Mr. Navarro no good whatsoever and will cause him additional suffering.

The case of Mr. Navarro pits the principle of autonomy against the principle of nonmaleficence. Mr. Navarro's rightful surrogate decision maker, his wife, wants a particular course of treatment, but the neurosurgeon knows that this treatment will cause Mr. Navarro considerable harm and do him no good. In this case, nonmaleficence triumphs. Whereas patient autonomy allows the right to refuse treatment, it does not include the right to demand a harmful or ineffectual treatment.

Prominent ethical dilemmas often feature beneficence or nonmaleficence in conflict with autonomy. In two famous ethical dilemmas, the families of Karen Ann Quinlan and Nancy Cruzan, young women with severe brain damage (persistent vegetative state) asked that physicians discontinue a respirator (in the Quinlan case) and a feeding tube (in the Cruzan case). Both cases were adjudicated in the courts. The Quinlan decision promoted the right of patients or their surrogate decision makers to withdraw treatment, even if the treatment is necessary to sustain life. The outcome of the Cruzan case placed limits on autonomy by requiring that life-supporting treatment can be withdrawn only when a patient has stated his or her wishes clearly in advance (Annas, 2005).

In 2005, the case of Terri Schiavo, for 15 years in a persistent vegetative state similar to the situations of Karen Ann Quinlan and Nancy Cruzan, made national headlines. In spite of multiple decisions of state and federal courts—up to the Supreme Courts of Florida and the United States—supporting the right of Terri Schiavo's husband to discontinue Ms. Schiavo's feeding tube, the US Congress, encouraged by President George Bush, passed legislation reopening the option of reinserting the feeding tube. Eventually, based on the precedents of the Quinlan and Cruzan cases, the courts prevailed and Ms. Schiavo died (Annas, 2005).

Overall, medical ethics has moved in the direction of giving priority to the principle of autonomy over that of beneficence.

In the late 20th century, a new generation of ethical dilemmas emerged, moving beyond the individual physician–patient relationship to involve the broader society. These social–ethical problems derive from the new reality that money may not be available to pay for a reasonable level of medical services for all people. When money and resources are bountiful, the issue of distributive justice refers to equality in medical care access and health outcomes (see Chapter 3). Is it fair that some people are unable to receive needed care because they lack money and insurance? When money and resources become scarce, the issue of justice takes on a new twist. Should limits be set on treatments given to people with high-cost medical needs, so that other people can receive basic services? If not, might health care consume so many resources that other social needs are sacrificed? If limits should be set, who decides these limits?

Angela and Amy Lakeberg [actual names] were Siamese twins sharing one heart. Without surgery, they would die shortly. With surgery, Amy

would die and Angela's chance of survival would be less than 1%. On August 20, 1993, a team of 18 physicians and nurses at Children's Hospital of Philadelphia performed an all-day operation to separate the twins. Amy died. The cost of the treatment was $1 million. The Medicaid program covered $700 to $1,000 per day, and the hospital underwrote the balance of the costs. On June 9, 1994, Angela died; she had spent her brief life on a respirator in the hospital.

The new fiscal reality has spawned two related dilemmas.

1. The first involves a conflict between the duty of the physician to follow the principles of beneficence and nonmaleficence and the growing sentiment that physicians should pay attention to issues of distributive justice. In the case of the Lakeberg twins, the hospital and surgeons adhered strictly to the principle of beneficence: Even a remote chance of aiding one twin was seen as worthwhile. The hospital could have balked, arguing that its funding of the surgery would be unfairly shifted to other payers. The surgeons could have declined to operate on the grounds that the money spent on the Lakebergs could have been better used by patients with a greater chance of survival. But, the surgeons could argue, who can guarantee that the money saved would have gone to better use?

2. The second category of social–ethical dilemma is the conflict between the individual patient's right to autonomy and society's claim to distributive justice. In the Lakeberg case, individual autonomy won out. The Lakeberg parents could have decided that spending $1 million of society's money on a less than 1% chance of saving one of two infants was excessive and could indirectly harm other patients.

Health professionals have a duty to help and not harm their patients. Individuals claim a right to health care and do not want others to restrict that care. Yet the principle of distributive justice (recognizing that resources for health care are limited and should be fairly allocated among the entire population) might lead to physicians denying legitimate services or patients setting aside rightful claims to treatment.

The basis for the principle of justice is the desire shared by many human beings to live in a civilized society. To live in a state of harmony, each person must balance the concerns of the individual with the needs of the larger community. There is no right or wrong answer to the question of whether the Lakeberg surgery should have been done, but the surgery must be seen as a choice. The $1 million spent on the twins might have been spent on immunizing 10,000 children, with greater overall benefit. When health resources are scarce, the principle of justice creates ethical dilemmas that touch many people beyond those involved in an individual physician–patient relationship. The imperatives of cost control have thrust the principle of justice to the forefront of health policy in the debate over rationing.

WHAT IS RATIONING?

Dr. Everett Wall works for a medical group that participates in an Accountable Care Organization (ACO). Betty Ailes came to him with a headache and wanted a magnetic resonance imaging (MRI) scan. After a complete history and physical examination, Dr. Wall prescribed medication and denied the scan. Ms. Ailes wrote to the medical director, complaining that Dr. Wall was rationing services to her.

Perry Hiler arrives at Vacant Hospital with fever and severe cough. His chest x-ray shows an infiltrate near the hilum of the lung consistent with pneumonia or tumor. Since Mr. Hiler has no insurance, the emergency department physician sends him to the county hospital. At the time, Vacant Hospital has 35 empty beds and plenty of staff. When he recovers, Mr. Hiler calls the newspaper to complain. The next day, a headline appears: "Vacant Hospital Rations Care."

Jim Delacour is a 50-year-old man with terminal cardiomyopathy. His physician sends him to a transplant center, where an evaluation concludes that he is an ideal candidate for a heart transplant. Because the number of transplant candidates is larger than the supply of donor hearts available, Mr. Delacour is placed on the waiting list. After waiting 6 weeks, he dies.

When the emergency department called, Dr. Marco Intensivo's heart sank. The eight-bed intensive care unit is filled with extremely ill patients, all capable of full recovery if they survive their acute illnesses. He has worried all day about another patient needing intensive care: a 55-year-old with a heart attack complicated by unstable arrhythmias. Which one of the nine needy cases will not get intensive care? Dr. Intensivo needs to make a decision, and fast.

The general public and the media often view rationing as a limitation of medical care such that "not all care expected to be beneficial is provided to all patients" (Aaron & Schwartz, 1984). Such a view only partially explains the concept of rationing. More precisely, rationing means a conscious policy of equitably distributing needed resources that are in limited supply (Reagan, 1988) (Table 13–2). Under this definition, only the last two cases presented above can be considered rationing. In the first case, Dr. Wall did not feel that the MRI was a resource needed by Betty Ailes. In the second, Vacant Hospital's refusal to care for Perry Hiler was simply a decision on the part of a private institution to place its financial well-being above a patient's health; there was no scarcity of health care resources. In the heart transplant and intensive care unit cases, in contrast, donor hearts and intensive care unit beds were in fact scarce. For Mr. Delacour, the scarcity was nationwide and prolonged; for Dr. Intensivo, the scarcity was within a particular hospital at a particular time. In both cases, decisions had to be made regarding the allocation of those resources.

During World War II, insufficient gasoline was available to both power the military machine and satisfy the demands of automobile owners in the United

Table 13–2. Two definitions of rationing

Popular usage of the term "rationing":
A limitation of medical care such that not all care expected to be beneficial is provided to all patients.
Precise usage of the term "rationing":
The limitation of resources, including money, going to medical care such that not all care expected to be beneficial is provided to all patients; and the distribution of these limited resources in a fair manner.

States. The government rationed gasoline, giving priority to the military, yet allowing each civilian to obtain a limited amount of fuel. In a rural area, there may be a shortage of health care providers; in an overcrowded urban public hospital, there may be an insufficient number of beds; in the transplant arena, donor organs are truly in short supply. These are cases of commodity scarcity, wherein specific items are in limited supply.

The United States is a nation with an adequate supply of hospital beds and physicians in most communities; commodity scarcity in health care is the exception (e.g., scarcity of primary care resources is a reality). But a different kind of health resource is becoming scarce, and that is money. Those who pay the bills are insistent that the flow of money into the health sector be restricted. Most discussions of health care rationing presume fiscal scarcity, not commodity scarcity.

In summary, rationing in medical care means the limitation of resources, including money, going to health care such that not all care expected to be beneficial is provided to all patients, and the fair distribution of these limited resources.

COMMODITY SCARCITY

While fiscal scarcity is the more common form of resource limitation, commodity scarcity provides an instructive example of the interaction of ethics and rationing. Resources may be scarce throughout an entire nation or within a small hospital. *Macroallocation* refers to the amount and distribution of resources within an entire society or among large populations, whereas *microallocation* refers to resource constraints at the level of an individual physician or institution.

▶ Macroallocation and Rationing at the System Level: Organ Transplants

Mr. George Elder is a 76-year-old nonsmoking retired business executive with end-stage heart failure. He has good pulmonary and renal function and is not diabetic; thus, he is medically a good candidate for a heart transplant. His life expectancy without a transplant is 1 month. He has a loving family, with the resources to pay the $300,000 cost of the procedure.

Mr. Matt Younger is a 46-year-old divorced man who is unemployed, having lost his job as an auto worker 3 years ago. He has a history of smoking and alcohol use. He suffers a heart attack, develops intractable heart failure, and will die within 1 month without a heart transplant. He has good pulmonary and renal function and is not diabetic, making him a good candidate for the procedure.

Mr. Elder and Mr. Younger are in the same hospital and cared for by the same cardiologist, who applied for donor hearts on behalf of both patients on the same day. The cardiologist receives a call that one donor heart—histocompatible with both patients—has become available. Who should receive it?

In 1951, the first kidney transplant was performed in Massachusetts. But it was in 1967, when Dr. Christiaan Barnard sewed a living heart into the chest of a person suffering end-stage cardiac disease, that modern medicine fully entered the age of transplantation. Since that time, many patients have dramatically benefited from transplantation of the kidneys, hearts, lungs, and livers of their fellow human beings. In 2018, 21,000 kidney, 3,400 heart, 8,200 liver, and 2,500 lung transplants were performed in the United States. Transplants are truly lifesaving in most cases. Seventy to eighty percent of patients receiving heart, liver, or kidney transplants survive at least 5 years after transplantation.

Transplantation of organs is both a medical miracle and an ethical watershed. It has generated debate on such questions as these: When are people really dead (so that their organs can be harvested for use in transplantation)? What is the responsibility of the families of brain-dead people to allow their organs to be harvested? Who pays and who is paid for organ transplants? Who should receive organs that are in short supply? We will focus only on the last of these issues.

The number of persons on the national waiting list for organ transplants rose from 16,000 in 1988 to 114,000 in 2019. The number of organs that could be harvested each year falls far short of the number needed. On average in 2017, 18 patients in the United States died each day awaiting organs.

Transplantation presents a classic case of commodity scarcity: there is insufficient supply to meet demand.

Explicit rationing, which is a system that determines who gets organs and who does not, is inevitable. Given the supply and demand imbalance, which potential transplant patients actually receive new organs? In the early 1980s, the major heart transplant center at Stanford University excluded people with "a history of alcoholism, job instability, antisocial behavior, or psychiatric illness," and required transplant recipients to enjoy "a stable, rewarding family and/or vocational environment." Stanford's recipients had a better than 50% chance of surviving 5 years, signifying that acceptance or rejection from the program was a matter of life and death. The US Department of Health and Human Services was concerned about Stanford's selection criteria, which favored those middle-class or wealthy people with satisfying jobs. Moreover, the $100,000 cost restricted heart transplants to those with insurance coverage or ability to pay out of pocket. Both the social and economic criteria for access to this lifesaving surgery raised serious issues of distributive justice.

Following the passage of the National Organ Transplantation Act of 1984, the federal government designated the United Network for Organ Sharing (UNOS) as a national system for matching donated organs and potential recipients (www.unos.org). According to the Task Force on Organ Transplantation (1986), organ allocation should be governed by medical criteria, with the major factors being urgency of need and probability of success. The Task Force recommended that if two or more patients are equally good candidates for an organ according to the medical criteria, length of time on the waiting list is the fairest way to make the final selection. Overall, UNOS follows these recommendations, placing potential recipients of organ transplants on its computerized waiting list. Recipients are prioritized according to a point scale based on severity of illness, time on the waiting list, and probability of a successful outcome. A serious attempt has been made to allocate scarce organs on the basis of justice criteria. But haunting the ethics of the prioritization process is the issue of ability to pay. In 2017, the average kidney transplant cost $260,000 and heart transplant $998,000. Persons needing a transplant are often rejected if they lack health insurance coverage (Ansell et al., 2014).

▶ Microallocation and Rationing at the Institutional Level

Ms. Wilson is a 71-year-old woman with a recently diagnosed lung cancer. Obstructing a bronchus, the tumor causes pneumonia, and Ms. Wilson is admitted to the hospital in her rural town. She deteriorates and becomes comatose, requiring a respirator. By the eighth hospital day, she is no better. On that day, Louis Ford, a previously healthy 27-year-old, is brought to the hospital with a crushed chest and pneumothorax suffered in an automobile accident. Mr. Ford is in immediate need of a respirator. None of the six patients in the intensive care unit can be removed from respirators without dying; of the six, Ms. Wilson has the poorest prognosis. She has no family. No other respirators exist within a 50-mile radius (Jonsen et al., 2010). Should Ms. Wilson be removed from the respirator in favor of Mr. Ford?

Whereas macroallocation decisions may be based on a set of rules governing rationing, as for organ transplant, microallocation choices typically operate in a less formal way, bringing ethical dilemmas into stark, uncompromising focus and placing issues of resource allocation squarely in the lap of the practicing physician. The microallocation choice involving Ms. Wilson incorporates all four ethical principles, which must be weighed and acted on within minutes: (1) Beneficence: For whom? This ideal cannot be realized for both patients. (2) Nonmaleficence: If Ms. Wilson is removed from the respirator, harm is done to her, but the price of not harming her is great for Mr. Ford. (3) Autonomy: Withdrawal of therapy requires the consent of the patient or family, which is impossible in Ms. Wilson's case. (4) Justice: Should resources be distributed on a first-come first-served basis or according to need?

These are tragic decisions. Many physicians would remove Ms. Wilson from the respirator and make all efforts to save Mr. Ford. The main consideration would be medical effectiveness: Ms. Wilson's chance of living more than a few months is slim, while Mr. Ford could be cured and live for many decades.

Less stark but similar decisions face physicians on a daily basis. On a busy day, which patients get more of the physician's time? In a public hospital with an MRI waiting list, when should a physician call the radiologist and argue for an urgent scan, thereby pushing other people down on the waiting list? Situations involving microallocation demonstrate why in daily practice health care professionals are often forced to balance the interests of one patient against those of another and the interests of the larger group.

FISCAL SCARCITY AND RESOURCE ALLOCATION

During the 1980s, technologic advances in medicine combined with the rapid rise in health care costs led to the belief that medical care rationing was upon us. However, great differences separate the case of organ transplants from that of medical care as a whole.

1. Medical care in general is not a scarce resource; in most population centers, facilities and personnel are abundant.
2. Whereas a nationwide structure is in place to decide who will receive a transplant, no such structure exists for medical care as a whole.

Dr. Ernest, who works for a multispecialty group practice, wants to do her part to keep medical costs down. She prescribes low-cost amoxicillin at 50 cents per capsule rather than ciprofloxacin, which is priced at $3 for each dose. She teaches back pain patients home exercises at no cost rather than sending them to physical therapy visits at $125 per session. At the end of each year, she enjoys calculating how many thousands of dollars she has saved compared with one of her colleagues, who ignores costs in making medical decisions. Because of her efforts and those of other cost-conscious physicians, the practice's pharmacy bill goes down, and practice management is able to lay off one physical therapist, thereby raising its profit margin.

While Dr. Ernest can be praised for attempting to reduce costs without sacrificing quality, her cost savings had no impact on overall national health care expenditures. Nor were the savings used to provide more childhood immunizations or to hire a physician assistant for a nearby rural community without any health care provider. In the United States, there is no national structure within which to effect a trade-off between savings in one area and benefits in another. According to analyst Joshua Wiener (1992),

In countries that have a socially determined health budget, cuts in one area can be justified on the grounds that the money will be spent on other, higher-priority services. This closed system of funding provides a moral underpinning for resource allocation across a range of potentially unlimited demands. In the United States, it is difficult to refuse additional resources for patients, because there is no certainty that the funds will be put to better use elsewhere.

In the United States, persuading physicians to save money on one patient in order to improve services for someone else is as illogical as telling a child to eat all the food on the plate because children in Africa are starving (Cassel, 1985).

For health care providers like Dr. Ernest to make their cost savings socially useful, two things are needed: a closed system of health care funding, whether governmental or private, and a decision-making structure with responsibility to allocate budgets to health care interventions in a fair manner.

For the purposes of the following discussion, let us assume that the United States is in a position of fiscal scarcity and that a mechanism exists to fairly allocate medical care resources from one individual or population group to another. Which ethical conflicts arise between beneficence, nonmaleficence, and autonomy on the one hand and justice (equitable distribution of resources) on the other?

THE RELATIONSHIP OF RATIONING TO COST CONTROL

Assume that Limittown, USA, has a fixed budget of $400 million for medical care in 2018. Limittown has three imaging centers, each with an MRI scanner that is used only 4 hours each weekday. None of the medical facilities perform bone marrow transplantation, a procedure that can prolong the lives of some leukemia patients. In 2018, Limittown spent $10 million to pay for bone marrow transplants at a university hospital 50 miles away.

Limittown's health commissioner projects that 2019 medical care expenditures will be $5 million over budget; she must implement cost savings. She considers two choices: (1) Two of the three

MRI scanners could be closed, allowing the remaining scanner's cost per procedure to be drastically reduced or (2) Limittown could stop paying for bone marrow transplantation for leukemia patients.

Is rationing the same as cost containment? We have defined rationing in medical care as the limitation of resources, including money, going to medical care such that not all care expected to be beneficial is provided to all patients, and the fair distribution of these limited resources. While the limitation of money going to medical care is cost containment, not all cost containment reduces beneficial care to patients. In the case of Limittown, both options for saving $5 million can be considered cost containment, but only denial of coverage for bone marrow transplants requires rationing. Consolidating MRI scanning at a single facility would allow the same number of scans to be performed, but at a substantially lower cost. Rationing is associated with painful cost control (reducing effective medical care), but cost containment (see Chapter 8) can be either painful or painless (not reducing effective medical care) (Table 13–3). The extent of unnecessary care and administrative waste strongly suggests that the United States does not need to ration effective medical services (Berwick & Hackbarth, 2012). To maximize beneficence and autonomy without violating distributive justice, no rationing of beneficial services should take place until all wasteful practices are curtailed; painless cost control should precede painful cost control.

▶ Care Provided to Profoundly Ill People

Lula Rogers is an 84-year-old diabetic woman with amputations of both legs; multiple strokes have rendered her unable to move, swallow, understand, or speak. She has been in a nursing

home for 3 years during which time her medical condition has slowly deteriorated. Ms. Rogers' son wishes to remove her feeding tube, but her physician and the nursing staff feel it is cruel to cause her death by malnutrition and dehydration. Ms. Rogers continues to live for 3 more years, costing $400,000.

A hotly debated issue is the amount of health care that should be provided to the profoundly and incurably ill. Were Lula Rogers' caregivers right to prolong her life? Or were they prolonging Ms. Rogers' suffering and denying her a peaceful death? Should cost be a factor in such decisions, or should such matters of life and death be governed by autonomy, beneficence, and nonmaleficence alone?

Of people dying in 2014, about 60% died in the hospital or nursing home; 40% died at home or in hospice (CDC, 2016). Patients in hospice programs have lower end-of-life costs than those not in hospice programs (Obermeyer et al., 2014), and family members of patients with cancer receiving hospice care reported better quality care compared with those not in hospice care (Kumar et al., 2017). Thus, reduced expenditures can go hand in hand with better care.

RATIONING BY MEDICAL EFFECTIVENESS AND COST-EFFECTIVENESS

Cost containment does not equal rationing, and eliminating administrative waste, medical waste, and unwanted interventions for the profoundly and incurably ill before rationing needed services best realizes the principles of beneficence and justice. However, if rationing of truly beneficial services were needed, the issues become more difficult. If a health care system or program must compromise beneficence because of true fiscal scarcity, how can this compromise be made in a manner that yields the least harm and allocates the harm in the fairest possible way?

Joy Fortune develops Hodgkin's disease, or cancer of the lymphatic system; she receives chemotherapy and is cured. Jessica Turner is moribund from advanced metastatic cancer of the pancreas. She undergoes chemotherapy and dies within 3 days.

In the event of rationing, science is the best guide: the providing or withholding of care is ideally

---

Table 13–3. Rationing and cost control

Not all cost control is rationing.
Painless cost control is not rationing, because no limitation is placed on medical care expected to be beneficial.
Painful cost control may require rationing because limits are placed on medical care expected to be beneficial.

determined by the probability that the treatment will maximize benefits and minimize harm, that is by the criterion of medical effectiveness. Chemotherapy can often cure Hodgkin's disease, but chemotherapy is unlikely to provide prolonged benefit to people with advanced pancreatic cancer. If rationing is needed and only one of these therapies can be offered, a decision based on the criterion of medical effectiveness would allow for the treatment of Hodgkin's disease but not of terminal pancreatic cancer.

If intervention A increases person-years of reasonable-quality life more than intervention B, intervention A is more medically effective. The cost of the two interventions is not considered. Cost-effectiveness adds dollars to the equation: If intervention A increases person-years of reasonable-quality life per dollar spent more than intervention B, it is more cost-effective.

▶ Rationing by Effectiveness: The Oregon Health Plan Model

One example of a systematic approach by a health insurance plan facing fiscal scarcity to ration services on the basis of medical effectiveness was the program implemented by the Oregon Health Plan in the 1990s (Bodenheimer, 1997). In 1994, Oregon added 100,000 poor uninsured Oregonians to its Medicaid program. To control costs, a prioritized list of services was developed, and the state legislature decided how many services would be covered. The prioritized list was based on how much improvement in quantity and quality of life the treatment was likely to produce; costs were not factored into the ranking. The final list contained 745 condition–treatment pairs, and the State of Oregon paid for items above line 574 on the list; conditions below that line were not covered (Kilborn, 1999). What are some of the Oregon Health Plan's ethical implications?

1. The plan was more than a rationing proposal; its chief feature was to extend Medicaid coverage to 100,000 more people. That aspect of the Oregon plan promoted the principle of justice.
2. Another positive feature of the plan was its attempt to prioritize medical care services on the basis of effectiveness, which, if rationing is needed, is a reasonable method for deciding which services to eliminate.

Other features of the Oregon plan must be viewed as negatively impacting distributive justice, or equal access to care without regard for ability to pay.

1. In 1996, 12% of beneficiaries reported being denied services because they were below the line on the priority list. Of those, 78% reported that the denial had worsened their health (Mitchell & Bentley, 2000). Medical services were rationed for Oregon's poor—those on Medicaid—but not for anyone else.
2. The plan targeted beneficial medical services in a state with considerable medical waste. In 1988, many areas of Oregon had average hospital occupancy rates below 50%. The closing of unneeded hospital beds could have saved $50 million per year, enough to pay for some of the treatments eliminated in the plan (Fisher et al., 1992). Oregon did not exhaust its options for painless cost control before proceeding to potentially painful rationing.

By 2004, the Oregon Health Plan had unraveled (Oberlander, 2006). The state entered a period of budgetary woes, new premiums and copays were instituted, and Oregon Health Plan enrollees responded by dropping out of the program. But the bold experiment in rational rationing remains alive in the minds of health care policymakers.

▶ Rationing by Cost Effectiveness

One additional criticism of the Oregon model is that it prioritized services only on the basis of effectiveness without considering cost-effectiveness. If money were not scarce, medical effectiveness (maximizing benefit and minimizing harm) would be the ideal standard upon which to ration care (i.e., the less effective the therapy, the lower its priority on the list of treatments to be offered). But it is unrealistic to pretend that costs can be ignored (Garber & Sox, 2010). Suppose that a bone marrow transplantation saves as many person-years of life by treating an advanced cancer as does doxycycline by curing pneumonia. The former costs $500,000, while the latter can be obtained for $25. There is no reason to ration doxycycline, as its cost is negligible, whereas to make bone marrow transplantation similarly accessible is costly.

Policymakers and health systems in the United States have demonstrated a distinct aversion to explicitly using cost-effectiveness to guide rationing on the basis of fiscal scarcity. For example, the Affordable Care Act established a new national organization, the Patient Centered Outcomes Research Institute (PCORI), to fund research on the relative effectiveness of different approaches to treating and managing illnesses. The legislation explicitly prohibits research funded by PCORI from including cost-effectiveness analysis; investigators are only allowed to compare the effectiveness of different interventions without regard to relative costs. When considering what new technologies or other interventions to approve for Medicare coverage, the Center for Medicare and Medicaid Services considers only evidence of whether the intervention is reasonable and necessary without regard to cost-effectiveness. Similarly, the Food and Drug Administration (FDA) bases approval of new drugs and devices solely on the criteria of safety and effectiveness. Many nations other than the United States do explicitly consider cost-effectiveness when deciding what services are to be covered under a universal health financing and coverage program. The British National Health Service relies on cost-effectiveness analyses produced the National Institute for Health and Care Excellence (known as NICE) for coverage determinations.

Some of the reluctance in the United States to formally incorporate cost-effectiveness into resource allocation policies reflects an inclination among politicians and health care stakeholders to evade the entire matter of whether rationing on the basis of fiscal scarcity is occurring. Other controversial aspects of cost-effectiveness analysis are discussed in Chapter 8. But the ethical aspects also pose challenges. In 1991, Dr. David Eddy (1991a) published a compelling article entitled "The individual vs society: Is there a conflict?" Dr. Eddy posed the case of Mrs. Smith, a woman with widely metastatic breast cancer, and noted that the cost-effectiveness of screening mammography was eight times as cost-effective as intensive treatment for metastatic breast cancer. If medical care must be rationed, it seems logical to spend funds on mammography rather than intensive treatment of metastatic disease because the former intervention is more cost-effective. Dr. Eddy (1991a) did not confine his analysis to cost-effectiveness, however, but moved on to the ethical issues.

Each of us can be in two positions when we make judgments about the value of different health care activities. We are in one position when we are healthy, contemplating diseases we might get, and writing out checks for taxes and insurance premiums. Call this the "first position." We are in a different position when we actually have a disease, are sitting in a physician's office, and have already paid our taxes and premiums (the "second position") . . . . Imagine that you are a 50-year-old woman employed by Mrs. Smith's corporation . . . . [The company] is considering two options: (1) cover screening for breast cancer . . . . or (2) cover [treatment of metastatic cancer] . . . . Now imagine you are in the first position . . . . as long as you do not yet have the disease (the first position), option 1 will always deliver greater benefit at lower cost than option 2 . . . . Now, let us switch you to the second position. Imagine that you already have breast cancer and have just been told that it has metastasized and is terminal . . . . The value to you of the screening option has plummeted because you already have breast cancer and can no longer benefit from screening . . . .

Maximizing care for individual patients attempts to maximize care for individuals when they are in the second position. Maximizing care for society expands the scope of concern to include individuals when they are in the first position. As this example illustrates, the program that delivers the most benefit for the least cost for society (option 1) is not necessarily best for the individual patient (option 2), and vice versa. But as this example also illustrates, individual patients and society are not distinct entities. Rather, they represent the different positions that each of us will be in at various times in our lives. When we serve ourselves in the second position, we can harm ourselves in the first.

Physicians generally care for patients in Dr. Eddy's second position—when they are sick. But if the cost of treating those in the second position reduces resources available to prevent illness for the far larger number of people in the first position (who may not be seeing physicians because they feel fine), the individual principles of beneficence and autonomy are superseding the societal principle of justice. One could even say that choosing for individuals in the second position violates beneficence for those in the first position. On the other hand, if all resources go to those in the first position (e.g., to cost-effective screening rather than expensive treatment for those with life-threatening disease), injustice is committed in the other direction by ignoring the costly needs of the very ill.

Clearly, no ideal method of rationing medical care exists. Rationing worsens health inequity with more vulnerable people usually receiving less care (Bauchner, 2019). All efforts should be made to control costs painlessly before resorting to the painful limitation of effective medical care. But if rationing is inevitable, a balance must be struck among many legitimate needs: the concerns of healthy people for illness prevention, the imperative for acutely sick people to obtain diagnosis and treatment, and the obligation to provide care and comfort to those with untreatable chronic illness.

A BASIC LEVEL OF GUARANTEED MEDICAL BENEFITS

Don Rich is a bank executive who receives his care through a New York City ACO. He develops angina pectoris, which remains stable for over a year. An exercise treadmill test suggests mild coronary artery disease. Although this evaluation indicates that Mr. Rich's condition can be safely managed with medications, he asks his cardiologist to arrange a coronary angiogram with stenting or coronary bypass if indicated. He is told that the ACO has finite resources for such procedures and limits their use to patients with unstable angina or highly abnormal treadmill tests, for whom the procedures are more efficacious. Mr. Rich flies to Texas, consults with a private cardiac surgeon, and receives a coronary angiogram at his own expense.

Most people in the United States believe that health care should be a right. But how much health care? If every person has a right to all beneficial health care, the nation may be unable to pay the bill or may be forced to limit other rights such as education or fire and police protection. One approach to this problem is to limit the health care right to a basic package of services. (In the case of Don Rich's ACO, angiography for stable angina pectoris is not within the basic package.) Any services

beyond the basics can be purchased by individuals who choose to spend their own money. This solution creates an ethical problem. If a service that does produce medical benefit is not included in the basic package or is denied by an insurance company medical director, that service becomes available only to those who can afford it. Where should society draw the line between a basic level of care that should be equally available to all, and "more than basic" services that may be purchased according to individual ability and willingness to pay (Eddy, 1991b)? Unless the basic package covers all beneficial health services, the principle of distributive justice, that all people equally receive a reasonable level of medical services without regard to ability to pay, will be compromised.

THE ETHICS OF HEALTH CARE FINANCING

The principle of distributive justice holds that young and healthy people should pay more in health costs than they use in health services so that older and less healthy people can receive health services at a reasonable cost. Even from the perspective of one's own long-term self-interest, it makes sense to pay more for health care while young and healthy, and to benefit when advanced age creates a greater risk of becoming sick.

A much-discussed issue involves individuals whose behavior, particularly smoking, eating unhealthy diets, and drinking alcohol in excess, is seen as contributing to their ill health.

Jim Butts, a heavy smoker, develops emphysema and has multiple hospitalizations for respiratory failure, including many days on the respirator. Randy Schipp, a former shipyard worker, develops work-related asbestosis and has multiple hospitalizations for respiratory failure, including many days on the respirator. Should Jim pay more for health insurance than Randy?

Gene eats a healthy diet, exercises regularly, but has a strong family history of heart disease; he suffers a heart attack at age 44. Mac eats fast food, does not exercise, and has a heart attack at age 44. Should Mac pay more for health care coverage than Gene?

One view holds that individuals who fall sick as a result of high-risk behavior such as smoking, substance abuse including use of alcohol, and consumption of unhealthy foods are entirely responsible for their behavior and should pay higher health insurance premiums. Opponents of this idea see it as "blaming the victim" and argue that high-risk behaviors have a complex causation that may involve genetic, social, and environmental factors. They cite a number of facts to support their position. The food industry spends billions of dollars each year on television advertising; the average child sees thousands of food commercials each year, most of them for products with poor nutritional value. The tobacco industry heavily advertises to teenagers. Some evidence finds a genetic predisposition to alcoholism. To the extent that individuals are not entirely at fault for high-risk behaviors, it would be unfair to charge them more for health insurance. On the other hand, it seems sensible that users of tobacco and alcohol pay through taxes on those products.

WHO ALLOCATES HEALTH CARE RESOURCES?

The predicament of limited resources has been likened to a herd of cattle grazing on a common pasture. The total grazing area may be regarded as the entirety of economic resources in the United States. A smaller pasture, the *medical commons*, comprises that portion of the grazing area dedicated to health care. The herd represents the nation's physicians, using the resources of the commons in the process of providing care to patients. Physicians, guided by medicine's moral imperative to "do everything possible for the patient," continually attempt to extend the borders of the medical commons. But communities outside the medical commons have legitimate claims to societal resources and view the herd as encroaching on resources needed for other pursuits (Grumbach & Bodenheimer, 1990).

Who decides the magnitude of the medical commons, that is, the resources devoted to health care? Physicians and other health care providers, whose interventions on behalf of their patients add up to the totality of medical resources used? The sum of individual consumer choices operating through a free market? Health insurance plans, watching over their particular piece of the commons? Or government, using the political process to set budgetary limits on the entire health care system?

Traditionally, physicians and patients have had a great deal to say about the size of the medical commons. In the United States, the medical commons traditionally has been an open range. The quantity and price of medical visits, hospital days, surgeries, diagnostic studies, and pharmaceuticals determine the total costs of medical care. This is not the case in other nations, where government health care budgets constitute a "fence" around the medical commons, setting a clear limit on the quantity of resources available. Some advocates of fence-building in the United States have considered parceling the medical commons into numerous subpastures, each representing an integrated health system or Accountable Care Organization (see Chapter 6) working within the constraints of fixed, prepaid budgets. Not all pastures would be equal in size, and the fences might have holes, allowing patients to purchase additional services outside the organized systems of care.

Ethical considerations play a role in both open and closed medical care systems. In the United States open range, the principles of beneficence and autonomy have the upper hand, tending toward an expanding, though not equitable, system. Fenced-in systems, in contrast, balance the more expansive principles of beneficence and autonomy with the demands of distributive justice in order to allocate resources within the medical commons.

If the United States moves toward a more fenced-in medical commons, decisions will be needed about who gets what. Do all 90-year-old people with multiple organ failure receive kidney dialysis that may extend their lives only a few months? Are very low-birth-weight infants afforded neonatal intensive care even with a small chance of leading a normal life? Do individual physicians, interacting with their patients, have the final say in making these decisions? Should societal bodies such as government, commissions of interested parties, or professional associations set the rules?

Microallocation issues come down to daily clinical decisions about which individual patients will receive what types of care (Lo, 2013). Physicians and other caregivers may well recoil from the prospect of "bedside rationing," believing that allocative decision making unduly compromises their commitment to the principles of beneficence and autonomy. Levinsky

(1984) has argued that physicians must maintain their single-mindedness in maximizing care for each patient:

> *There is increasing pressure on doctors to serve two masters. Physicians in practice are being enjoined to consider society's needs as well as each patient's needs in deciding what type and amount of medical care to deliver . . . . When practicing medicine, doctors cannot serve two masters. It is to the advantage both of our society and of the individuals it comprises that physicians retain their historic single-mindedness. The doctor's master must be the patient.*

Yet if physicians abstain from the arena of macroallocation decision making, who is to decide? Currently, these decisions are often made by medical directors of private insurance companies and the leaders of the Medicare and Medicaid programs. Studies have documented that such decisions vary from plan to plan, and even within a single insurance plan, a medical director may make different decisions on different days for similar patients (Light, 1994). If physicians refuse to accept two masters, then medicine will be granting allocation decisions to insurance company and governmental officials. Physicians and other health professionals will continue to face individual patient responsibilities but will find it difficult to escape the obligation to balance the wishes of individual patients against the larger needs of society.

If physicians are to serve two masters (i.e., to maintain their dedication to individual patients while at the same time responsibly managing resources), they need rules to assist them. These rules should operate at both a population and an individual level. At the population level, society should ideally decide which general treatments are to be collectively paid for through the process of universal health insurance. At the individual level, rules are needed to guide decisions about the prioritization of resources for specific patients. The workings of organ transplantation provide a model of how physicians can serve two masters: they do everything possible to procure organs for their transplant patients, but also accept the rules of the system that attempt to allocate organs in a fair manner (Benjamin et al., 1994). The modern health care professional is caught in a global ethical dilemma. On the one hand, patients and their families expect the best that modern technology can offer, paid for through private or public insurance. The imperatives of beneficence, nonmaleficence, and autonomy rule the bedside. On the other hand, grave injustices take place on a daily basis. An uninsured young person with a curable illness is unable to pay for care, while an insured, bedridden individual who had a stroke incurs vast medical bills during the last weeks of her ebbing life. Should not the physician at the stroke patient's bedside be concerned about both patients? However this dilemma is resolved, the principle of justice will relentlessly peek at the physician from under the bed.

REFERENCES

Aaron HJ, Schwartz WB. *The Painful Prescription.* Washington, DC: The Brookings Institution; 1984.

Annas GJ. "Culture of life" politics at the bedside—the case of Terri Schiavo. *N Engl J Med.* 2005;352:1710–1715.

Ansell D, et al. When the only cure is a transplant. *Health Affairs Blog.* February 21, 2014.

Bauchner H. Rationing of health care in the United States. *JAMA.* 2019;321:751–752.

Beauchamp TL, Childress JF. *Principles of Biomedical Ethics.* 7th ed. New York, NY: Oxford University Press; 2013.

Benjamin M, et al. What transplantation can teach us about health care reform. *N Engl J Med.* 1994;330:858–860.

Berwick DM, Hackbarth AD. Eliminating waste in US health care. *JAMA.* 2012;307:1513–1516.

Bodenheimer T. The Oregon Health Plan: lessons for the nation. *N Engl J Med.* 1997;337:651–655, 720–723.

Cassel CK. Doctors and allocation decisions: a new role in the new Medicare. *J Health Polit Policy Law.* 1985;10:549–564.

CDC. Percentage Distribution of Deaths, by Place of Death — United States, 2000–2014. *MMWR Morb Mortal Wkly Rep.* 2016;65:357.

Eddy DM. Comparing benefits and harms: the balance sheet. *JAMA.* 1990;263:2493.

Eddy DM. Clinical decision making: from theory to practice. The individual vs society: is there a conflict? *JAMA.* 1991a;265(11):1446–1450.

Eddy DM. What care is "essential?" What services are "basic?" *JAMA.* 1991b;265:782, 786–788.

Fisher ES, et al. Prioritizing Oregon's hospital resources. *JAMA.* 1992;267:1925–1931.

Garber AM, Sox HC. The role of costs in comparative effectiveness research. *Health Aff (Millwood).* 2010;29:1805–1811.

Grumbach K, Bodenheimer T. Reins or fences: a physician's view of cost containment. *Health Aff (Millwood).* 1990;9:120–126.

Jonsen AR, et al. *Clinical Ethics: A Practical Guide to Ethical Decisions in Clinical Medicine.* 7th ed. New York, NY: McGraw-Hill; 2010.

Kilborn PT. Oregon falters on a new path to health care. *New York Times.* January 3, 1999.

Kumar P, et al. Family perspectives on hospital care experiences of patients with cancer. *J Clin Oncology.* 2017;35:432–439.

Levinsky NG. The doctor's master. *N Engl J Med.* 1984;311:1573–1575.

Light DW. Life, death, and the insurance companies. *N Engl J Med.* 1994;330:498–500.

Lo B. *Resolving Ethical Dilemmas. A Guide for Clinicians.* 5th ed. Baltimore, MD: Lippincott Williams & Wilkins; 2013.

Mitchell JB, Bentley F. Impact of Oregon's priority list on Medicaid beneficiaries. *Med Care Res Rev.* 2000;57:216–234.

Oberlander J. Health reform interrupted: the unraveling of the Oregon Health Plan. *Health Aff (Millwood).* 2006;26:w96–w105.

Obermeyer Z, et al. Association between the Medicare hospice benefit and health care utilization and costs for patients with poor-prognosis cancer. *JAMA.* 2014;312:1888–1896.

Reagan MD. Health care rationing: what does it mean? *N Engl J Med.* 1988;319:1149–1151.

Task Force on Organ Transplantation. *Issues and Recommendations.* Washington, DC: US Department of Health and Human Services; 1986.

Wiener JM. Rationing in America: overt and covert. In: Strosberg MA, et al., eds. *Rationing America's Medical Care: The Oregon Plan and Beyond.* Washington, DC: The Brookings Institution; 1992.

Health Care in Four Nations

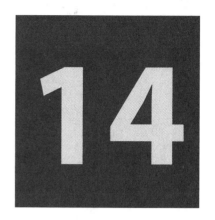

The financing and organization of medical care throughout the developed world spans a broad spectrum. In most countries, the preponderance of medical care is financed or delivered (or both) in the public sector; in others, like the United States, most people both pay for and receive their care through private institutions.

In this chapter, we describe the health care systems of four nations: Germany, Canada, the United Kingdom, and Japan. Each of these nations resides at a different point on the international health care continuum. Examining their diverse systems may aid us in our search for an improved health care system for the United States.

Recall from Chapter 2 the four varieties of health care financing: out-of-pocket payments, individual private insurance, employment-based private insurance, and government financing. Germany, Canada, the United Kingdom, and Japan emphasize the last two modes of payment. Germany finances medical care through government-mandated, employment-based private insurance, though German private insurance is a world apart from that found in the United States. Canada and the United Kingdom feature government-financed systems. Japan's financing falls between the German method of financing and the government model of Canada and the United Kingdom. Regarding the delivery of medical care, the German, Japanese, and Canadian systems are predominantly private, while the United Kingdom's is a mixture of private and public delivery.

Although these four nations demonstrate great differences in their manner of financing and organizing medical care, in one respect they are identical: They all provide universal health care coverage, thereby guaranteeing to their populations financial access to medical services.

GERMANY

▶ Health Insurance

Hans Deutsch is a bank teller living in Germany. He and his family receive health insurance through a sickness fund that insures other employees and their families at his bank and at other workplaces in his city. When Hans went to work at the bank, he was required by law to join the sickness fund selected by his employer. The bank contributes 7.3% of Hans's salary to the sickness fund, and 7.3% is withheld from Hans's paycheck and sent to the fund. Hans's sickness fund collects the same 14.6% employer–employee contribution for all its members.

Germany was the first nation to enact compulsory health insurance legislation. Its pioneering law of 1883 required certain employers and employees to make payments to existing voluntary sickness funds, which would pay for the covered employees' medical care. Initially, only industrial wage earners with incomes less than $500 per year were included; the eligible population was extended in later years.

Eighty-six percent of Germans now receive their health insurance through the mandatory sickness funds, with 11% covered by voluntary insurance plans (Fig. 14–1). The remaining 3% are covered under special programs. Some sickness funds are organized

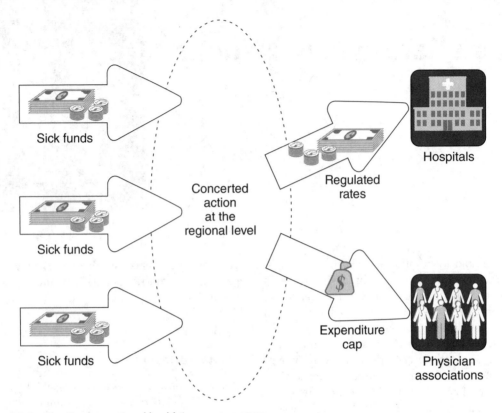

▲ **Figure 14–1.** The German national health insurance system.

by geographic area, some by employer or occupation, and some are nationally based (Blumel & Busse, 2017).

In 2018, the proportion of earnings going to a sickness fund was set at 14.6%, with employers and employees each paying half. These contributions formerly went directly to the sickness funds, which are nonprofit, closely regulated entities that lie somewhere between the private and public sectors. Since 2009, employee and employer contributions are collected by a government-run health fund, which then distributes the money to health funds based on a risk-adjusted (more for older and sicker people) amount per insured person. The number of sickness funds is shrinking, down from 1,000 to about 110 in 2017. The funds are not allowed to exclude people because of illness, or to raise contribution rates according to age or medical condition; that is, they may not use experience rating. The funds are required to cover a broad range of benefits, including hospital and physician services,

prescription drugs, and dental, preventive, and maternity care (Blumel & Busse, 2017).

Hans's father, Peter Deutsch, is retired from his job as a machinist in a steel plant. When he worked, his family received health insurance through a sickness fund set up for employees of the steel company. The fund was run by a board, half of whose members represented employees and the other half the employer. On retirement, Peter's family continued its coverage through the same sickness fund with no change in benefits. The sickness fund continues to pay approximately 60% of his family's health care costs (subsidized by the contributions of active workers and the employer), with 40% paid from Peter's retirement pension fund.

Hans has a cousin, Georg, who formerly worked for a gas station in Hans's city, but is now unemployed. Georg remained in his sickness fund after losing his job. His contribution to the fund is paid by the government. Hans's best friend at the bank was diagnosed with lymphoma and became permanently disabled and unable to work. He remained in the sickness fund, with his contribution paid by the government.

Upon retiring from or losing a job, people and their families retain membership in their sickness fund. Health insurance in Germany, as in the United States, is employment based, but German health insurance, unlike in the United States, must continue to cover its members whether or not they change jobs or stop working for any reason.

Hans's Uncle Karl is an assistant vice president at the bank. Because he earns more than 57,600 Euros per year, he is not required to join a sickness fund, but can opt to purchase private health insurance. Many higher-paid employees choose a sickness fund; they are not required to join the fund selected by the employer for lower-paid workers but can join one of 15 national "substitute" funds.

Eleven percent of Germans, those with higher incomes, choose voluntary private insurance. Private insurers pay higher fees to physicians than do sickness funds, often allowing their policyholders to receive preferential treatment.

In summary, Germany finances health care through a merged social insurance and public assistance structure (see Chapters 2 and 15 for discussion of these concepts), such that no distinctions are made between employed people who contribute to their health insurance, and unemployed people, whose contribution is made by the government.

Medical Care

Hans Deutsch develops chest pain while walking, and it worries him. He does not have a physician, and a friend recommends a general practitioner (GP), Dr. Helmut Arzt. Because Hans is free to see any ambulatory care physician he chooses, he indeed visits Dr. Arzt, who diagnoses angina pectoris—coronary artery disease. Dr. Arzt prescribes some medications and a healthy diet, but the pain persists. One morning, Hans awakens

with severe, suffocating chest pain. He calls Dr. Arzt, who orders an ambulance to take Hans to a nearby hospital. Hans is admitted for a heart attack and is cared for by Dr. Edgar Hertz, a cardiologist. Dr. Arzt does not visit Hans in the hospital. Upon discharge, Dr. Hertz sends a report to Dr. Arzt, who then resumes Hans's medical care. Hans never receives a bill.

German medicine maintains a separation of ambulatory care physicians and hospital-based physicians. Most ambulatory care physicians are prohibited from treating patients in hospitals, and most hospital-based physicians do not have private offices for treating outpatients. People often have their own primary care physician but are allowed to make appointments to see ambulatory care specialists without referral from the primary care physician. Over 40% of Germany's physicians are generalists compared with 33% in the United States. The German system tends to use a dispersed model of medical care organization (see Chapter 5), with little coordination between ambulatory care physicians and hospitals.

Paying Physicians and Hospitals

Dr. Arzt bills his regional association of physicians and receives a fee for each patient visit and for each procedure done during the visit, but is aware that total regional association payments are subject to a spending cap. If in the first quarter of the year, the physicians in his regional association bill for more patient services than expected, each fee is proportionally reduced during the next quarter. If the volume of services continues to increase, fees drop again in the third and fourth quarters of the year. Dr. Arzt's colleague Dr. Hertz, as a hospital physician, receives a salary and is not affected by the spending cap.

Ambulatory care physicians are required to join their regional physicians' association. Rather than paying physicians directly, sickness funds pay a global sum each year to the physicians' association in their region, which in turn pays physicians on the basis of a detailed fee schedule. These sums have been based on the number of patients cared for by the physicians in each regional association, but in 2007, a risk-adjustment factor was introduced that increases payments for populations with greater health problems. Physicians' associations, in an attempt to stay within their global budgets, can reduce fees if the volume of services delivered by their physicians is too high. Sickness funds pay hospitals on a basis similar to the diagnosis-related groups used in the United States Medicare program. Included within this payment is the salary of hospital-based physicians—essentially a form of the episode-based bundled payment method that Medicare in the United States is now beginning to implement (see Chapter 4) (Blumel & Busse, 2017).

▶ Cost Control

The 1977 German Cost Containment Act created a body called Concerted Action, made up of representatives of the nation's health providers, sickness funds, employers, unions, and different levels of government. Concerted Action is convened twice each year, and every spring, it sets guidelines for physician fees, hospital rates, and the prices of pharmaceuticals and other supplies. Based on these guidelines, negotiations are conducted at state, regional, and local levels between the sickness funds in a region, the regional physicians' association, and the hospitals to set physician fees and hospital rates that reflect Concerted Action guidelines. Since 1986, not only have physician fees been controlled, but as described in the above vignette about Dr. Arzt, the total amount of money flowing to physicians has been capped. As a result of these efforts, Germany's health expenditures as a percentage of the gross domestic product actually fell between 1985 and 1990 from 8.7% to 8.3%.

In 1991, however, German health care costs resumed an upward surge, paving the way for a 1993 cost-control law restricting the growth of sickness fund budgets. However, Germany's health care expenditures as a percent of GDP have continued to rise, to 11.3% in 2017.

CANADA

▶ Health Insurance

The Maple family owns a small grocery store in Outer Snowshoe, a tiny Canadian town. Grandfather Maple has a heart condition for which he sees Dr. Rebecca North, his family physician, regularly. The rest of the family is healthy and goes to Dr. North for minor problems and preventive care, including children's immunizations. Neither as employers nor as health consumers do the Maples worry about health insurance. They receive a plastic card from their provincial government and show the card when they visit Dr. North.

The Maples do worry about taxes. The federal personal income tax, the goods and services tax, and the various provincial taxes take a significant amount of family income. But the Maples would never let anyone take away their health insurance system.

In 1947, the province of Saskatchewan initiated the first publicly financed universal hospital insurance program in North America. Other provinces followed suit, and in 1957, the Canadian government passed the Hospital Insurance Act, which was fully implemented by 1961. Hospital, but not physician, services were covered. In 1963, Saskatchewan again took the lead and enacted a medical insurance plan for physician services. The Canadian federal government passed universal medical insurance in 1966. The Canada Health Act of 1984 enumerates the responsibilities of the federal and provincial governments in providing universal health care.

Canada has a tax-financed, public, single-payer health care system. In each Canadian province, the single payer is the provincial government (Fig. 14–2), with funding of the provincial programs coming from both federal and provincial tax revenues. During the 1970s, federal taxes financed 50% of health services, but the federal share has since declined and in 2016 constituted 24% of provincial health program expenditures (Allin & Rudoler, 2017). Provincial taxes vary in type from province to province and include income taxes, payroll taxes, and sales taxes. Some provinces, for example, British Columbia and Alberta, charge a health care premium—essentially an earmarked tax—to finance a portion of their health budgets.

Unlike Germany, Canada has severed the link between employment and health insurance. Wealthy or poor, employed or jobless, retired or younger than 18, every Canadian receives the same health insurance. No Canadian would even imagine that leaving, changing, retiring from, or losing a job has anything to do with

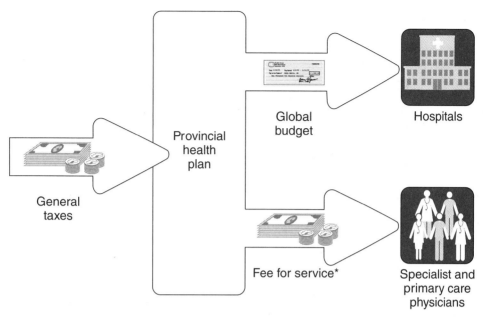

▲ **Figure 14–2.** The Canadian national health insurance system. *Some primary care physicians are paid capitation or salary.

health insurance. In Canada, no distinction is made between the two public financing mechanisms of social insurance (in which only those who contribute receive benefits) and public assistance (in which people receive benefits based on need rather than on having contributed). Everyone contributes through the tax structure and everyone receives benefits.

The benefits provided by Canadian provinces are broad, including hospital, physician, and ancillary services, with no deductibles or copayments. Provincial plans also pay for outpatient drugs, although the scope of drug coverage varies across provinces and some patients pay part of the cost. Most provinces also provide limited long-term care benefits. In 2016, 16% of Canadians reported cost-related access problems compared with 33% in the United States (Osborn et al., 2016).

The Canadian health care system is unique in its prohibition of private health insurance for coverage of services included in the provincial health plans. Hospitals and physicians that receive payments from the provincial health plans are not allowed to bill private insurers for such services, thereby avoiding the

preferential treatment of privately insured patients that occurs in many health care systems. Canadians can purchase private health insurance policies for gaps in provincial health plan coverage, such as pharmaceutical benefits, home care, vision and dental care, and private hospital rooms.

▷ **Medical Care**

Grandfather Maple has had intermittent sensations of palpitations in his chest for a few weeks. He calls Dr. North, who tells him to come right over. An electrocardiogram reveals rapid atrial fibrillation, an abnormal heart rhythm. Because Mr. Maple is tolerating the rapid rhythm, Dr. North starts treatment in the office with a blood thinner to prevent a stroke and metoprolol to gradually slow his heart rate, tells him to return the next day, and writes out a referral slip to see Dr. Jonathan Hartwell, a cardiologist in a nearby small city.

Dr. Hartwell arranges a stress echocardiogram at the local hospital to evaluate Mr. Maple's arrhythmia, finds evidence of coronary ischemia and recommends a coronary angiogram and possible coronary artery bypass surgery. Because Mr. Maple's condition is not urgent, Dr. Hartwell arranges for his patient to be placed on the waiting list at the University Hospital in the provincial capital 50 miles away. One month later, Mr. Maple awakens at 2 AM in a cold sweat, gasping for breath. His daughter calls Dr. North, who urgently sends for an ambulance to transport Mr. Maple to the University Hospital. There Mr. Maple is admitted to the coronary care unit, his condition is stabilized, and he undergoes emergency coronary artery bypass surgery the next day. Ten days later, Mr. Maple returns home, complaining of pain in his incision but otherwise feeling well.

In 2015, half of Canadian physicians were family physicians (contrasted with the United States, where only 33% of physicians are generalists). Canadians have free choice of physician. As a rule, Canadians see their family physician for routine medical problems and visit specialists only through referral by the family physician. Specialists are allowed to see patients without referrals, but only receive the higher specialist fee if they specify the referring primary care physician in their billing; for that reason, most specialists will not see patients without a referral. Unlike the European model of separation between ambulatory and hospital physicians, Canadian family physicians are allowed to care for their patients in hospitals. Because of the close scientific interchange between Canada and the United States, the practice of Canadian medicine is similar to that in the United States; the differences lie in the financing system and the far greater use of primary care physicians. The treatment of Mr. Maple's heart condition is not significantly different from what would occur in the United States, with the exception that high-tech procedures such as cardiac surgery and magnetic resonance imaging (MRI) scans are regionalized in a limited number of facilities and performed far less frequently than in the United States. In 2017, Canada had 10 MRI scanners per million inhabitants compared with 37.5 in the United States. In 2010–2012, Canada performed 56 coronary artery bypass graft surgeries per 100,000 population per year compared with 79 in the United States (Head et al., 2017; The Statistics Portal, 2017).

For Canadians, prompt access to some types of services is more difficult than for people in the United States (Osborn et al., 2016). Canadians on average wait longer for elective operations than do insured people in the United States. In 2018, between 60% and 80% of patients in Canada scheduled for elective hip replacement received their operations within 6 months. For urgent surgery such as hip fracture repair, 80% to 90% receive surgery within 2 days. Waits vary greatly among provinces; in Ontario and Quebec which make up 60% of Canada's population, elective wait times are shorter (Canadian Institute for Health Information, 2018).

Canada's universal insurance program has created a fairer system for distributing health services. Canadians are much less likely than their counterparts in the United States to report experiencing financial barriers to medical care (Commonwealth Fund, 2017). Nonetheless, serious inequities in care remain for low-income families despite universal insurance coverage, particularly for indigenous populations (Martin et al., 2018).

▶ Paying Physicians and Hospitals

For Dr. Rebecca North, collecting fees is a simple matter. Each week she electronically bills the provincial government, listing the patients she saw and the services she provided. Within a month, she is paid in full according to a fee schedule. Dr. North wishes the fees were higher, but loves the simplicity of the billing process. Her staff spends 2 hours per week on billing, compared with the 30 hours of staff time her friend Dr. South in Michigan needs for billing purposes.

Dr. North is less happy about the global budget approach used to pay hospitals. She often begs the hospital administrator to hire more physical therapists, to speed up the reporting of laboratory results, and to institute a program of diabetic teaching. The administrator responds that he receives a fixed payment from the provincial government each year, and there is no extra money.

Until relatively recently, almost all physicians in Canada—family physicians and specialists—were paid on a fee-for-service basis, with fee levels negotiated between provincial governments and provincial medical associations (Fig. 14–2). Physicians participating in the provincial programs must accept the government rate as payment in full and cannot bill patients directly for additional payment. Because fee-for-service payment emphasizes volume over quality of care and makes cost control difficult (see Chapter 9), Canadian provinces are experimenting with alternative forms of payment such as salary or capitation, particularly for family physicians. In 2017–2018, 73% of physician payments were fee-for-service and 27% were alternative payment models (Canadian Institute for Health Information, 2019).

Canadian hospitals, most of which are private nonprofit institutions, negotiate a global budget with the provincial government each year. Hospitals have no need to prepare the itemized patient bills that are so administratively costly in the United States. Hospitals must receive approval from their provincial health plan for new capital projects such as the purchase of expensive new technology or the construction of new facilities. Canada also regulates pharmaceutical prices and provincial plans maintain formularies of drugs approved for coverage.

▶ Cost Control

The Canadian system has attracted the interest of many people in the United States because in contrast to the United States, the Canadians have found a way to deliver comprehensive care to their entire population at far less cost. In 1970, the year before Canada's single-payer system was fully in place, Canada and the United States spent approximately the same proportion of their gross domestic products on health care—7.2% and 7.4%, respectively. By 1990, Canada's health expenditures had risen to 9% of the gross domestic product, compared with 12% for the United States. In 2017, Canada dedicated 10.4% of its gross domestic product to health care while the United States reached 17.1% (OECD, 2019). The differences in cost between the United States and Canada are primarily accounted for by four items: (1) administrative costs, which are more than 300% greater per capita in the United States; (2) more widespread use of expensive high-tech services in the United States; (3) cost per patient day in hospitals; and (4) physician fees and pharmaceutical prices, which are much higher in the United States

(Woolhandler et al., 2003; Reinhardt, 2008; Squires & Anderson, 2015).

While 2017 Canadian per capita health care costs ($4,826) were far lower than those in the United States ($10,209), Canada became concerned with cost increases in the 1990s, when Canadian provinces instituted caps on physician payments similar to those used in Germany (Barer et al., 1996). However, the Canadian federal government's fiscal austerity policies of the 1990s appear to have shaken the public's traditionally high level of confidence in the Canadian health care system. In 2010, about one-quarter of Canadians were not confident that they would receive the care they needed (Schoen et al., 2010). In a 2017 comparison of overall health system performance, the United States ranked last and Canada ranked third to last among 11 developed nations (Schneider et al., 2017). From 2010 to 2017, Canada's health expenditures as percent of gross domestic product actually went down, but reducing health care spending has consequences.

THE UNITED KINGDOM

▶ Health Insurance

Roderick Pound owns a small bicycle repair shop in the north of England; he lives with his wife and two children. His sister Jennifer is a lawyer in Scotland. Roderick's younger brother is a student at Oxford, and their widowed mother, a retired saleswoman, lives in London. Their cousin Anne is totally and permanently disabled from a tragic automobile accident. A distant relative, who became a US citizen 15 years before, recently arrived to help care for Anne.

Simply by virtue of existing on the soil of the United Kingdom—whether employed, retired, disabled, or a foreign visitor—each of the Pound family members is entitled to receive tax-supported medical care through the National Health Service (NHS).

In 1911, Great Britain established a system of health insurance similar to that of Germany. Approximately half the population was covered, and the insurance arrangements were highly complex, with contributions flowing to "friendly societies," trade union and employer funds, commercial insurers, and county insurance committees. In 1942, the world's most renowned treatise on social insurance was published by Sir William Beveridge. The Beveridge Report proposed that Britain's diverse and complex social insurance and public assistance programs, including retirement, disability and unemployment benefits, welfare payments, and medical care, be financed and administered in a simple and uniform system. One part of Beveridge's vision was the creation of a national health service for the entire population. In 1948, the NHS began.

The great majority of NHS funding comes from taxes. As in Canada, the United Kingdom completely separates health insurance from employment, and no distinction exists between social insurance and public-assistance financing. Unlike Canada, the United Kingdom allows private insurance companies to sell health insurance for services also covered by the NHS. Eleven percent of the population in 2015 purchased private insurance or had private insurance provided as an employment benefit. Private insurance may be used to pay for care at private hospitals and allows patients to "hop over" the queues that exist for some NHS services and receive expedited treatment at private facilities. People with private insurance are also paying taxes to support the NHS (Thorlby & Arora, 2017) (Fig. 14–3).

▶ Medical Care

Dr. Timothy Broadman is an English GP, whose list of patients numbers 1,750. Included on his list is Roderick Pound and his family. One day, Roderick's son broke his leg playing soccer. He was brought to the NHS district hospital by ambulance and treated by Dr. Pettibone, the hospital orthopedist, without ever seeing Dr. Broadman.

Roderick's mother has severe degenerative arthritis of the hip, which Dr. Broadman cares for. A year ago, Dr. Broadman sent her to Dr. Pettibone to be evaluated for a hip replacement. Because this was not an emergency, Mrs. Pound required a referral from Dr. Broadman to see Dr. Pettibone. The orthopedist examined and x-rayed her hip and agreed that she needed a hip replacement, but not on an urgent basis. Mrs. Pound has been

on the waiting list for her surgery for more than 6 months. Mrs. Pound has a wealthy friend with private health insurance who got her hip replacement within 3 weeks from Dr. Pettibone, who has a private practice in addition to his employment with the NHS.

Prior to the NHS, most primary medical care was delivered through GPs. The NHS maintained this tradition and formalized a gatekeeper system by which specialty and hospital services (except in emergencies) are available only by referral from a GP. Every person in the United Kingdom who wants to use the NHS must be enrolled on the list of a GP. There is free choice of GP (unless the GP's list of patients is full), and people can switch from one GP's list to another.

Whereas the creation of the NHS in 1948 left primary care essentially unchanged, it revolutionized Britain's hospital sector. As in the United States, hospitals had mainly been private nonprofit institutions or were run by local government; most of these hospitals were nationalized and arranged into administrative regions. Because the NHS unified the United Kingdom's hospitals under the national government, it was possible to institute a true regionalized plan (see Chapter 5).

Patient flow in a regionalized system tends to go from GP (primary care for common illnesses) to local hospital (secondary care for more serious illnesses) to regional or national teaching hospital (tertiary care for complex illnesses). Traditionally, most specialists have had their offices in hospitals. As in Germany, GPs do not provide care in hospitals. GPs have a tradition of working closely with social service agencies in the community, and home care is highly developed in the United Kingdom.

▶ Paying Physicians and Hospitals

Dr. Timothy Broadman does not think much about money when he goes to his surgery (office) each morning. He receives a payment from the NHS to cover part of the cost of running his office, and every month he receives a capitation payment for each of the 1,750 patients on his list. Ten percent of his income has been coming from extra fees he receives when he gives vaccinations to the kids; does Pap smears, family planning, and

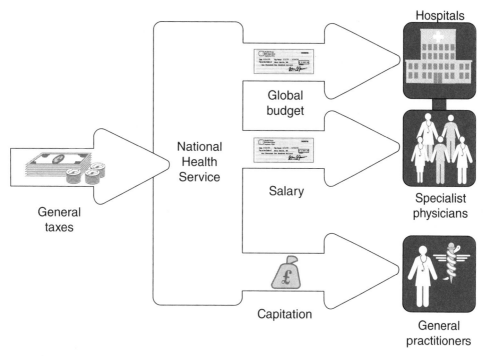

▲ **Figure 14–3.** The British National Health Service: traditional model.

other preventive care; and makes home visits after hours. He also receives additional payments from the pay-for-performance system for GPs.

Since early in the 20th century, the major method of payment for British GPs has been capitation (see Chapter 4). This mode of payment did not change when the NHS took over in 1948. The NHS did add some fee-for-service payments as an encouragement to provide certain preventive services and home visits during nights and weekends. Consultants (specialists) are salaried employees of the NHS, although some consultants are allowed to see privately insured patients on the side, whom they bill fee-for-service.

In 2004, a major new payment mode began for GPs: pay for performance (P4P) (see Chapter 10), known in the United Kingdom as the Quality and Outcomes Framework (QOF). NHS management negotiated the program with the British Medical Association (BMA), and the success of the negotiations was in large part because of the government's policy of increasing payment to GPs, whose average income rose by 60% from 2002 to 2007, with GP incomes approaching those of hospital specialists (Doran & Roland, 2010). The NHS and BMA agreed on dozens of clinical indicators measuring quality for preventive services and common chronic illnesses such as coronary heart disease, hypertension, diabetes, and asthma. In addition, physician practices are measured on practice organization—involving such measures as documentation in medical records, ability of patients to access the practice by phone, computerization, and safe management of medications—and on the patient experience as measured by patient surveys. Physician practices were awarded points for GPs who performed well on these measures with each point worth a sum of money. In 2005, GP practices achieving maximum quality could increase earnings by approximately $77,000 per physician, though the size of performance-related payments has since declined (Roland & Campbell, 2014) and by 2014, GP incomes had slid back to their pre-QOF level (Roland & Guthrie, 2016).

In the first year of the program, quality appeared to improve, largely due to nurse-run chronic disease management. An analysis of performance improvement prior to and following the introduction of P4P suggests that performance had been increasing before P4P, but that quality increased slightly faster after P4P for some chronic conditions.

In 2014, financial incentives were removed from some of the quality indicators, resulting in quality reductions for the measures with financial incentives removed with no change in measures with incentives maintained. Scotland abolished the QOF altogether in 2016 (Minchin et al., 2018).

▶ Cost Control

Health expenditures in the United Kingdom accounted for 7.0% of the gross domestic product (GDP) in 2000, far below the US figure of 13.4%. Believing that the NHS needed more resources, the government of Prime Minister Tony Blair infused the NHS with a major increase in funds. Between 1999 and 2004, the number of NHS physicians increased by 25%. In addition, the QOF channeled the equivalent of several billion new dollars into physician practices. By 2017, health expenditures as a proportion of the GDP had risen to 9.6% and per capita spending had increased from $1,837 (2000) to $4,245 (2017) (Table 14–2). As a result, the NHS scaled back its funding; since 2010, tight budgets have created stress throughout the NHS. Queues have lengthened for some nonemergency consultant visits and elective surgeries.

Two major factors allow the United Kingdom to keep its health care costs low: the power of the governmental single payer to limit budgets and the mode of payment of physicians. While Canada also has a single payer of health services, it had traditionally paid most physicians fee-for-service. In contrast, the United Kingdom relies chiefly on capitation and salary to pay physicians; payment can more easily be controlled by limiting increases in capitation payments and salaries. Moreover, because consultants (specialists) in the United Kingdom are NHS employees, the NHS can restrict the number of consultant slots, including those for surgeons. Overall, the United Kingdom controls costs by controlling the supply of personnel and facilities; for example, in 2017, the United Kingdom had 7.2 MRI scanners per million population compared with the US rate of 37.5 (OECD, 2019).

The United Kingdom is often viewed as a nation that rations certain kinds of health care. In fact, primary and preventive care are not rationed, and average waiting times to see a GP in the United Kingdom are similar to those for people in the United States seeking medical appointments (Schneider et al., 2017). A striking characteristic of British medicine is its economy. British physicians traditionally do less of nearly everything—perform fewer surgeries, prescribe fewer medications, order fewer x-rays, and are more skeptical of new technologies than US physicians (Payer, 1988).

▶ Reforms of the English National Health Service

Since 1991, England has diverged from the classic NHS model that remains largely in effect in Scotland and Wales, and implemented a series of structural changes. Currently, GPs are required to belong to one of the 211 local "clinical commissioning groups" which in 2014 controlled about half the NHS budget (Fig. 14–4). These groupings of GPs use these funds to pay for primary care and buy specialty care for their patients. The formerly strict regionalization of specialist and hospital services has been weakened as GPs and patients have some choice in which specialists and hospitals will provide their care (Thorlby & Arora, 2017). Hospitals are organized into trusts which contract with local commissioning groups to provide services. Critics of these reforms have questioned whether the revised structures in England are superior to the traditional structure in Scotland and Wales.

JAPAN

▶ Health Insurance

Akiko Tanino works in the accounting department of the Mazda car company in Tokyo. Like all Mazda employees, she is enrolled in the health insurance plan directly operated by Mazda. Each month, a percentage of Akiko's salary is deducted from her paycheck and paid to the Mazda health plan. Mazda makes an additional equal payment to its health plan for Akiko.

Akiko's father Takeshi recently retired after working for many years as an engineer at Mazda. When he retired, his health insurance changed from the Mazda company plan to the community-based health insurance plan administered by the municipal government where he lives. Mazda makes payments to this health insurance plan to help pay for the health care costs of the company's retirees. In addition, the health insurance plan requires that Takeshi pay the plan a premium indexed to his income.

Akiko's brother Kazuo is a mechanic at a small auto repair shop in Tokyo. He is automatically enrolled in the government-managed health insurance plan operated by the Japanese national government. Kazuo and his employer each contribute equal percentages of Kazuo's salary to the government plan.

Although Japanese society has a cultural history distinct from the other nations discussed in this chapter, its health care system draws heavily from European and North American traditions. Similar to Germany, Japan's modern health insurance system is rooted in an employment-linked social insurance program. Japan first legislated mandatory employment-based social insurance for many workers in 1922, building on preexisting voluntary mutual aid societies. The system was gradually expanded until universal coverage was achieved in 1961 with passage of the National Health Insurance Act (Fig. 14–5).

Every large employer is required to operate its own self-insured plan for employees and dependents, known as "society-managed insurance" plans. Hundreds of employer-based plans exist. The boards of directors of society plans comprise 50% employee and 50% employer representatives. Employees and their dependents are required to enroll in their company's society plan, and the employee and the employer must contribute a premium to fund the society. Society-managed insurance plans cover 24% of the Japanese population (Tatara & Okamoto, 2009).

Employees and dependents in smaller companies are compulsorily enrolled in a single national health insurance plan for small businesses operated by the national government. This government-managed insurance plan, primarily financed by a compulsory premium equally shared between employer and employee, covers 28% of the population. The federal government also uses general tax revenues to subsidize the government-managed insurance plan. A third type of health insurance, called national health insurance or citizen's health insurance, covers self-employed workers and retirees (39% of the population). Each municipal government in Japan administers a national health insurance plan and levies a compulsory premium on the self-employed

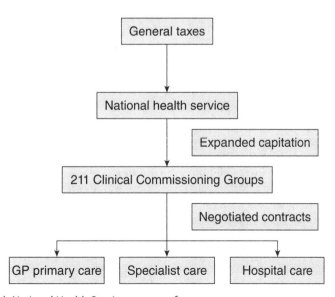

▲ **Figure 14–4.** The British National Health Service: recent reforms.

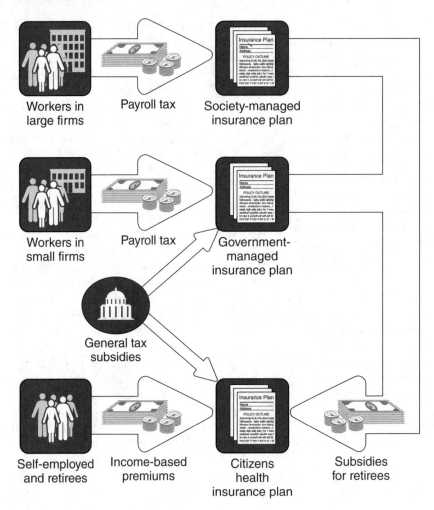

▲ **Figure 14–5.** The Japanese health system.

workers and retirees in its jurisdiction. The premiums are augmented by general tax revenues and subsidies from employers to cover their retirees' costs (Tatara & Okamoto, 2009). A smattering of smaller insurance programs exists for government employees and other special categories of workers, and resemble the society-managed insurance plans (Matsuda, 2017).

All plans are required to provide standard comprehensive benefits, including payment for hospital and physician services, prescription drugs, maternity care, and dental care. In addition, in 2000 Japan implemented a long-term insurance plan, financed by general tax revenues and an earmarked income tax, which provides

comprehensive benefits to disabled adults, including payment for home care, case management, and institutional services. To reduce the premium burden for the elderly, cross-subsidies exist among the different health insurance plans. Except for children, the elderly, and those with low incomes, all plans require cost-sharing at the point of service, with patients paying 30% of the costs of their care and the health insurance plan paying 70% (Matsuda, 2017).

In summary, Japan—like Germany—builds on an employment-based social insurance model, using additional general tax subsidies to create a universal insurance program. Compared with Germany, the national and local governments in Japan are more involved in directly administering health plans and a majority of Japanese are covered by government-run or government-managed plans rather than by employer-managed private plans.

Medical Care

Takeshi Tanino's knee has been aching for several weeks. He makes an appointment at a clinic operated by an orthopedic surgeon. At the clinic Takeshi has a medical examination, an x-ray of the knee, and is scheduled for regular physical therapy. During the examination, the orthopedist notes that Takeshi's blood pressure is high and recommends that Takeshi see an internist at a different clinic about this problem.

Six months later, Takeshi develops a cough and fever. He makes an appointment at the medical clinic of a nearby hospital run by Dr. Suzuki, is diagnosed with pneumonia, and is admitted to the medical ward. He is treated with intravenous antibiotics for 2 weeks and remains in the hospital for an additional 2 weeks after completing antibiotics for further intravenous hydration and nursing care.

Health plans place no restrictions on choice of hospital and physician and do not require preauthorization before using medical services. Most medical care is provided in three types of settings: (1) independent clinics, each owned by a physician and staffed by the physician and other employees, with many clinics also having small inpatient wards; (2) small hospitals with inpatient and outpatient departments, owned by a physician with employed physician staff; and (3) larger public and private hospitals with outpatient and inpatient departments and salaried physician staff. Larger hospitals offer a wide range of specialties while smaller hospitals and clinics have a more limited selection of specialty departments. Care is delivered in a specialty-specific manner, with a few organizations using a primary care-oriented gatekeeper model (Matsuda, 2017).

Physician entrepreneurship is a strong element in the organization of health care in Japan. Many clinics and small hospitals are family-owned businesses founded and operated by independent physicians,

often passed down within a family from one generation to another. Many physicians expanded their clinics to become small hospitals; larger hospitals are often operated by the government. The distinction between clinics and hospitals in Japan is not as great as in most nations. Clinics are permitted to operate inpatient beds and only become classified as hospitals when they have more than 20 beds. Although many physician-owned clinics and hospitals are modest facilities, others are larger institutions offering a wide array of outpatient and inpatient services featuring the latest biomedical technology, electronic medical records, and automated dispensing of medications.

Rates of hospital admission and surgery are relatively low in Japan; yet when hospitalized, patients remain unusually long compared with most developed nations. Average length of stay was 17 days in 2015 compared with 6 days in the United States (OECD, 2017).

Paying Physicians and Hospitals

One month after returning home from the hospital, Takeshi Tanino develops stomach pain that awakens him several nights. He makes an appointment at a general medical clinic run by Dr. Sansei. Dr. Sansei performs an endoscopy, which reveals gastritis. Dr. Sansei prescribes an proton pump inhibitor and arranges for Takeshi to return to the clinic every 4 weeks for the next 6 months. Takeshi's stomach ache improves after a few days of using the medication. At each follow-up visit, Dr. Sansei questions Takeshi about his symptoms and dispenses a new 4-week supply of medications.

In the past, insurance plans paid both physicians and hospitals on a fee-for-service basis. In 2003, a per diem hospital payment based on diagnosis was introduced while physicians continue to be paid fee-for-service. The government strictly regulates physician fees, hospital payments, and medication prices, which are low by US standards, and also attempts to control the volume of expensive services. Services such as MRI scans that had shown large increases in volumes have had substantial cuts in fees (Ikegami & Anderson, 2012). Physicians make up for low fees with high volume, at times seeing 60 patients per day. In 2017, the number

Table 14–1. Total health expenditures as a percentage of gross domestic product (GDP), 1970–2017

	1970	1980	1990	2000	2010	2017
Germany	5.5	7.9	8.3	10.3	11.0	11.3
United Kingdom	4.5	5.8	6.0	7.0	8.5	9.6
Canada	7.2	7.4	8.9	8.8	10.6	10.4
Japan	4.1	6.5	6.0	7.7	9.2	10.7
United States	7.4	9.2	11.9	13.4	16.4	17.1

Source: Organisation for Economic Co-operation and Development. Health Statistics, 2019 https://www.oecd.org/OECD › health › health-data.
Note: 2017 US Government data differs from OECD data, placing US health expenditures at 17.9% of GDP.

of physician visits per capita was approximately 13, compared with 4 for the United States. Physicians are permitted to directly dispense medications, not just to prescribe them, and make a profit from the sale of pharmaceuticals, and many physician visits are solely for the purpose of refilling medications. Recently, pharmacists have begun to fill an increasing number of prescriptions (Matsuda, 2017).

▶ Cost Control

Health care costs in Japan were 10.7% of GDP in 2017, up from 7.7% in 2000. Concerns are mounting due to Japan's demographics. The health care system relies heavily on payroll taxes and thus requires a large employed population. But with a low birth rate and the longest life expectancy in the world, Japan's population is aging faster than that of other developed nations. The proportion of Japanese older than 65 years was 27% in 2017 compared with 15% for the United States.

Through its fee schedule, the government has kept medical prices low, which is the main cost-containment strategy. But physicians work at a fast pace seeing many patients for short visits, while many hospitals are old and underfunded. The stresses resulting from Japan's demographic reality make for an uncertain future.

CONCLUSION

Key issues in evaluating and comparing health care systems are access to care, level of health expenditures, public satisfaction with health care, and the overall quality of care as expressed by the health of the population. Germany, Canada, the United Kingdom, and Japan provide universal financial access to health care through government-run or government-mandated programs. These four nations have controlled health care costs more successfully than has the United States (Tables 14–1 and 14–2), though all four face challenges in containing their spending.

In 2017, data from international surveys of 11 developed nations showed that the United States ranked last in overall health system performance. The United Kingdom ranked first, Germany eighth, and Canada ninth. Adults in the United States were much more likely than adults in Germany, the United Kingdom, and Canada to report problems with access to medical services due to costs (Fig. 14–6) (Commonwealth Fund, 2017).

Crossnational comparisons of health care quality are treacherous since it is difficult to disentangle the impacts of socioeconomic factors and medical care

Table 14–2. Per capita health spending in US dollars, 2017

Germany	$5,729
United Kingdom	$4,245
Canada	$4,826
Japan	$4,717
United States	$10,209

Source: Data from the Organisation for Economic Co-operation and Development, 2019. www.oecd.org.
Note: 2017 US Government data differs from OECD data, placing per capita health spending at $10,739.

Table 14–3. Health outcome measures

	Infant Mortality, per 1,000 Live Births[a]	Life Expectancy at Birth (years)[a]		Life Expectancy at Age 65 (years)[a]		Mortality Amenable to Health Care, 2013, Deaths per 100,000 Population[b]
		Men	Women	Men	Women	
Germany	3.4	78.3	83.1	17.9	21.0	83
United Kingdom	3.8	79.2	82.8	18.6	20.8	85
Canada	4.7	79.8	83.9	19.2	22.0	78
Japan	2.0	80.8	87.0	19.4	24.2	66 (2007)
United States	5.9	76.3	81.1	18.0	20.5	112

Infant mortality data are for 2016; life expectancy data are for 2015.
[a]Data from the Organisation for Economic Co-operation and Development, 2019. www.oecd.org; Commonwealth Fund, International Health System Profiles, 2017.
[b]Premature deaths that effective health care could avoid.

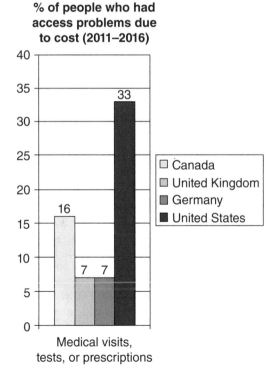

% of people who had access problems due to cost (2011–2016)

Legend:
☐ Canada
☐ United Kingdom
☐ Germany
■ United States

Medical visits, tests, or prescriptions

▲ **Figure 14–6.** Problems accessing medical services due to costs. (Source: Commonwealth Fund. Mirror, Mirror 2017: International Comparison Reflects Flaws and Opportunities for Better U.S. Health Care, July 2017.)

on the health status of the population. But such comparisons can convey rough impressions of whether a health care system is functioning at a reasonable level of performance. From Table 14–3, it is clear that the United States has an infant mortality rate higher than Germany, Canada, the United Kingdom, and Japan, with the Japanese rate being the lowest. Japan also has the highest male and female life expectancy rates at birth. The life expectancy rate at age 65 is believed by some observers to measure the impact of medical care, especially its more high-tech component, more than it measures underlying socioeconomic influences. Even by this standard, the United States ranks below the other four nations (Table 14–3). Researchers have developed another metric intended to assess the functioning of national health care systems, known as "mortality amenable to health care"; the United States performs poorly on this metric as well, relative to other nations (Table 14–3).

Just as epidemiologic studies often derive their most profound insights from comparisons of different populations (see Chapter 11), research into health services can glean insights from the experience of other nations. As the United States confronts the challenge of achieving universal access to high-quality health care at an affordable cost, lessons may be learned from examining how other nations have addressed this challenge.

REFERENCES

Barer ML, et al. Re-minding our Ps and Qs: medical cost controls in Canada. *Health Aff (Millwood)*. 1996;15(2):216–234.

Blumel M, Busse R. The German Health System. In Commonwealth Fund. International Profiles of Health Care Systems. May 2017. https://www.commonwealthfund.org/publications/fund-reports/2017/may/international-profiles-health-care-systems. Accessed October 22, 2019.

Allin S, Rudoler D. The Canadian Health Care System. In Commonwealth Fund. International Profiles of Health Care Systems. May 2017. https://www.commonwealthfund.org/publications/fund-reports/2017/may/international-profiles-health-care-systems. Accessed October 22, 2019.

Canadian Institute for Health Information. Physicians in Canada, 2018. CIHI 2019. https://www.cihi.ca/en/physicians-in-canada. Accessed October 23, 2019.

Canadian Institute for Health Information. Access Data and Reports, 2018. https://www.cihi.ca/en. Accessed October 22, 2019.

Commonwealth Fund. Health Care System Performance Rankings. 2017. https://www.commonwealthfund.org/chart/2017/health-care-system-performance-rankings. Accessed October 23, 2019.

Doran T, Roland M. Lessons from major initiatives to improve primary care in the United Kingdom. *Health Aff (Millwood)*. 2010;29:1023–1029.

Head SJ, et al. Current practice of state-of-the-art surgical coronary revascularization. *Circulation*. 2017;136:1331–1345.

Ikegami N, Anderson GF. In Japan, all-payer rate setting under tight government control has proved to be an effective approach to containing costs. *Health Aff (Millwood)*. 2012;31:1049–1056.

Martin D, et al. Canada's university health-care system: achieving its potential. *Lancet*. 2018;391:1718–1735.

Matsuda R. The Japanese Health Care System. In Commonwealth Fund. International Profiles of Health Care Systems. May 2017. https://www.commonwealthfund.org/publications/fund-reports/2017/may/international-profiles-health-care-systems. Accessed October 23, 2019.

Minchin M, et al. Quality of care in the United Kingdom after removal of financial incentives. *N Engl J Med*. 2018;379:948–957.

Organisation for Economic Co-operation and Development (OECD). Health at a Glance, 2017. http://www.oecd.org/health/health-systems/health-at-a-glance-19991312.htm. Accessed October 23, 2019.

Organisation for Economic Co-operation and Development (OECD). Health Statistics, 2019. https://www.oecd.org/OECD › health › health-data. Accessed October 23, 2019.

Osborn R, et al. In new survey of 11 countries, US adults still struggle with access to and affordability of health care. *Health Aff (Millwood)*. 2016;35:2327–2336.

Payer L. *Medicine and Culture*. New York, NY: Henry Holt; 1988.

Reinhardt U. Why does US health care cost so much? Economix. November 14, 2008. http://economix.blogs.nytimes.com. Accessed October 23, 2019.

Roland M, Campbell S. Successes and failures of pay for performance in the United Kingdom. *N Eng J Med*. 2014;370:1944–1949.

Roland M, Guthrie B. Quality and Outcomes Framework: what have we learnt? *BMJ*. 2016;354:i4060.

Schneider EC, et al. Mirror Mirror 2017: International Comparison Reflects Flaws and Opportunities for Better US Health Care. Commonwealth Fund, July 2017.

Schoen C, et al. How health insurance design affects access to care and costs, by income, in eleven countries. *Health Affairs*. 2010;29:2323–2334.

Squires D, Anderson C. US Health Care from a Global Perspective. Commonwealth Fund, October 2015. https://www.commonwealthfund.org/.../2015/oct/us-health-care-global-perspective. Accessed October 23, 2019.

Tatara K, Okamoto E. Japan: Health System Review. *Health Syst Transit*. 2009;11(5):1–164.

The Statistics Portal. Number of MRI units in selected countries as of 2017. 2018. https://www.statista.com/statistics/282401/density-of-magnetic-resonance-imaging-units-by-country/. Accessed October 23, 2019.

Thorlby R, Arora S. The English Health Care System. In Commonwealth Fund. International Profiles of Health Care Systems. May 2017. https://www.commonwealthfund.org/publications/fund-reports/2017/may/international-profiles-health-care-systems. Accessed October 23, 2019.

Woolhandler S, et al. Costs of health care administration in the United States and Canada. *N Engl J Med*. 2003;349:768–775.

Health Care Reform and National Health Insurance

For more than 100 years, reformers in the United States argued for the passage of a national health insurance program, a government guarantee that every person is covered for basic health care. Finally in 2010, the United States took a major, though incomplete, step forward toward universal health insurance with the passage of the Affordable Care Act (ACA). In 2019, the ACA had survived numerous attempts to repeal it, but the law's future is uncertain.

The subject of national health insurance has seen six periods of intense activity, alternating with times of political inattention. From 1912 to 1916, 1946 to 1949, 1963 to 1965, 1970 to 1974, 1991 to 1994, and 2009 to 2019, it was the topic of major national debate. In 1916, 1949, 1974, and 1994, national health insurance was defeated and temporarily consigned to the nation's back burner. Guaranteed health coverage for two groups—the elderly and some of the poor—was enacted in 1965 through Medicare and Medicaid. In 2010, with the passage of the ACA or "Obamacare," the stage was set for the expansion of coverage to millions of uninsured people. National health insurance means the guarantee of health insurance for all the nation's residents—what is commonly referred to as "universal coverage." Much of the focus, as well as the political contentiousness, of national health insurance proposals concern how to pay for universal coverage. National health insurance proposals may also address provider payment and cost containment.

The controversies that erupt over universal health care coverage become simpler to understand if one returns to the four basic modes of health care financing outlined in Chapter 2: out-of-pocket payment, individual private insurance, employment-based private insurance, and government financing. There is general agreement that out-of-pocket payment does not work as a sole financing method for costly contemporary health care. National health insurance involves the replacement of out-of-pocket payments by one, or a mixture, of the other three financing modes.

Under government-financed national health insurance plans, funds are collected by a government or quasigovernmental fund, which in turn pays hospitals, physicians, and other health care providers. Under private individual or employment-based national health insurance, funds are collected by private insurance companies, which then pay providers of care.

Historically, health care financing in the United States began with out-of-pocket payment and progressed through individual private insurance, then employment-based insurance, and finally government financing for Medicare and Medicaid (see Chapter 2). In the history of US national health insurance, the chronologic sequence is reversed. Early attempts at national health insurance legislation proposed government programs; private employment-based national health insurance was not seriously entertained until 1971, and individually purchased universal coverage was not suggested until the 1980s (Table 15–1). Following this historical progression, we shall first discuss government-financed national health insurance, followed by private employment-based and then individually purchased coverage. The ACA represents a pluralistic approach that draws on all three of these

Table 15–1. Attempts to legislate national health insurance

1912–1919	American Association for Labor Legislation
1946–1949	Wagner–Murray–Dingell bill supported by President Truman
1963–1965	Medicare and Medicaid passed as a first step toward national health insurance
1970–1974	Kennedy and Nixon proposals
1991–1994	A variety of proposals introduced, including President Clinton's Plan
2010	Patient Protection and Affordable Care Act signed into law by President Obama

financing models: government financing, employment-based private insurance, and individually purchased private insurance.

GOVERNMENT-FINANCED NATIONAL HEALTH INSURANCE

▶ The American Association for Labor Legislation Plan

In the early 1900s, 25% to 40% of people who became sick did not receive any medical care. In 1915, the American Association for Labor Legislation (AALL) published a national health insurance proposal to provide medical care, sick pay, and funeral expenses to lower-paid workers—those earning less than $1,200 a year—and to their dependents. The program would be run by states rather than the federal government and would be financed by a payroll tax–like contribution from employers and employees, perhaps with an additional contribution from state governments. Government-controlled regional funds would pay physicians and hospitals. Thus, the first national health insurance proposal in the United States was a government-financed program (Starr, 1982).

In 1910, Edgar Peoples worked as a clerk for Standard Oil, earning $800 a year. He lived with his wife and three sons. Under the AALL proposal, Standard Oil and Mr. Peoples would each pay $13 per year into the regional fund, with the state government contributing $6. The total of $32 (4% of wages) would cover the Peoples family.

The AALL's road to national health insurance followed the example of European nations, which often began their programs with lower-paid workers and gradually extended coverage to other groups in the population. Key to the financing of national health insurance was its compulsory nature; mandatory payments were to be made on behalf of every eligible person, ensuring sufficient funds to pay for people who fell sick.

The AALL proposal initially had the support of the American Medical Association (AMA) leadership. However, the AMA reversed its position and the conservative branch of labor, the American Federation of Labor, along with business interests, opposed the plan (Starr, 1982). The first attempt at national health insurance failed.

▶ The Wagner–Murray–Dingell Bill

In 1943, Democratic Senators Robert Wagner of New York and James Murray of Montana, and Representative John Dingell of Michigan introduced a health insurance plan based on the social security system enacted in 1935. Employer and employee contributions to cover physician and hospital care would be paid to the federal social insurance trust fund, which would in turn pay health providers. The Wagner–Murray–Dingell bill had its lineage in the New Deal reforms enacted during the administration of President Franklin Delano Roosevelt.

In the 1940s, Edgar Peoples' daughter Elena worked in a General Motors plant manufacturing trucks to be used in World War II. Elena earned $3,500 per year. Under the 1943 Wagner–Murray–Dingell bill, General Motors would pay 6% of her wages up to $3,000 into the social insurance trust fund for retirement, disability, unemployment, and health insurance. An identical 6% would be taken out of Elena's check for the same purpose. One-fourth of this total amount ($90) would be dedicated to the health insurance portion of social security. If Elena or her children became sick, the social insurance trust fund would reimburse their physician and hospital.

Edgar Peoples, in his seventies, would also receive health insurance under the Wagner–Murray–Dingell bill, because he was a social security beneficiary.

Elena's younger brother Marvin was permanently disabled and unable to work. Under the Wagner–Murray–Dingell bill he would not have received government health insurance unless his state added unemployed people to the program.

As discussed in Chapter 2, government-financed health insurance can be divided into two categories. Under the social insurance model, only those who pay into the program, usually through social security contributions, are eligible for the program's benefits. Under the public assistance (welfare) model, eligibility is based on a means test; those below a certain income may receive assistance. In the welfare model, those who benefit may not contribute, and those who contribute (usually through taxes) may not benefit (Bodenheimer & Grumbach, 1992). The Wagner–Murray–Dingell bill, like the AALL proposal, was a social insurance proposal. Working people and their dependents were eligible because they made social security contributions, and retired people receiving social security benefits were eligible because they paid into social security prior to their retirement. The permanently unemployed were not eligible.

In 1945, President Truman, embracing the general principles of the Wagner–Murray–Dingell legislation, became the first US president to strongly champion national health insurance. After Truman's surprise election in 1948, the AMA succeeded in a massive campaign to defeat the Wagner–Murray–Dingell bill. In 1950, national health insurance returned to obscurity (Starr, 1982).

▶ Medicare and Medicaid

In the late 1950s, fewer than 15% of the elderly had health insurance (see Chapter 2) and a strong social movement clamored for the federal government to come up with a solution. The Medicare law of 1965 took the Wagner–Murray–Dingell approach to national health insurance, narrowing it to people 65 years and older. Medicare was financed through social security contributions, federal income taxes, and individual premiums. Congress also enacted the Medicaid program in 1965, a public assistance or "welfare" model of government insurance that covered a portion of the low-income population. Medicaid was paid for by federal and state taxes.

In 1966, at age 66, Elena Peoples was automatically enrolled in the federal government's Medicare Part A hospital insurance plan, and she chose to sign up for the Medicare Part B physician insurance plan by paying a $3 monthly premium to the Social Security Administration. Elena's son, Tom, and Tom's employer helped to finance Medicare Part A; each paid 0.5% of wages (up to a wage level of $6,600 per year) into a Medicare trust fund within the social security system. Elena's Part B coverage was financed in part by federal income taxes and in part by Elena's monthly premiums. In case of illness, Medicare would pay for most of Elena's hospital and physician bills.

Elena's disabled younger brother, Marvin, age 60, was too young to qualify for Medicare in 1966. Marvin instead became a recipient of Medicaid, the federal–state program for certain groups of low-income people. When Marvin required medical care, the state Medicaid program paid the hospital, physician, and pharmacy, and a substantial portion of the state's costs were picked up by the federal government.

Medicare is a social insurance program, requiring individuals or families to have made social security contributions to gain eligibility to the plan. Medicaid, in contrast, is a public assistance program that does not require recipients to make contributions but instead is financed from general tax revenues. Because of the rapid increase in Medicare costs, the social security contribution has risen substantially. In 1966, Medicare took 1% of wages, up to a $6,600 wage level (0.5% each from employer and employee); by 2019, the payments had risen to 2.9% of all wages, higher for wealthy people. The Part B premium has jumped from $3 per month in 1966 to $135.50 per month in 2019, higher for wealthy people.

▶ The 1970 Kennedy Bill and the Single-Payer Plan of the 1990s

Many people believed that Medicare and Medicaid were a first step toward universal health insurance. European nations started their national health insurance programs by covering a portion of the population and later extending coverage to more people. Medicare and Medicaid seemed to fit that tradition. Shortly after Medicare and Medicaid became law, the labor movement, Senator Edward Kennedy of Massachusetts, and Representative Martha Griffiths of Michigan drafted legislation to cover the entire population through a national health insurance program. The 1970 Kennedy–Griffiths Health Security Act followed in the footsteps of the Wagner–Murray–Dingell bill, calling for a single federally operated health insurance system that would replace all public and private health insurance plans.

Under the Kennedy–Griffiths 1970 Health Security Program, Tom Peoples, who worked for Great Books, a small book publisher, would continue to see his family physician as before. Rather than receiving payment from Tom's private insurance company, his physician would be paid by the federal government. Tom's employer would no longer make a social security contribution to Medicare (which would be folded into the Health Security Program) and would instead make a larger contribution of 3% of wages up to a wage level of $15,000 for each employee. Tom's employee contribution was set at 1% up to a wage level of $15,000. These social insurance contributions would pay for approximately 60% of the program; federal income taxes would pay for the other 40%.

Tom's Uncle Marvin, on Medicaid since 1966, would be included in the Health Security Program, as would all residents of the United States. Medicaid would be phased out as a separate public assistance program.

The Health Security Act went one step further than the AALL and Wagner–Murray–Dingell proposals: It combined the social insurance and public assistance approaches into one unified program. In part because of the staunch opposition of the AMA and the private insurance industry, the legislation went the way of its predecessors: political defeat.

In 1989, Physicians for a National Health Program offered a new government-financed national health insurance proposal. The plan came to be known as the "single-payer" program, because it would establish a single government fund within each state to pay hospitals, physicians, and other health care providers, replacing the multipayer system of private

insurance companies (Himmelstein & Woolhandler, 1989). Several versions of the single-payer plan were introduced into Congress in the 1990s, each bringing the entire population together into one health care financing system, merging the social insurance and public assistance approaches (Table 15–2). The California Legislature passed a single-payer plan in 2006 and 2008, but the proposals were vetoed by the Governor.

THE EMPLOYER-MANDATE MODEL OF NATIONAL HEALTH INSURANCE

In response to Democratic Senator Kennedy's introduction of the 1970 Health Security Act, President Nixon, a Republican, countered with a plan of his own, the nation's first employment-based, privately administered national health insurance proposal. For 3 years, the Nixon and Kennedy approaches competed in the congressional battleground; however, because most of the population was covered under private insurance, Medicare, or Medicaid, there was relatively little public pressure on Congress. In 1974, the momentum for national health insurance collapsed, not to be seriously revived until the 1990s. The essence of the Nixon proposal was the employer mandate, under which the federal government requires (or mandates) employers to purchase private health insurance for their employees.

Table 15–2. Categories of national health insurance plans

1. Government-financed health insurance plans	Money is collected through taxes or premiums by a public or quasipublic fund that pays health care providers
2. Employer-mandated private health insurance plans	The government requires employers to pay for all or part of private health insurance policies for their employees
3. Individual-mandated private health insurance plans	The government requires individuals to purchase private health insurance, with subsidies for low-income people
4. Hybrid plans	Government-financed insurance for the elderly and the poor, employer-mandated private insurance for employees of larger businesses and their dependents, individual-mandated private insurance for employees of smaller businesses or the unemployed

Tom Peoples' cousin Blanche was a receptionist in a physician's office in 1971. The physician did not provide health insurance to his employees. Under Nixon's 1971 plan, Blanche's employer would be required to pay 75% of the private health insurance premium for his employees; the employees would pay the other 25%.

Blanche's boyfriend, Al, had been laid off from his job in 1970 and was receiving unemployment benefits. He had no health insurance. Under Nixon's proposal, the federal government would pay a portion of Al's health insurance premium.

No longer was national health insurance equated with government financing. Employer mandate plans preserve and enlarge the role of the private health insurance industry rather than replacing it with tax-financed government-administered plans. The Nixon proposal changed the entire political landscape of national health insurance, moving it toward the private sector.

Between 1980 and 2010, the number of people in the United States without health insurance rose from 25 million to 50 million (see Chapter 3). Approximately three-quarters of the uninsured were employed or dependents of employed persons. In response to this crisis, President Clinton submitted legislation to Congress in 1993 calling for universal health insurance through an employer mandate. Like the Nixon proposal, the essence of the Clinton plan was the requirement that employers pay for most of their employees' private insurance premiums. The proposal failed.

A variation on the employer mandate type of national health insurance is the voluntary approach. Rather than requiring employers to purchase health insurance for employees, employers are given incentives such as tax credits to cover employees voluntarily. The attempt of some states to implement this type of voluntary approach failed to significantly reduce the numbers of uninsured workers.

THE INDIVIDUAL-MANDATE MODEL OF NATIONAL HEALTH INSURANCE

In 1989, a new species of national health insurance appeared, sponsored by the conservative Heritage Foundation: the individual mandate. Just as many states require motor vehicle drivers to purchase automobile insurance, the Heritage plan called for the federal government to require all US residents to purchase individual health insurance policies. Tax credits would be made available on a sliding scale to individuals and families too poor to afford health insurance premiums (Butler, 1991). Under the most ambitious versions of the individual mandate, employer-sponsored insurance and government-administered insurance would be dismantled and replaced by a universal, individual mandate program. Ironically, the individual insurance mandate shares at least one feature with the single-payer, government-financed approach to universal coverage: Both would sever the connection between employment and health insurance, allowing portability and continuity of coverage as workers moved from one employer to another or became self-employed.

Tom Peoples received health insurance through his employer, Great Books. Under an individual mandate plan, Tom would be legally required to purchase health insurance for his family. Great Books could offer a health plan to Tom and his coworkers but would not be required to contribute anything to the premium. If Tom purchased private health insurance for his family at a cost of $10,000 per year, he would receive a tax credit of $4,000 (i.e., he would pay $4,000 less in income taxes). Tom's Uncle Marvin, formerly on Medicaid, would be given a voucher to purchase a private health insurance policy.

With individual mandate health insurance, the tax credits may vary widely in their amount depending on characteristics such as household income and how much of a subsidy the architects of individual mandate proposals build into the plan. Under most proposals, a family might receive a $4,000 tax credit for a $10,000 premium, subsidizing less than half of the premium's cost. Another version of individual health insurance expansion is the voluntary concept, supported by President George W. Bush during his presidency. Uninsured individuals would not be required to purchase individual insurance but would receive a tax credit if they chose to purchase insurance. The tax credits in the Bush plan were small compared to the cost of most health insurance policies, with the result that these voluntary approaches would have convinced few uninsured people to purchase coverage.

▶ The Massachusetts Individual Mandate Plan of 2006

Nearly 20 years after the Heritage Foundation's individual mandate proposal, Massachusetts enacted a state-level health coverage bill implementing the nation's first individual mandate. The Massachusetts plan, enacted under Republican Governor Mitt Romney, mandated that every state resident must have health insurance meeting a minimum standard set by the state or pay a penalty. The law provided state subsidies for purchase of private health insurance coverage to individuals with incomes below 300% of the federal poverty level if they are not covered by Medicaid or through employment-based insurance. The law did not eliminate existing employer-based or government insurance programs for those already covered by those mechanisms.

Following enactment of the Massachusetts Plan, the uninsurance rate among nonelderly adults in the state dropped from 14% in 2006 to 3.7% in 2014 (Skopec & Long, 2015). Some residents of Massachusetts continued to have trouble affording private insurance even with some degree of state subsidy, and the high levels of cost-sharing allowed under the minimum benefit standards left many insured individuals with substantial out-of-pocket payments. The Massachusetts Plan set the stage for a national plan enacted under the sponsorship of Barack Obama after his election as President in 2008.

THE PLURALISTIC REFORM MODEL: THE AFFORDABLE CARE ACT OF 2010

Following a year-long bitter debate, the Democrat-controlled House of Representatives and Senate passed the Affordable Care Act (ACA) without a single Republican vote in favor. President Obama, on March 23, 2010, signed the most significant health legislation since Medicare and Medicaid in 1965 (Morone, 2010). Although the ACA was attacked as "socialized medicine" and a "government takeover of health care," its policy pedigree derives much more from the proposals of a Republican President (Nixon), a Republican Governor (Romney), and a conservative think tank (the Heritage Foundation) than from the single-payer national health insurance tradition of Democratic Presidents Roosevelt and Truman. The pluralistic

financing model of the ACA includes individual and employer mandates for private insurance and an expansion of the publicly financed Medicaid program (see Chapter 2).

In 2013, Mandy Must, a single mother of 2 children working for a small shipping company in Houston that did not offer health insurance benefits, was uninsured. In 2014, Mandy earned $35,000 per year and was required by the ACA to obtain private insurance coverage. She received a federal subsidy of $9,000 toward her purchase of an individual insurance policy with an annual premium cost of $12,000.

Mandy's older sister Dorothy Woent was a self-employed accountant with no dependents living in Dallas and earning $48,000 a year. She did not have health insurance, and at her income level was not eligible for a federal subsidy to purchase an individual insurance policy. She would have to pay $5,500 annually to purchase a qualifying health plan that included a $5,000 annual deductible. In 2014, Dorothy was in good health and having trouble paying the mortgage on her house. She decided not to enroll in a health insurance plan and instead paid a $695 fine to the federal government for not complying with the ACA's individual mandate. In 2019, she was relieved to learn that these fines had been discontinued.

In 2013, Walter Groop worked full-time as a salesperson for a large department store in Miami which did not offer health insurance benefits to its workers. In 2014, he began to apply for an individual policy to meet the requirements of the ACA, but his employer informed him that the department store would start contributing toward group health insurance coverage for its employees to avoid paying penalties under the ACA.

In 2013, Job Knaught had been an unemployed construction worker in Chicago for over 18 months and, aside from an occasional odd job, had no regular source of income. Because he was not disabled, he did not qualify for Medicaid prior to the ACA despite being poor. In 2014, Job became eligible for Illinois' expanded Medicaid program.

As a result of the ACA, the number of uninsured Americans dropped from 50 million in 2010 to 28 million in 2017 (see Chapter 3). Yet the ACA has weathered recurring storms since its enactment.

2017–2019: Undermining the ACA

From 2011 to 2017, the Republican-controlled House of Representatives voted 70 times to repeal all or parts of the law. The final legislative attempt to cripple the ACA was a bill passed in the House in the summer of 2017. In a dramatic 2 AM July 27, 2017, 51–49 vote in the Senate, moderate Republican Senator John McCain, soon to die from brain cancer, cast the deciding vote against the bill.

One legislative effort to undermine the ACA succeeded: the December 2017 passage of the Tax Cuts and Jobs Act eliminated the tax penalty to be paid by uninsured persons who failed to enroll in an individual health insurance plan. This effectively ended the individual insurance mandate because the requirement to purchase health insurance could no longer be enforced. As a result, healthy people whose enrollment is important to keep down insurance premiums will increasingly forgo health insurance which could make insurance less affordable. The Trump Administration made it easier for healthy people to reject ACA insurance by allowing low-cost, low-benefit plans to complete with the ACA insurance exchanges. These plans can deny insurance to people with pre-existing illnesses.

When the 2018 election gave Democrats control over the House of Representatives, legislative efforts to repeal the ACA ended. However, the Trump Administration, which came to power in 2017, has continued to undermine Obamacare administratively. On his first day in office, the new President issued an executive order to Federal agencies to waive, defer, and delay implementation of the law. Information and outreach to assist people to sign up for Obamacare was curtailed resulting in half a million fewer people enrolling in health insurance plans. The 2018 open enrollment period was cut in half. The government launched videos detailing problems patients were having with the ACA (Rovner, 2018). Between 2016 and 2018, the number of children with health insurance dropped by 400,000 (Goodnough and Sanger-Katz,

2019). The federal subsidies to reduce deductibles and copayments for low-income people ended. The proposed 2020 budget would drastically cut Medicaid funds, thereby forcing states to disenroll millions of Medicaid beneficiaries. A Senate bill supported by the President would end the ACA's insurance subsidies and Medicaid expansion.

The attack on the ACA has also been active in the courts. In June 2012, the Supreme Court failed to declare the entire law unconstitutional, but did rule that the ACA could not require states to expand their Medicaid programs, making Medicaid expansion optional for states. Most states with Republican governors and/or Republican controlled legislatures refused to expand Medicaid, leaving millions of low-income Americans uninsured. A new legal attack was mounted in 2018 when 20 states filed a lawsuit again alleging that the entire ACA is unconstitutional. A Texas judge ruled in favor of the lawsuit, which is likely to arrive at the Supreme Court sometime in 2020.

Fifty-three percent of the public had a favorable opinion of the ACA in November 2018, with 40% unfavorable, a substantial increase in support for the ACA. Whether the increasing premiums, deductibles, and copayments will erode this support remains to be seen. Whatever the public thinks, the fate of the ACA depends on the decisions of the Supreme Court and the outcome of the 2020 election. The ACA could survive or come to an end.

2017–2019: Resurgence of the Single Payer Concept

While all national health insurance proposals prior to 1971 were government-financed "single-payer" plans, these plans were largely relegated to the sidelines until the era of the ACA. Because the ACA increasingly burdens its enrollees with high deductibles and copayments, and because the ACA's future is in jeopardy, many political figures in the Democratic Party are proclaiming that the ACA is only a first step and now is the time to take the next step toward government-financed health insurance. In 2019, the single-payer concept has taken on a more popular name: Medicare for All, since the public knows and overwhelmingly supports Medicare. Under this proposal, the entire population would become enrolled in the Medicare program over time, perhaps starting the process by reducing the Medicare eligibility age from 65 to 55. In April 2019 public opinion polling, 56% favored Medicare for All with 38% opposed. However, most people want to retain the choice to keep their private insurance, which a pure Medicare for All plan would not allow (Kaiser Family Foundation, 2019).

A compromise between improving the ACA vs Medicare for All is the "public option," which allows people to choose between their existing private insurance and a government-run plan, which likely would be Medicare. Individuals through the ACA, or individuals or families with employer-based insurance, could choose to enroll in Medicare rather than in a private insurance plan. Through the ACA, lower-income families would continue to receive a premium subsidy whether they opted for private insurance or Medicare. The 2020 presidential election is highlighting a major debate over these proposals (Sanger-Katz, 2019).

SECONDARY FEATURES OF NATIONAL HEALTH INSURANCE PLANS

The primary distinction among national health insurance approaches is the mode of financing: government versus employment-based versus individual-based health insurance, or a mixture of all three. But while the overall financing approach is the headline news of reform proposals, details in the fine print are important in determining whether a universal coverage plan will be able to deliver true health security to the public (Table 15–3). What are some of these secondary features?

▶ Benefit Package

An important feature of any health plan is its benefit package. Most national health insurance proposals cover hospital care, physician visits, laboratory, x-rays, physical and occupational therapy, pharmacy, and other services usually emphasizing acute care. Mental health services were often not fully covered, a situation in part addressed by the Mental Health Parity Act of 1996 and Mental Health Parity and Addiction Equity Act of 2008 which apply to group private health insurance plans. Neither the ACA nor most previous reform proposals include comprehensive benefits for dental

Table 15–3. Features of national health insurance plans

Primary Feature	
How the plan is financed	Government, employer mandate, and/or individual mandate?
Secondary Features	
Benefit package	Which services are covered?
Patient cost-sharing	Will there still be considerable amounts of out-of-pocket payments in the form of patient share of premiums, and deductibles and copayments at the point of service?
Effect on existing programs	Do Medicare, Medicaid, and private insurance arrangements continue in their current form or are they largely dismantled?
Cost containment	Are cost controls introduced, and, if so, what type of controls?
Delivery system reform	Is only health care financing addressed, or does the plan call for changes in the organization and structure for delivering care?

care, long-term care, or complementary medicine services such as acupuncture.

▶ Patient Cost-Sharing

Patient cost-sharing involves payments made by patients at the time of receiving medical care. It is sometimes broadened to include the amount of health insurance premium paid directly by an individual. The breadth of the benefit package influences the amount of patient cost-sharing: the more the services are not covered, the more the patients must pay out of pocket. Many plans impose patient cost-sharing requirements on covered services, usually in the form of deductibles (a lump sum each year), coinsurance payments (a percentage of the cost of the service), or copayments (a fixed fee, e.g., $20 per visit or per prescription). In general, single payer proposals restrict cost-sharing to minimal levels, financing most benefits from taxes. In comparison, the individual mandate provisions of the ACA include high levels of cost-sharing (Chapter 3). Critics have argued that this degree of out-of-pocket payment raises questions about whether the "Affordable" Care Act (ACA) is a misnomer and that people of modest incomes are seriously underinsured. The arguments against cost-sharing as a cost-containment tool are discussed in Chapter 9.

Effects on Medicare, Medicaid, and Private Insurance

Any national health insurance program must interact with existing health care programs, whether Medicare, Medicaid, or private insurance plans. Single-payer proposals make far-reaching changes: Medicaid and private insurance are eliminated in their current form and melded into a single insurance program that resembles a Medicare-type program for all Americans. The most sweeping versions of individual mandate plans, proposed by the Heritage Foundation, would dismantle both employment-based private insurance and government-administered insurance programs. Employer mandates, which extend rather than supplant employment-based coverage, have the least effect on existing dollar flows in the health care system, as do pluralistic models such as the ACA that preserve and extend existing financing models through the employer mandates and broadened Medicaid eligibility.

Cost Containment

By increasing access to medical care, national health insurance has the capacity to cause a rapid rise in national health expenditures, as did Medicare and Medicaid (see Chapter 2). By the 1990s, policymakers recognized that access gains must be balanced with cost control measures.

National health insurance proposals have vastly disparate methods of containing costs (see Chapter 9). As noted above, individual- and employment-based proposals tend to use patient cost-sharing as their chief cost-control mechanism. In contrast, government-financed plans look to global budgeting and regulation of fees to keep expenditures down. Single-payer plans, which concentrate health care funds in a single public insurer, can more easily establish a global budgeting approach than can approaches with multiple private insurers.

Proposals that build on the existing pluralistic financing model of US health care, such as the ACA, face challenges in taming the unrelenting increases in

health expenditures endemic to a fragmented financing system. An item contributing to the demise of President Bill Clinton's health reform proposal was a measure to cap annual increases in private health insurance premiums. President Obama eschewed such a regulatory approach in developing the ACA, resulting in weak language about private insurance plans needing to "justify" premium increases to participate in health insurance exchanges. In an effort to control costs, the ACA limits the percentage of health insurance premiums that can be retained by an insurance company in the form of overhead and profits (a concept known as the "medical loss ratio," whereby a greater loss ratio means more premium dollars being "lost" by the company in payments for actual health care services). The ACA also intended to cap the amount that an employer can contribute toward a health insurance premium as a nontaxable benefit to the employee ($10,200 for an individual policy and $27,500 for a family policy), in an attempt to discourage enrollment in the most expensive plans, but this provision has been delayed until at least 2022. Many savings in the ACA are expected to come from slowing the rate of growth in expenditures for Medicare through measures such as reducing payments to Medicare Advantage plans. The architects of the ACA put most of their cost-containment hopes in proposals to redesign health care delivery to achieve better value, discussed next.

Reform of Health Care Delivery

Throughout the history of US national health insurance proposals, reformers viewed their primary goal as modifying the methods of financing health care to achieve universal coverage. Addressing how providers were paid often emerged as a closely related consideration because of its importance for making universal coverage affordable. However, intervening in health care delivery did not feature prominently in reform proposals. Reformers were loath to antagonize the AMA and hospital associations by challenging professional sovereignty over health care organization and delivery. Even advocates of single payer reform in the United States looked to the lessons of government insurance in Canadian provinces, where until recently government took great pains to focus on insurance financing and payment rate regulation and not on care delivery reform.

The ACA goes farther than previous reform efforts in proposing measures to shape health care delivery. The ACA created and funded an Innovation Center in the Centers for Medicare and Medicaid Services to spearhead care redesign, including the promotion of Accountable Care Organizations. As discussed in Chapter 6, Accountable Care Organizations are intended to be provider-organized systems for delivering care that seek the ideal of higher quality at lower cost by emphasizing more integrated and coordinated models of care for defined populations of patients, along with financial incentives rewarding higher value care. However, up through 2014, Medicare ACOs authorized by the ACA had not achieved the cost reductions they hoped for (Markovitz et al., 2019).

WHICH FINANCING MODEL FOR NATIONAL HEALTH INSURANCE PLAN IS BEST?

Historically, in the United States, the government-financed single payer road to national health insurance is the oldest and most traveled of the three approaches. Advocates of government financing cite its universality: Everyone is insured in the same plan simply by virtue of being a US resident. Its simplicity creates a potential cost saving: The 31% of health expenditures spent on administration could be reduced, thus making available funds to extend health insurance to the uninsured (Woolhandler et al., 2003). Employers would be relieved of the burden of providing health insurance to their employees. Employees would regain free choice of physician, choice that is being lost as employers are choosing which health plans (and therefore which physicians) are available to their employees. Health insurance would be delinked from jobs, so that people changing jobs or losing a job would not be forced to change or lose their health coverage. Single-payer advocates, citing the experience of other nations, argue that cost control works only when all health care moneys are channeled through a single mechanism with the capacity to set budgets (Woolhandler & Himmelstein, 2019). While opponents accuse the government-financed approach as an invitation to bureaucracy, single-payer advocates point out that private insurers have average administrative costs of 14%, far higher

than government programs such as Medicare with its 2% administrative overhead. A cost-control advantage intrinsic to tax-financed systems in which a public agency serves as the single payer for health care is the administrative efficiency of collecting and dispensing revenues under this arrangement.

Single-payer detractors charge that one single government payer would have too much power over people's health choices, dictating to physicians and patients which treatments they can receive and which they cannot, resulting in waiting lines and the rationing of care. Millions of people would lose the private insurance that they like. Opponents also state that the shift in health care financing from private payments (out of pocket, individual insurance, and employment-based insurance) to taxes would be unacceptable in an antitax society. Moreover, the United States has a long history of politicians and government agencies being overly influenced by wealthy private interests, and this has contributed to making the public mistrustful of the government.

The employer mandate approach—requiring all employers to pay for the health insurance of their employees—is seen by its supporters as the most logical way to raise enough funds to insure the uninsured without massive tax increases (though employer mandates have been called hidden taxes). Because most people younger than 65 years now receive their health insurance through the workplace, it may be less disruptive to extend this process rather than change it.

The conservative advocates of individual-based insurance and the liberal supporters of single-payer plans both criticize employer mandate plans, saying that forcing small businesses—many of whom do not insure their employees—to shoulder the fiscal burden of insuring the uninsured is inequitable and economically disastrous; rather than purchasing health insurance for their employees, many small businesses may simply lay off workers, thereby pitting health insurance against jobs. Moreover, because millions of people change their jobs in a given year, job-linked health insurance is administratively cumbersome and insecure for employees, whose health security is tied to their job. Finally, critics point out that under the employer mandate approach, "Your boss, not your family, chooses your physician"; changes in the health plans offered by employers often force employees and their families to change physicians, who may not belong to the health plans being offered.

Advocates of the individual mandate assert that their approach, if adopted as the primary means of financing coverage, would free employers of the obligation to provide health insurance, and would grant individuals a stable source of health insurance whether they are employed, change jobs, or become disabled. There would be no need either to burden small businesses with new expenses and thereby disrupt job growth or to raise taxes substantially. While opponents argue that low-income families would be unable to afford the mandatory purchase of health insurance, supporters claim that income-related subsidies (as in the ACA) are a fair and effective method to assist such families.

The individual mandate approach is criticized as inefficient, with each family having to purchase its own health insurance. To enforce a requirement that every person buy coverage could be even more difficult for health insurance than for automobile insurance. Moreover, to reduce the price of their premiums, many families would purchase high-deductible plans with high cost-sharing, leaving lower- and middle-income families with unaffordable out-of-pocket costs.

CONCLUSION

The concept of national health insurance rests on the belief that everyone should contribute to finance health care and everyone should benefit. People who pay more than they benefit are likely to benefit more than they pay years down the road when they face an expensive health problem. In the years during and after the passage of the ACA, national health insurance took center stage in the United States with fierce debate over "Obamacare." This debate revealed a wide gulf between those who believe that all people should have financial access to health care and those who do not share this belief. The fate of the ACA, still in question in 2019, will determine which of those two beliefs holds sway in the United States.

REFERENCES

Bodenheimer T, Grumbach K. Financing universal health insurance: taxes, premiums, and the lessons of social insurance. *J Health Polit Policy Law*. 1992;17:439–462.

Butler SM. A tax reform strategy to deal with the uninsured. *JAMA*. 1991;265:2541–2544.

Goodnough A, Sanger-Katz M. Number of uninsured children rose 400,000, eroding gains. *New York Times*. October 23, 2019.

Himmelstein DU, Woolhandler S. A national health program for the United States: a physicians' proposal. *N Engl J Med*. 1989;320:102–108.

Kaiser Family Foundation. Tracking Public Opinion on National Health Plan. April 24, 2019. https://www.kff.org/health-costs/poll-finding/kff-health-tracking-poll-april-2019/. Accessed October 25, 2019.

Markovitz AA, et al. Performance in the Medicare Shared Savings Program after accounting for nonrandom exit. *Ann Intern Med*. 2019;171:27–36.

Morone J. Presidents and health reform: from Franklin D. Roosevelt to Barack Obama. *Health Aff (Millwood)*. 2010;29:1096–1100.

Rovner J. Timeline: despite GOP's failure to repeal Obamacare, the ACA has changed. *Kaiser Health News*. April 5, 2018.

Sanger-Katz M. The difference between a public option and Medicare for all. *New York Times*. February 19, 2019.

Skopec L, Long SK. Findings from the 2014 Massachusetts Health Insurance Survey, May 2015. SHADAC › sites › default › files › MA_2014_HH_findings. Accessed October 25, 2019.

Starr P. *The Social Transformation of American Medicine*. New York, NY: Basic Books; 1982.

Woolhandler S, et al. Costs of health care administration in the United States and Canada. *N Engl J Med*. 2003;349:768–775.

Woolhandler S, Himmelstein DU. Single-payer reform—"Medicare for all". *JAMA*. 2019;321:2399–2400.

Conflict and Change in America's Health Care System

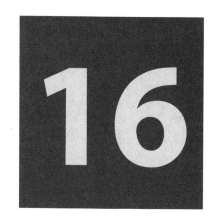

As this book enters its closing chapters, we step back from the details of the US health care system to view the system as a larger whole. Who are the major actors? How have they interacted over the past few decades? What might the future bring?

THE FOUR MAJOR ACTORS

The health care sector of the nation's economy is a 3.5 trillion dollar system that finances, organizes, and provides health care services for the people of the United States. Four major actors can be found on this stage (Table 16–1).

1. The *purchasers* supply the funds. These include individual health care consumers, businesses that pay for the health insurance of their employees, and the government, which pays for care through public programs such as Medicare and Medicaid and through various tax subsidies. All purchasers of health care are ultimately individuals, because individuals finance businesses by purchasing their products and fund the government by paying taxes. Nonetheless, businesses and the government assume special importance as the nation's *organized* purchasers of health care.

2. The *insurers* receive money from the purchasers and pay the providers. Traditional insurers take money from purchasers (individuals or businesses), assume risk, and pay providers when policyholders require medical care. Yet some insurers are the same as purchasers; the government can be viewed as an insurer or purchaser in the Medicare and Medicaid programs, and businesses that self-insure their employees can similarly occupy both roles. (In previous chapters, the term "payer" refers to both purchasers and insurers.)

3. The *providers*, including hospitals, physicians, Accountable Care Organizations (ACOs), nurses, nurse practitioners, physician assistants, pharmacists, social workers, nursing homes, home care agencies, and pharmacies, among others, actually provide the care.

4. The *suppliers* are the pharmaceutical, medical supply, and computer industries, which manufacture equipment, supplies, electronic health records, and medications used by providers to treat patients.

Insurers, providers, and suppliers make up the health care industry. Each dollar spent on health care represents an expense to the purchasers and income to the health care industry. In the past, purchasers viewed this expense as an investment, money spent to improve the health of the population and thereby the economic and social vitality of the nation. But over the past 40 years, a fundamental conflict has intensified between the purchasers and the health care industry: The purchasers wish to reduce, and the health care industry to increase, the number of dollars spent on health care. We will now explore the changing relationships among purchasers, insurers, providers, and suppliers (Table 16–2).

Table 16–1. The four major actors

Purchasers
- Individuals
- Employers
- Government

Insurers

Providers
- Hospitals
- Nursing homes
- Home care agencies
- Pharmacies
- Physicians
- Other caregivers

Suppliers
- Pharmaceutical companies
- Pharmacy benefit managers (PBMs)
- Medical supply companies
- Computer equipment and software vendors

Table 16–2. Historical overview of US health care

1945–1970: provider–insurer pact
- Independent hospitals and small private practices
- Many private insurers
- Providers tended to dominate the insurers, especially in Blue Cross and Blue Shield
- Purchasers (individuals, businesses, and, after 1965, government) had relatively little power
- Payments for providers were generous

The 1970s: tensions develop
- Purchasers (especially government) become concerned about costs of health care
- Under pressure from purchasers, insurers begin to question generous payments of providers

The 1980s: revolt of the purchasers
- Purchasers (business joining government) become very concerned with rising health care costs
- Attempts are made to reduce health cost inflation through Medicare DRGs, fee schedules, capitated HMOs, and selective contracting

The 1990s: breakup of the provider–insurer pact
- Spurred by the purchasers, selective contracting spreads widely as a mechanism to reduce costs
- Price competition is introduced
- Large integrated health networks are formed
- Large physician groups emerge
- Insurance companies dominate many managed care markets
- For-profit institutions increase in importance
- Insurers gain increasing power over providers, creating conflict and ending the provider–insurer pact

The new millennium: resurgence of provider and supplier power
- HMOs fade in importance
- Hospitals consolidate into hospital systems, forcing insurers to pay them more
- Insurers respond by consolidating, with a few large national insurers dominating many markets
- Many specialists form single specialty groups
- Specialists move profitable procedures out of hospitals into specialist-owned centers
- Pharmaceutical companies and pharmacy benefit managers earn huge profits
- Less uninsurance and more underinsurance

Approaching 2020: The four actors lose their identity
- Cross-sector vertical consolidation brings insurers, providers, and suppliers together into huge conglomerates.

THE YEARS 1945 TO 1970: THE PROVIDER–INSURER PACT

Independent hospitals and small private physician offices populated the US health delivery system (see Chapter 6). Some large institutions combined hospital and physician care (e.g., the Kaiser–Permanente system, the Mayo Clinic, and urban medical school complexes) (Starr, 1982). Competition among health care providers was minimal because most geographic areas did not have an excess of facilities and personnel. The health care financing system included hundreds of private insurance companies, joined by the governmental Medicare and Medicaid programs enacted in 1965. The United States had a relatively dispersed health care industry.

Bert Neighbor was a 63-year-old man, who developed abdominal pain in 1962. Because he was well insured under Blue Cross, his physician placed him in Metropolitan Hospital for diagnostic studies. On the sixth hospital day, a colon cancer was surgically removed. On the 15th day, Mr. Neighbor went home. The hospital sent its $1,200 bill to Blue Cross, which paid the entire bill. In calculating Mr. Neighbor's bill, Metropolitan Hospital included

part of the cost of the 80-bed new building under construction.

At a subsequent meeting of the Blue Cross board of directors, the hospital administrator (also a Blue

*Cross director) was asked whether it was reason-
able to include the cost of capital improvements
when preparing a bill. Other Blue Cross directors, also hospital administrators with construction plans, argued that it was proper, and the
matter was dropped. In the same meeting, the
directors voted a 34% increase in Blue Cross premiums. Sixteen years later, a study revealed that
the metropolitan area had 300 excess hospital
beds, with hospital occupancy down from 82%
to 60%.*

A defining characteristic of the health care
industry was an alliance of insurers and providers.
This provider–insurer pact was cemented with the
creation of Blue Cross and Blue Shield, the nation's
largest health insurance system for half a century (see
Chapter 2). Blue Cross was formed by the American
Hospital Association, and Blue Shield was run by state
medical societies affiliated with the American Medical
Association. In the case of the Blues, the provider–
insurer relationship was more than a political alliance;
it involved legal control of insurers by providers. As in
the example of Metropolitan Hospital, the providers
set generous rules of payment, and the Blues made the
payments without asking too many questions (Law,
1974). Commercial insurers usually played by the same
payment rules.

By the 1960s, the power of the provider–insurer
pact was so great that the hospitals and Blue Cross
virtually wrote the provider payment provisions of
Medicare and Medicaid, guaranteeing that physicians
and hospitals would be well paid (Law, 1974). With
open-ended payment policies, the costs of health care
inflated at a rapid pace.

The disinterest of the chief organized purchaser
(business) stemmed from two sources: the healthy
economy and the tax subsidy for health insurance.
From 1945 through 1970, US business controlled
domestic and foreign markets with little foreign competition. Labor unions in certain industries had gained
generous wages and fringe benefits, and business could
afford these costs because profits were high and world
economic growth was robust (Kuttner, 1980; Kennedy,
1987). The cost of health insurance for employees was
a tiny fraction of total business expenses. Moreover,
payments by business for employee health insurance

were considered a tax-deductible business expense,
thereby cushioning any economic drain on business
(Reinhardt, 1993). For these reasons, increasing costs
generated by providers and paid by insurers were
passed on to business, which with few complaints paid
higher and higher premiums for employees' health
insurance, and thereby underwrote the expanding
health care system. No countervailing forces put the
brakes on the enthusiasm that united providers and the
public in support of a medical industry that strived to
translate the proliferation of biomedical breakthroughs
into an improvement in people's lives.

THE 1970S: TENSIONS DEVELOP

*Jerry Neighbor, Bert Neighbor's son, developed
abdominal pain in 1978. Because Blue Cross no
longer paid for in-hospital diagnostic testing, his
physician ordered outpatient x-ray studies. When
colon cancer was discovered, Jerry Neighbor was
admitted to Metropolitan Hospital on the morning
of his surgery. His total hospital stay was 9 days,
6 days shorter than his father's stay in 1962.
Since 1962, medical care costs had risen by
approximately 10% per year. Blue Cross paid
Metropolitan Hospital $460 for each of the 9 days
Jerry Neighbor spent in the hospital, for a total
cost of $4,140. The Blue Cross board of directors,
which in 1977 included for the first time more
business than hospital representatives, submitted
a formal proposal to the regional health planning
agency to reduce the number of hospital beds in
the region, in order to keep hospital costs down.
The planning agency board had a majority of
hospital and physician representatives, and they
voted the proposal down.*

In the early 1970s, the United States fell from its post-
war position of economic dominance, as Western
Europe and Japan gobbled up markets (not only abroad
but in the United States itself) formerly controlled by
US companies. The United States' share of world industrial production was dropping, from 60% in 1950 to
30% in 1980. Except for a few years during the mid-
1980s, inflation or unemployment plagued the United
States from 1970 until the early 1990s.

The new economic reality was a critical motor of
change in the health care system. With less money in

their respective pockets, individual health care consumers, business, and government became concerned with the accelerating flow of dollars into health care. Prominent business-oriented journals published major critiques of the health care industry and its rising costs (Bergthold, 1990). These developments produced tensions within the health industry itself.

Faced with Blue Cross premium increases of 25% to 50% in a single year, Blue Cross subscribers protested at state hearings in eastern and midwestern states and challenged hospital control over Blue Cross boards (Law, 1974). Some state governments began to regulate hospital construction, and a few states initiated hospital rate regulation. The federal government established a network of health planning agencies, in an attempt to slow hospital growth. Thus, the purchasers took on an additional role as health care regulators. But the health care industry resisted these attempts by purchasers to control health care costs. Medical inflation continued at a rate far above that of inflation in the general economy (Starr, 1982).

Nonetheless, these early initiatives from the purchasers made an impact on the provider–insurer pact. As pressure mounted on insurers not to increase premiums, insurers demanded that services be provided at lower cost. Blue Cross legally separated from the American Hospital Association in 1972 (Law, 1974). State medical societies were forced to relinquish some of their control over Blue Shield plans. Conflicts erupted between providers and insurers as the latter imposed utilization review procedures to reduce the length of hospital stays. Hospitals, which had hitherto purchased the newest diagnostic and surgical technology desired by physicians or their medical staff, began to deny such requests because insurers would no longer guarantee their reimbursement. Moreover, the glut of hospital beds and specialty physicians, which had been produced by the attractive payments of the 1960s and the influence of the biomedical model on medical education (see Chapter 5), turned on itself as half-empty hospitals and half-busy surgeons began to compete with one another for patients. Strains were showing within the provider–insurer pact. But major change was awaiting the arrival of the powerful purchaser: business.

THE 1980s: THE REVOLT OF THE PURCHASERS

In 1989, Ryan Neighbor, Jerry Neighbor's brother, became concerned when he noticed blood in his stools; he decided to see a physician. Six months earlier, his company had increased the annual health insurance deductible to $1,000, which could be avoided by joining one of the HMOs offered by the company. Ryan Neighbor opted for the Blue Cross HMO, but his family physician was not involved in that HMO, and Mr. Neighbor had to pick another physician from the HMO's list. The physician diagnosed colon cancer; Ryan Neighbor was not allowed to see the surgeon who had operated on his brother but was sent to a Blue Cross HMO surgeon. While Mr. Neighbor respected Metropolitan Hospital, his surgery was scheduled at Crosstown Hospital; Blue Cross had refused to sign a contract with Metropolitan when the hospital failed to negotiate down from its $1,800 per diem rate. Ryan Neighbor's entire Crosstown Hospital stay was 5 days, and the HMO paid the hospital $7,500, based on its $1,500 per diem contract.

The late 1980s produced a severe shock: The cost of employer-sponsored health plans jumped 18.6% in 1988 and 20.4% in 1989 (Cantor et al., 1991). Between 1976 and 1988, the percentage of total payroll spent on health benefits almost doubled from 5% to 9.7% (Bergthold, 1991). In another development, many large corporations began to self-insure. Rather than paying money to insurance companies to cover their employees, employers increasingly took on the health insurance function themselves and used insurance companies only for claims processing and related administrative tasks. In 1991, 40% of employees receiving employer-sponsored health benefits were in self-insured plans. Self-insurance placed employers at risk for health care expenditures and forced them to pay more attention to the health care issue (Bergthold, 1990). Business, the major private purchaser of health care, threw its clout behind managed care, particularly HMOs, as a cost-control device. By shifting from fee-for-service to capitated reimbursement, managed care could transfer a portion of the health expenditure risk from purchasers and insurers to providers (see Chapter 4).

Individual health care consumers, in their role as purchasers, also showed some clout during the late 1980s. Because employers were shifting health care payments to employees, labor unions began to complain about health care costs, and major strikes took place over the issue of health benefits. More than 70% of people polled in a 1992 Louis Harris survey favored health care cost controls. The growing tendency of private health insurers to reduce their risks by dramatic premium increases and policy cancellations for policyholders with chronic illnesses created a series of horror stories in the media that turned health insurance companies into unpopular institutions.

The government, facing a tax revolt and budget deficits, took measures to slow the rising costs of Medicare and Medicaid, with limited success. The 1983 Medicare Prospective Payment System (diagnosis-related groups [DRGs]) reduced the rate of increase of Medicare hospital costs, but outpatient Medicare costs and costs borne by private purchasers escalated in response. In 1989, Medicare physician payments were brought under tighter control (Davis & Burner, 1995). Numerous states scaled back their Medicaid programs, but because of the economic recession and the growing crisis of uninsurance (see Chapter 3), the federal government was forced to expand Medicaid eligibility, and Medicaid costs rose faster than ever before. Governments began to experiment with managed care for Medicare and Medicaid as a cost-control device.

The most significant development of the 1980s was the growth of selective contracting. Purchasers and insurers had usually paid any and all physicians and hospitals. Under selective contracting, purchasers and insurers choose which providers they would pay and which not (Bergthold, 1990). The message of selective contracting was clear: Purchasers and insurers will do business only with providers who keep costs down. Patients like Ryan Neighbor lost free choice of physician because employers could require employees to change health plans and therefore physicians. For the health care industry, selective contracting meant fierce competition for contracts and the crumbling of the provider–insurer pact.

As a result of the purchasers' revolt, managed care became a burgeoning movement in US health care. By 1990, 95% of insured employees were enrolled in some form of managed care plan, including fee-for-service plans with utilization management, preferred provider organizations (PPOs), and HMOs. The growth of managed care plans, especially HMOs, competing against one another for contracts with business and the government, changed the entire political topography of US health care.

THE 1990s: THE BREAKUP OF THE PROVIDER–INSURER PACT

In 1994, Pamela Neighbor, Ryan's cousin, developed constipation. Earlier that year, her law firm had switched from Blue Cross HMO to Apple a Day HMO because the premiums were lower; all employees of the firm were forced to change their physicians. Apple a Day contracted only with Crosstown Hospital, whose rates were lower than those of Metropolitan, resulting in Metropolitan losing patients and closing its doors. Ms. Neighbor's new physician diagnosed colon cancer and arranged for her admission to Crosstown Hospital for surgery. The physician's office was across the street from the now-closed Metropolitan Hospital. Four days before the procedure, a newspaper headline proclaimed that Apple a Day and Crosstown had failed to agree on a contract. The operation was canceled. Pamela Neighbor waited to see what would happen next.

During the 1990s, many metropolitan areas in the United States experienced upheavals of their medical care landscape. Independent hospitals began to merge into hospital systems. In mature managed care markets, three or four health care networks were competing for those patients with private insurance, Medicare, or Medicaid. Selective contracting allowed purchasers and insurers to set payment rates to health care providers. HMOs that demanded higher premiums from employers did not get contracts and lost their enrollees. Providers who demanded higher payment from insurers were cut out of contracts and lost many of their patients.

Selective contracting disorganized rather than organized medical care patterns. With most HMO growth occurring among network model HMOs rather than the structurally integrated prepaid group practice model such as Kaiser Permanente (see Chapter 6), physicians were forced to admit patients from one HMO to one hospital and those from another HMO to a different hospital. Laboratory, x-ray, and specialist services close to a primary care physician's office were sometimes not covered under contracts with that physician's patients' HMO, forcing referrals to be made across town (Anders, 1996).

The 1990s was a period of purchaser dominance over health care. The average annual growth in Medicare expenditures declined from 12% in the early 1990s to zero in 1999 and 2000. On the private side, employers bargained hard with insurers, causing insurance premium annual growth to drop from 13% in 1990 to 3% in 1995 and 1996. In California, the Pacific Business Group on Health, negotiating on behalf of large companies for 400,000 employees, and California Public Employee Retirement System (CalPERS), representing a million public employees, forced HMO premiums to go down during the 1990s. Enrollment in HMO insurance plans grew rapidly in the 1990s, expanding from 40 million enrollees in 1990 to 80 million in 1999.

THE NEW MILLENNIUM: RESURGENCE OF PROVIDER AND SUPPLIER POWER

In 2005, Pamela Neighbor, who was feeling well, made an appointment for her yearly colon cancer follow-up. The IPA in which her physician practiced had recently gone bankrupt and closed its doors. Ms. Neighbor's employer had switched its employees from Apple a Day Insurance Company's HMO product to Apple a Day PPO, allowing patients to access most of the physicians and all the hospitals in town. Ms. Neighbor had a difficult time finding a new primary care physician, and when she found one, it took several weeks to get an appointment. Eventually, a colonoscopy was scheduled at a diagnostic center owned by a group of gastroenterologists. She was diagnosed with a second colon cancer and her primary care physician arranged for her admission to Crosstown Hospital. Ms. Neighbor never saw her primary care physician in the hospital; a surgeon plus a
salaried inpatient physician called a hospitalist cared for Ms. Neighbor during her 4-day hospital stay. Apple a Day paid Crosstown Hospital $7,200, $1,800 per diem.

Several trends characterized the first decade of the 21st century: the counterrevolution by providers, consolidation in the health care market, less uninsurance and more underinsurance, growing power of specialists and specialty services, increasing physician–hospital tensions, an emerging crisis in primary care, and the growing power of the pharmaceutical industry and pharmacy benefit managers.

▶ The Provider Counter-Revolution

The first decade of the 21st century could be called the era of the provider counter-revolution. Hospitals consolidated into hospital systems and demanded large price increases from insurers. From 2000 to 2010, HMO enrollment dropped from 32% to 19% of insured employees and preferred provider organization (PPO) enrollment grew from about 30% to 60% (Claxton et al., 2010). Tightly managed care was faltering.

Negotiations between providers and insurers became increasingly hostile, with one side or the other often refusing to sign contracts. As hospitals and providers gained an upper hand in negotiations with health plans, costs accelerated. Insurance premiums for family coverage went from an average of $6,000 per year in 2000 to almost $14,000 in 2010 (Claxton et al., 2010). At the same time, individuals were stuck with a greater proportion of health care costs. Twenty percent of insured employees, up from 10% in 2006, had deductibles of $1,000 or more for individual coverage. In a typical high-deductible plan, employees paid over $3,000 for their portion of the premium plus a deductible of $4,000 (Claxton et al., 2010). Employees' out-of-pocket health care costs increased 34% from 2004 to 2007 (Gabel et al., 2009).

Large insurers bought up smaller ones and merged with one another. Three huge for-profit insurers—Anthem, UnitedHealthcare, and Aetna—dominated many metropolitan areas. Providers also consolidated. By 2001, 65% of hospitals were members of multi-hospital systems or networks (Bazzoli, 2004), and consolidation intensified in the ensuing two decades. Many cities had only two or three competing hospital systems. Private primary care and specialty practices were acquired by hospital systems hoping to increase their market clout (Iglehart, 2011). (See Chapter 6 for more discussion of the horizontal and vertical forms of provider consolidation.)

The Quest for Profitability and the Growing Power of Specialists and Specialty Services

For-profit insurers and providers increased their dominance in health care. Beginning with the rise in the 1970s of the "medical–industrial complex" (Relman, 2007), for-profits continued to expand their reach. In stark contrast with the consumer cooperative and nonprofit origins of HMOs, nine of the 10 largest HMOs were for-profit by 1994. Already in 1990, 77% of nursing homes and 50% of home health agencies were for-profit. Between 1993 and 1996, more than 100 nonprofit hospitals were taken over by for-profit hospital chains, though several financial scandals slowed down this trend. For-profit hospitals provide less charity care, treat fewer Medicaid patients, have higher administrative costs, and lower quality than nonprofit hospitals (Relman, 2007).

A growing proportion of profitable services—cataract surgery and orthopedic procedures, diagnostic studies such as colonoscopies, and CT or MRI studies—shifted from hospital facilities to physician-owned ambulatory centers. Physicians earn income from both the services they directly provide and the facility's profits. The common practice of physicians referring patients for imaging tests at a facility owned by the same physician is associated with higher volumes of imaging services, increasing costs, and exposing patients to unnecessary radiation (Relman, 2009; Sunshine & Bhargavan, 2010).

Specialists increasingly joined single-specialty groups, with the majority of cardiologists or orthopedists in some cities belonging to a dominant group (Liebhaber & Grossman, 2007). Organized specialists with market power in a local area negotiate for high payment rates from insurers. The income of specialists who offer procedural or imaging services far outpaced earnings for primary care physicians (Bodenheimer et al., 2007). Multispecialty groups, which include primary care physicians and tend to have the best scores on quality report cards, did not grow as much in part

because specialist physicians in multispecialty groups are expected to share their high revenues with primary care physicians who generate lower payments for the group (Casalino et al., 2004; Mehrotra et al., 2006). As discussed in Chapter 5, lucrative payment for procedurally oriented specialty care is one key factor shaping a physician workforce weighted toward nonprimary care fields and a hospital sector filled with tertiary care facilities.

Nonprofit community hospitals responded to competition from specialist physicians by creating "specialty service lines" to attract specialist physicians and well-insured patients to their institutions. To create capacity for these profitable service lines, hospitals de-emphasized traditional medical-surgical wards. Filling a hospital bed with a patient receiving an organ transplant or spine surgery is more financially rewarding than filling the same bed with an elderly patient with pneumonia or heart failure. Strategic planning by hospitals focused on how to maximize the most profitable service lines, rather than how to provide services most needed in the community (Berenson et al., 2006).

Surgeons, diagnostic cardiologists, gastroenterologists, ophthalmologists, and radiologists can successfully run a practice without ever setting foot in a hospital by performing their work in ambulatory centers of which these physicians are owners. Because these specialists no longer need the hospital, they feel little obligation to be on call for hospital emergency departments or for patients in intensive care. Hospitals are forced to pay specialists large sums to provide nighttime emergency department backup or are employing specialists to perform duties formerly done for free. The divorce of physicians from the community hospital is not limited to specialists. The new hospitalist specialty—physicians who care only for hospitalized patients—grew rapidly from 500 in 1997 to 30,000 in 2010. As a result, many primary care physicians are never seen in a hospital, making care coordination difficult (Bodenheimer, 2008).

Pharmaceutical Manufacturers and Pharmacy Benefit Managers

Mega Pharmaceutical Company developed Sugarlow, a new diabetes drug and set the list price as $1,000 for a month supply of 60 pills. Because many other excellent, low-cost diabetes drugs had been on the market for decades, Mega spent $300 *million advertising Sugarlow on TV and another $150 million persuading doctors on its benefits.*

Mega made a deal with Super PBM, a big pharmacy benefits manager company, to place Sugarlow as number 1 on the formularies of the largest insurance companies and Medicare Part D plans—which increased the odds that doctors would prescribe the medication. To pay Super PBM for giving Sugarlow such a favorable formulary placement, Mega offered a rebate to Super PBM of $200 for every 60 pills sold through Super PBM; pharmacies would receive a discount from $1,000 to $800 for the pills and SuperPBM could keep the $200. Mega and Super PBM made large profits within the first year of Sugarlow being on the market as Sugarlow became one of the most widely prescribed diabetic drugs. Mega soon increased the price of Sugarlow to $1,200 for a month supply for pharmacies not using Super PBM.

In 1988, prescription drugs accounted for 5.5% of national health expenditures, and 71% of drug costs were paid out of pocket by individuals. In contrast, by 2017, prescription drug costs had risen to $333.4 billion or 10% of total health expenditures, with 86% covered by employers, insurers, and governmental purchasers (Schulman et al., 2018). The growing cost of pharmaceuticals for the elderly became a major national issue, resulting in the passage of Medicare Part D in 2003 (see Chapter 2).

Companies developing a new brand-name drug enjoy a patent for 20 years from the date the patent application is filed, during which time no other company can produce the same drug. Once the patent expires, generic drug manufacturers can compete by selling the same product at lower prices. To fend off this competition, brand-name manufacturers can make minimal changes in a product and obtain a new patient for that product, thereby extending patents on their brand-name products (Tribble, 2018). Because 89% of drugs prescribed in 2016 were generic, brand-name manufacturers have been acquiring generic companies and generic companies have been merging with one another. The volume of these mergers and acquisitions skyrocketed from 2013 to 2016 (Gagnon & Volesky, 2017). One outcome of this consolidation has

been dramatic increases in prices for many generic drugs. Some generic price hikes became a national scandal; from 2012 to 2017, the cost of pyrimethamine, an important drug for treatment of the opportunistic infection toxoplasmosis, increased from $13.50 to $750 per pill, and nitroglycerin, a widely used medication for heart disease, from $15.91 to $91.76 for one bottle of pills (Wapner, 2019). Per capita spending on prescription drugs increased by 25% from 2014 to 2017 (Kamal et al., 2019).

For years, drug companies have been among the most profitable industries in the United States, in 2015 earning average profits between 15% and 20% of revenues compared with 4% to 9% for large nondrug companies (US Government Accountability Office, 2017). The pharmaceutical industry argues that high drug prices are justified by its expenditures on research and development of new drugs, yet in 2016, the industry spent $26.3 billion on marketing to physicians and TV advertising to patients and demonstrates high profits even after accounting for investment in research and development (Schwartz & Woloshin, 2019). Unlike many nations, the US government does not impose regulated prices on drugs; as a result of drug industry lobbying, the government is not allowed to regulate drug prices under Medicare Part D. In 2018, the industry spent an additional $27.5 million on lobbying (Scutti, 2019).

Pharmacy Benefit Managers

Contributing to the cost of medications is an entity that most health care consumers have never heard of. Pharmacy benefit management companies (PBMs), which appeared in the late 1960s, have become formidable players in the pharmaceutical supply chain.

As explained in the above vignette, insurers (including Medicare Part D plans) have given PBMs the authority to decide whether a particular medication will be on the insurer's formulary and thereby covered by insurance. Getting on formularies is crucial for manufacturers because medications not on formularies will not sell. To persuade PBMs to place their drugs on insurers' formularies, drug companies reduce the drug's price as a discount paid to the PBM. These discounts, which add up to billions of dollars annually, have turned PBMs into highly profitable companies. Moreover, PBMs are paid by insurers to reimburse pharmacies for medications the insurer's patients obtain, yet PBMs pay pharmacies less than what they receive from insurers; this "spread" also increases PBM profits. For example, in Ohio, a Medicaid insurer paid CVS's PBM $224 million more for prescription drugs than the PBM paid the pharmacists who provided the medications. The $224 million was the PBM's spread. In 2017, 3 PBMs—CVS Caremark, Express Scripts, and United Health's Optum—controlled over 85% of the PBM market (Royce et al., 2019; Schulman et al., 2018).

APPROACHING 2020: THE FOUR ACTORS LOSE THEIR IDENTITY

This chapter began by introducing the four major actors on the health care stage (Table 16–1). It was clear who was a purchaser, an insurer, a provider, or a supplier. This is no longer true. In the past, horizontal consolidation took place within each actor's sphere: insurers buying other insurers, hospitals merging into multi-hospital systems. Vertical consolidation took place within the sphere of one actor—providers—with hospitals buying physician practices. But by 2020, the lines separating the four actors were being erased as trans-sector vertical consolidations altered the health care landscape. Actors are merging with one another and non-health companies are entering the health care world.

Insurers Acquiring Providers

In 2017, the nation's largest health insurer, UnitedHealthcare, acquired the DaVita Medical Group for $4.9 billion. DaVita had previously engineered a major horizontal consolidation, acquiring 300 clinics, outpatient surgicenters and urgent care centers. The former DaVita practices are housed within the Optum Division of UnitedHealthcare. Smaller instances of insurers buying medical practices abound (Japson, 2019).

Providers Acquire Insurers

In 2018, the giant pharmacy chain CVS Health purchased Aetna, the nation's third largest health insurer, for $69 billion. This trans-sector vertical consolidation means that the millions of Aetna policyholders will be steered to CVS's 9,800 pharmacies and 1,100 walk-in clinics. CVS and its competitor Walgreens together control between 50% and 75% of the drugstore market in each of the country's 14 largest metropolitan areas, but pharmacy chains like CVS are worried that Amazon will start a lower-cost mail-order prescription business; Aetna could prevent its policyholders from choosing such an Amazon option. Prior to the Aetna deal, CVS was already in the insurance business, operating a stand-alone Medicare Part D prescription drug plan and a Medicare Advantage plan (Johnson & Why, 2017; Morris, 2017). In another possible provider-insurer deal, Walmart, whose stores house a large pharmacy chain and retail clinics, is engaged in talks to acquire Humana, the nation's fifth largest health insurer.

Providers Acquire Suppliers

In 2007, the pharmacy chain CVS acquired Caremark, a large PBM, to become CVS Health. Caremark had posed a threat to brick-and-mortar pharmacies with its mail-order pharmacy business. Today, CVS Caremark is one of the nation's leading pharmacy benefit management (PBM) companies; the PBM steers patients to CVS pharmacies including calling patients using independent drug stores to switch to CVS (Candisky, 2018).

Insurers Acquiring Suppliers

In 2018, the nation's fourth largest health insurer, CIGNA, merged with one of the largest PBMs, Express Scripts (Livingston, 2018). Anthem, the nation's second largest health insurer, announced in 2017 that it will start its own PBM. Anthem had previously used the Express Scripts PBM but broke off their contract claiming that Express Scripts was making windfall profits by not passing along to Anthem its savings from drug discounts (Morse, 2019).

Multiple Functions Within One Company

Optum is the rapidly growing health services company buried inside the nation's largest health insurer, UnitedHealthcare. Optum has built its own huge PBM and has acquired 200 ambulatory surgery centers and 280 urgent care centers. Optum reportedly has

20,000 affiliated physicians and added to its portfolio with UnitedHealthcare's acquisition of Da Vita. As the nation's largest health care consultant, Optum offers population health management, pharmacy benefit management, analytics, and other services to care providers, insurance plans, and government entities through its OptumRx, OptumInsight, and OptumHealth businesses. Optum touches 91 million health care consumers in 75 geographic markets (Morse, 2017).

Non-Health Companies Moving into Health Care

JPMorgan Chase, Berkshire Hathaway, and Amazon embarked in 2018 on a joint venture with the goal of a major overhaul of health care for their million-plus employees. Amazon may move into the online pharmacy business and place retail clinics in the 472 Whole Foods stores owned by Amazon.

In another development, private equity firms are buying physician practices. These firms, with little or no health care experience, are investment management companies that buy and invest in existing businesses. These firms have targeted profitable ophthalmology and orthopedic practices, horizontally merging smaller practices to increase the physicians' bargaining power with insurers. Hoping that shared savings from ACOs will increase primary care profitability, private equity firms are also buying primary care practices (Kutscher, 2015).

THE CHALLENGE

The US health care system is dominated by shifting power relationships among purchasers, insurers, providers, and suppliers. The unstoppable trend is consolidation and the emergence of health care oligopolies. Horizontal consolidation of hospitals and vertical integration of hospitals acquiring physician practices has caused many local areas to be dominated by one or two powerful health systems. Horizontal insurance company mergers have allowed the two largest insurers to control 70% of the market in one-half of all local insurance markets (Gaynor, 2018). The recent conglomeratization of health care with cross-sector vertical integration of insurers, providers, and suppliers, is producing a health care landscape populated by fewer, and much larger, companies. The long historical trend from the 1–2 doctor practice and neighborhood drug store

to the mega-corporation is nearing its apogee. Patients continue to be challenged as health care costs rise and as individuals bear a greater share of those costs.

The drive to make money—whether for physicians, for-profit and nonprofit hospitals, insurers, pharmaceutical companies, or health care conglomerates—increasingly determines what happens in health care. Although, as noted in Chapter 6, integrated health care structures may confer some benefit in promoting improved coordination of care under a population health–oriented model, the driving force behind the high degree of consolidation occurring in the United States is the desire among health care actors to wield greater economic power in the health care marketplace and generate financial returns to investors. The commitment of all health care professionals to the ethical principles of beneficence, nonmaleficence, patient autonomy, and distributive justice is tested on a daily basis in the profit-oriented environment of 21st century health care in America.

Chapter 1 introduced the paradox of excess and deprivation: some people get too little care while others receive too much, which is costly and may be harmful. The 21st century has seen a sharpening of this paradox, with growing income inequality in American society. As noted in Chapter 3, the top 10% of earners received 50% of the nation's total income in 2017 compared with 33% in 1965 (Saez, 2019). The top 10% also controls three-quarters of all the wealth in the United States (Khullar & Chokshi, 2018). Not only is there growing concentration of wealth in the United States, but wealthy individuals are consuming a larger share of health care services. Following enactment of Medicare and Medicaid, the average annual health care expenditures per capita for the poorest 20% of people in the United States increased to a level above that for high-income individuals—consistent with the greater health care needs among low income people. In recent years, average health care expenditures have flipped back to the pre-Medicare and Medicare pattern, with the wealthiest 20% of people in the United States now consuming more health care than individuals in lower income groups. Inequality in the larger society undergirds the paradox of excess and deprivation in health care. Overcoming this paradox remains the fundamental challenge facing the health care system of the United States.

REFERENCES

Anders G. *Health Against Wealth: HMOs and the Breakdown of Medical Trust*. Boston, MA: Houghton Mifflin Company; 1996.

Bazzoli GJ. The corporatization of American hospitals. *J Health Polit Policy Law*. 2004;29:885–905.

Berenson RA, et al. Specialty service lines: salvos in the new medical arms race. *Health Aff (Millwood)*. 2006;25(5): w337–w343.

Bergthold L. *Purchasing Power in Health*. New Brunswick, NJ: Rutgers University Press; 1990.

Bergthold L. The fat kid on the seesaw: American business and health care cost containment, 1970–1990. *Annu Rev Public Health*. 1991;12:157–175.

Bodenheimer T. Coordinating care—a perilous journey through the health care system. *N Engl J Med*. 2008;358:1064–1071.

Bodenheimer T, et al. The primary care-specialty income gap: why it matters. *Ann Intern Med*. 2007;146:301–306.

Candisky C. Three CVS actions raise concerns for some pharmacies, consumers. *The Columbus Dispatch*. April 15, 2018.

Cantor JC, et al. Business leaders' views on American health care. *Health Aff (Millwood)*. 1991;10(1):98–105.

Casalino L, et al. Growth of single-specialty medical groups. *Health Aff (Millwood)*. 2004;23(2):82–90.

Claxton G, et al. Health benefits in 2010: premiums rise modestly, workers pay more toward coverage. *Health Aff (Millwood)*. 2010;29:1942–1950.

Davis MH, Burner ST. Three decades of Medicare: what the numbers tell us. *Health Aff (Millwood)*. 1995;14(4):231–243.

Gabel JR, et al. Trends in underinsurance and the affordability of employer coverage, 2004–2007. *Health Aff (Millwood)*. 2009;28:w595–w626.

Gagnon M-A, Volesky KD. Merger mania: mergers and acquisitions in the generic drug sector from 1995 to 2016. *Global Health*. 2017;13:62–68.

Gaynor M. Examining the Impact of Healthcare Consolidation. Statement before the Committee on Energy and Commerce Oversight and Investigations Subcommittee, U.S. House of Representatives. February 14, 2018. https://docs.house.gov/meetings/IF/IF02/20180214/106855/HHRG-115-IF02-Wstate-GaynorM-20180214.pdf. Accessed October 27, 2019

Iglehart JK. Doctor-workers of the world, unite! *Health Aff (Millwood)*. 2011;30:556–558.

Japson B. UnitedHealth: DaVita medical deal progressing on path to close. *Forbes*. April 17, 2019.

Johnson CY. Why CVS Health would want to buy Aetna. *Washington Post*. October 26, 2017.

Kamal R et al. What are the recent and forecasted trends in prescription drug spending? *Kaiser Family Foundation*. February 20, 2019. https://www.healthsystemtracker.org/chart-collection/recent-forecasted-trends-prescription-drug-spending/. Accessed October 27, 2019.

Kennedy P. *The Rise and Fall of the Great Powers*. New York, NY: Random House; 1987.

Khullar D, Chokshi DA. Health, income and poverty: where we are and what could help. *Health Affairs Policy Brief*. October 4, 2018.

Kutscher B. Why private equity firms are buying up primary care practices. *Concierge Medicine Today*. April 18, 2015.

Kuttner R. *Revolt of the Haves*. New York, NY: Simon & Schuster; 1980.

Law SA. *Blue Cross: What Went Wrong?* New Haven, CT: Yale University Press; 1974.

Liebhaber A, Grossman JM. Physicians moving to mid-sized, single-specialty practices. Tracking Report No. 18. Washington, DC: Center for Studying Health System Change; August 2007. www.hschange.org/CONTENT/941/index.html. Accessed October 27, 2019.

Livingston S. Cigna and Express Scripts close on $67 billion merger. *Modern Healthcare*. December 20, 2018.

Mehrotra A, et al. Do integrated medical groups provide higher-quality medical care than individual practice associations? *Ann Intern Med*. 2006;145:826–833.

Morris C. Why did CVS buy Aetna for $69 billion? *Fortune*. December 4, 2017.

Morse S. Secret weapon: UnitedHealth's Optum business is laying waste to old notions about how payers make money. *Healthcare Finance*. May 10, 2017.

Morse S. Anthem accelerates start for pharmacy benefit manager IngenioRx. *Healthcare Finance*. January 31, 2019.

Reinhardt UE. Reorganizing the financial flows in US health care. *Health Aff (Millwood)*. 1993;12(suppl):172–193.

Relman AS. *A Second Opinion. Rescuing America's Health Care*. New York, NY: Public Affairs; 2007.

Relman AS. The health reform we need and are not getting. *New York Rev Books*. 2009;56(11):38–40.

Royce TJ, et al. Pharmacy benefit manager reform: lessons from Ohio. *JAMA*. 2019. [epub ahead of print.]

Saez E. Striking it richer: the evolution of top incomes in the United States. *UC Berkeley*. 2019. https://eml.berkeley.edu/~saez/saez-UStopincomes-2017.pdf. Accessed October 27, 2019.

Scutti S. Big Pharma spends record millions on lobbying amid pressure to lower drug prices. *CNN*. January 24, 2019. https://www.cnn.com/2019/01/23/health/phrma-lobbying-costs-bn/index.html.

Schulman KA, et al. The relationship between pharmacy benefit managers (PBMs) and the cost of therapies in the US pharmaceutical market. *Am Heart J*. 2018;206:113–122.

Schwartz LM, Woloshin S. Medical marketing in the United States, 1997–2016. *JAMA*. 2019;321:80-96.

Starr P. *The Social Transformation of American Medicine.* New York, NY: Basic Books; 1982.

Sunshine J, Bhargavan M. The practice of imaging self-referral doesn't produce much one-stop service. *Health Aff (Millwood)*. 2010;29:2237–2243.

Tribble SJ. Drugmakers play the patent game to lock in prices, block competitors. *Kaiser Health News.* October 2, 2018.

US Government Accountability Office. Drug Industry Profits, Research and Development Spending, and Merger and Acquisition Deals. November 2017. https://www.gao.gov/products/GAO-18-40. Accessed October 27, 2019.

Wapner J. Medication keeps getting more expensive—and Big Pharma won't explain why. *Newsweek*. May 30, 2019.

Conclusion: Tensions and Challenges

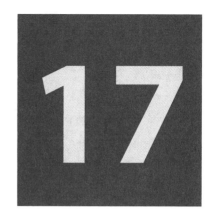

The perfect health care system is like perfect health—a noble aspiration but one that is impossible to attain. In the preceding chapters, we have discussed many fundamental issues and principles involved in formulating health care policy. A recurrent theme has been the notion that "magic bullets" are hard to come by. As stated in Chapter 2, policies tend to evolve in a cyclic process of finding solutions that create new problems that require new solutions. Policy changes may offer a degree of relief for a pressing problem, such as inadequate access to care, but frequently also give rise to various side effects, such as stimulating health care cost inflation.

All health care systems face the same challenges: improving health, controlling costs, prioritizing allocation of resources, enhancing the quality of care, and distributing services fairly. These challenges require the management of various tensions that pull at the health care system (O'Neil & Seifer, 1995). The goal of health policy is to find the points of equilibrium that produce the optimal system of health care (Table 17–1).

Dr. Madeleine Longview is chief resident in critical care medicine and supervises the intensive care unit of a large municipal hospital. It's 5:30 AM, and the intensive care unit team has finally stabilized the condition of a 15-year-old admitted the previous evening with gunshot wounds to the abdomen and chest. Dr. Longview sits by the nursing desk and surveys the other patients in the unit: a 91-year-old woman admitted from a nursing home with sepsis from a urinary tract infection, a
50-year-old man with shock lung caused by drugs ingested in a suicide attempt, and a 32-year-old woman with lupus erythematosus who is rejecting her second kidney transplant. Dr. Longview feels personally responsible for the care of every one of these patients. She tells herself that she will do her best to help each of them survive.

As Dr. Longview gazes out of the windows of the intensive care unit, the apartment houses surrounding the hospital take shape in the breaking dawn. She wonders: Which block will be the scene of the next drive-by shooting or episode of spouse abuse? Which window shade hides a homebound elder lying on the floor dehydrated and unable to move, waiting for someone to find him and bring him to the emergency department? Which one of the unvaccinated kids in the neighborhood will one day be rushed into the unit limp with meningitis? In which room is someone lighting up the first cigarette of the day? Dr. Longview somehow feels responsible for all those patients-to-be, as well as for the patients lying in the hospital beds around her. After these sleepless nights on duty, the doubts about the value of all the work she does in the intensive care unit creep into her thoughts. She has visions of shutting down the unit and putting all the money to work hiring public health nurses in the community, or maybe just paying for a better grammar school in the neighborhood. But then what would happen to the patients needing her care right now?

Table 17–1. Major tensions in health care

Health of the individual patient	Health of the population
Tertiary care	Primary care
Acute care	Chronic and preventive care
Cost unawareness in medical practice	Cost awareness
Unlimited expectations for care	Affordability of care
Individual physician	Organized health care team
Professional management	Corporate management
Market competition	Government regulation
Inequity in distribution	Fair distribution

Source: Data from O'Neil E, Seifer S. Health care reform and medical education: forces towards generalism. *Acad Med.* 1995;70(1 suppl):S37–S43.

One of the most basic tensions affecting physicians and other caregivers is the tension between caring for the individual patient and caring for the larger community or population. Many of the most important decisions to be made in health policy—decisions such as allocating health care resources, addressing the social context of health and illness, and augmenting activities in prevention and public health—depend on broadening the practitioner's view to encompass the population health perspective. The challenge for physicians and other clinicians will be to make room for this broader perspective while preserving the ethical duty to care for the individual patients under their charge.

Like Dr. Longview, the health care system as a whole will continue to struggle over finding the proper balance between the provision of acute care services and preventive and chronic care services, as well as striking the right balance between the levels of tertiary and primary care. Few observers would encourage Dr. Longview to succumb to her despair, close all the intensive care units, and expel all the critical care subspecialists from the health care system. Yet most would agree that health care in the United States has drifted too far away from the primary care end of the tertiary care–primary care axis.

Dr. Tom Ransom has performed what he believes to be a reasonably thorough workup for Zed's abdominal pain and decreased appetite, including

a detailed history and physical examination, blood tests, and abdominal ultrasound—all of which were normal. When Dr. Ransom tells Zed that they will have to work together to manage Zed's symptoms, Zed tells Dr. Ransom that he wants one more test, an abdominal CT scan. Zed says that he had a cousin with similar symptoms who was eventually diagnosed with advanced-stage lymphoma after complaining of pain for over a year.

Dr. Ransom is in a quandary. He believes it extremely unlikely that Zed has serious pathologic changes in his abdomen that will be detected on CT scan. He could order the scan, but then there's the issue of the cost. He can't recall whether Zed is covered by a fee-for-service plan or by one of the health maintenance organization (HMO) plans that pay on a capitated basis and puts Dr. Ransom at financial risk for all radiologic tests ordered. He starts to ask Zed about his coverage but feels a pang of guilt that he should allow these economic considerations to intrude into his clinical judgment.

The desire (and in many instances, expectation) of patients to receive all potentially beneficial care, and the unwillingness of these same individuals in their role as purchasers to spend unlimited amounts to finance health care, creates a strain for all caregivers and systems of care. Physicians increasingly are being called upon to incorporate considerations of costs when making clinical decisions. Debate will continue about the best ways to encourage physicians to be more accountable for the costs of care in a manner that is socially responsible and does not unduly intrude on the physician's ability to serve the individual patient. Is it necessary to use payment methods that place physicians at financial risk for their treatment decisions in order to control costs? Are more global methods available to induce physicians and other caregivers to practice in a more cost-conscious manner? If Zed does not get a CT scan, does that constitute painless or painful cost control?

On the eve of his retirement, Dr. Melvin Steadman reminisces with his son, Dr. Kevin Steadman. The elder Dr. Steadman has practiced as a solo pediatrician for more than 40 years in the same town.

The only boss he has known in his professional life has been himself. He has served as president of the local medical society, helped spearhead efforts to build a special children's wing of the local hospital, and antagonized several of his colleagues when he pushed for a change in hospital policy that required physicians to attend extra continuing medical education courses in order to maintain their hospital privileges. Mel swore that he'd never retire; but he also swore that he'd never let the insurance companies "tell me how to practice medicine." He has refused to sign any managed care contracts. Facing a dwindling supply of patients, Mel has decided to call it quits.

His son Kevin is also a pediatrician, working as a staff physician for a large for-profit multispecialty group that recently opened up an office in town. Kevin remembers the many nights when his father didn't get home from work until after he had gone to bed. Kevin's work hours are more regular at the group practice, and he is on call for only one weekend every 2 months. He considers his father's approach to medicine old-fashioned in many ways—excessively paternalistic toward patients and irrationally scornful of the pediatric nurse practitioners who work with Kevin. He does, however, envy his father's professional independence. Just this week, the group practice notified Kevin that he would have to divide his time between his current office and a new site that would soon open in a suburban mall. His schedule will be limited to 10-minute drop-in appointments at the new site, rather than the style of practice that promotes a sense of continuity, one that allows him to get to know his patients over time.

A system of health care formerly managed according to a professional model by independent practitioners is being pulled toward a corporate model of care featuring large organizations managed by executives and administrators. As the role of corporate entities expands, traditional responsibilities toward patients and local communities are vying with new obligations to shareholders. Power relationships are changing, with health care conglomerates challenging the dominance of the medical profession. A shift toward multidisciplinary group practice may provide more opportunity for health care professionals to work collegially and implement new approaches to quality improvement to elevate the competence of all health care providers. At the same time, a competitive, for-profit health care environment may induce physicians to compromise their humanity and base their clinical decisions in part on personal monetary considerations.

Aurora can't wait any longer in the crowded county hospital emergency department. She's already been there for 6 hours, and the physician hasn't seen her yet. Her lower abdomen still hurts, but she figures she'll just have to put up with it for a few more days. She really doesn't have much choice. Poor, uninsured, and without legal documents, where else could she go? Aurora has two young children at home who need to be put to bed. In half an hour, their father has to get to his night job as a security officer. As she enters her apartment, she collapses, the pregnancy in her fallopian tube having ruptured, producing internal hemorrhage. Her husband frantically dials 911, praying that his wife won't die.

Over the years, no tension within the US health care system has been as far from reaching a point of satisfactory equilibrium as the achievement of a basic level of fairness in the distribution of health care services and the burden of paying for those services. The Affordable Care Act has taken a step toward resolving that tension. But because financial barriers remain for millions of people, both insured and uninsured, not all patients benefit from early detection of potentially curable cancers, patients with chronic diseases are hospitalized because of lack of timely primary care, hypertensive patients forego the medications that might avert strokes and kidney failure, and babies are born prematurely and spend their first weeks of life in a neonatal intensive care unit. The poor continue to pay a greater proportion of their income for health care than do more affluent families.

People providing and receiving care in the United States must work together to achieve a brighter future for the nation's health care system. Changing the future will require that people look beyond their immediate self-interest to view the common good of a health care system that is accessible, affordable, and of high quality for all. A heightened level of public discourse will be needed, with a populace that is better informed and more actively engaged in shaping the future of their health care system. Concepts in health policy based on established facts rather than ideologically driven myths will need to be discussed and debated in a manner that connects with the daily realities experienced by patients and caregivers. The attitudes and actions of physicians and other health care professionals will play a major role in determining the future of health care in the United States. With leadership and foresight among the community of health care professionals, our nation may yet achieve a system that allows the most honorable features of the healing professions to flourish.

REFERENCE

O'Neil E, Seifer S. Health care reform and medical education: forces towards generalism. *Acad Med*. 1995;70:S37.

Questions and Discussion Topics

CHAPTER 2: PAYING FOR HEALTH CARE

1. What are the four modes of financing health care? Describe each.

2. Describe regressive, proportional, and progressive financing. Explain how each of the following is regressive, proportional, or progressive: out-of-pocket payments, experience-rated individual private insurance, community-rated individual private insurance, health insurance purchased 100% by the employer (assuming that employees actually pay for health insurance as explained in the text), and the federal income tax.

3. Harvey, who has worked all his life for General Electric, reaches 65 years of age. He does not retire. Is he eligible for Medicare Part A? Part B? Six months later, his wife, who has never worked, reaches 65 years of age. Is she eligible for Medicare Part A? Part B? How are Parts A and B paid for?

4. Hubert has received social security disability for 24 months because he has AIDS. Is he eligible for Medicare?

5. Rena developed chronic renal failure and started renal dialysis 2 weeks ago. She feels fine and is working. Is she eligible for Medicare?

6. Heidi, aged 72 years, on Medicare Part A and B without Medicaid or a Medigap policy, is hospitalized for a stroke complicated by a deep vein thrombosis of the leg and a pulmonary embolus. She is in the acute hospital for 70 days and cared for by a family practitioner and a neurologist. She improves somewhat and is then transferred to the skilled nursing facility (SNF) for rehabilitation. She remains in the SNF for 30 days and is still severely disabled and unable to go home. She is sent to a nursing home for custodial care, where she stays for 3 months. Surprisingly, she improves and goes home, where she receives skilled physical therapy services from a home care agency and also has a homemaker come in for 4 hours a day to buy food, cook, and clean the house. She is on three prescription medications at home. What does Heidi pay and what does Medicare pay? Acute hospital? SNF? Nursing home? Home care? Physicians? Prescriptions while in hospital? Prescriptions while at home?

▶ Discussion Topics

1. Discuss your experiences with health insurance that was provided through a job. How did you obtain the insurance? Did you pay part of the premium? Were there deductibles or copayments? How many choices of plans did you have? What happened if you left your job?

2. Divide into two groups: one insurance company selling community-rated health insurance policies and the other selling experience-rated policies. Each side should try to convince the instructor to buy its policy, first with the instructor as a young, healthy person, and then with the instructor as an older person with diabetes. Which policy is the young person more likely to choose, and which the older person?

CHAPTER 3: ACCESS TO HEALTH CARE

1. What are the main features of the ACA that expand health insurance coverage?
2. Compare access to health care for people with private insurance, for Medicaid recipients, and for people without insurance. Give examples.
3. Compare health outcomes for people with private insurance, for Medicaid recipients, and for people without insurance. Give examples.

▶ Discussion Topics

1. What are some explanations as to why Ace Banks was healthy at age 48 while Bill Downes died at that age?
2. Discuss possible reasons why minority patients have poorer outcomes than white patients for many diseases.
3. What is the relationship between socioeconomic status (including factors such as income, education, and occupation) and health? Why does such a relationship exist?
4. What would be the best strategies to improve the health status of African-Americans in the United States?

CHAPTER 4: PAYING HEALTH CARE PROVIDERS

1. Explain each mode of physician payment: fee-for-service, episode-of-illness, capitation, and salary. Explain each mode of hospital payment: fee-for-service, per diem, episode-of-illness (diagnosis-related group [DRG]), and global budget.
2. How does capitation payment free insurers of risk? How does capitation payment shift risk to providers of care?
3. What are the arguments for risk-adjusting capitation payments?

▶ Discussion Topics

1. You are a primary care physician (PCP) caring for a young woman with new onset of severe headaches and amenorrhea and a normal physical examination. What are the financial incentives and disincentives that would lead you to order or not to order a magnetic resonance imaging (MRI) scan in a case in which the need for the MRI was equivocal?

(a) under traditional fee-for-service practice;
(b) under fee-for-service practice with utilization review;
(c) under an independent practice association (IPA)-model health maintenance organization (HMO) in which you receive a capitation payment that places you at risk for laboratory and x-ray studies and specialty referrals; and
(d) under a staff model HMO that has a two-month waiting list for elective MRI scans?

In the case of the staff model HMO, what would you do if you felt you needed to obtain the MRI within 48 hours?

2. You are a hospital administrator and your hospital is in financial difficulty. You are about to address the medical staff, imploring them to help the hospital financially. In the old days, all you had to say was, in effect: "Admit as many patients as possible and keep them in the hospital as long as you can," but times have changed. For some methods of payment, you want physicians to admit more patients; for others, you don't. For some methods, you want patients to stay long, for others, you don't. What do you tell the medical staff regarding the following:
(a) Medicare (DRG) patients;
(b) Medicaid (per diem) patients;
(c) HMO (per diem) patients; and
(d) HMO (capitated) patients.

For each of these categories of patients, does it help or hurt the hospital for physicians to
(a) admit more patients;
(b) keep them in the hospital more days; and
(c) order more diagnostic studies?

CHAPTER 5: HOW HEALTH CARE IS ORGANIZED—I: PRIMARY, SECONDARY, AND TERTIARY CARE

▶ Discussion Topics

1. You are 63 years old and you begin to experience chest pain when walking. You do not have a physician. A friend suggests that you need a coronary artery bypass and recommends a cardiac surgeon at the medical school. What do you do
(a) under a dispersed model of health care delivery?
(b) under a regionalized model?

2. Give some examples of the statement, "Common disorders commonly occur and rare ones rarely happen." What are the implications of this statement for the ratio of generalist to specialist physicians in the United States?

3. In Great Britain and Canada, about 50% of physicians are generalists. In the United States, approximately one-third of physicians are generalists (general and family practitioners, general internists, and general pediatricians). Assume you are Chair of the Health Subcommittee of the US House of Representatives Ways and Means Committee. What legislation might you propose to increase the proportion of generalist physicians?

4. Discuss the pros and cons of requiring everyone to enter the health care system through a "gatekeeper" health care provider (generalist physician, nurse practitioner, or physician assistant).

5. What are some advantages of a primary care–based health system?

CHAPTER 6: HOW HEALTH CARE IS ORGANIZED—II: HEALTH DELIVERY SYSTEMS

1. What is vertical integration? What is virtual integration?

2. What is an ACO?

3. What is a medical home and a medical neighborhood? Is a medical neighborhood the same as an ACO?

CHAPTER 7: THE HEALTH CARE WORKFORCE AND THE EDUCATION OF HEALTH PROFESSIONALS

Describe past and future trends in the physician, nursing, and pharmacist workforce.

CHAPTER 8: PAINFUL VERSUS PAINLESS COST CONTROL

1. Give examples of medical interventions that lie on the steeper portions of the cost–benefit curve, and interventions that lie on the flatter portions.

2. Give examples of painless cost control. Are these painless for everyone?

▶ Discussion Topics

1. CABGville has four cardiac surgery units; one unit performs 300 coronary artery bypass graft (CABG) surgeries each year, and the other units perform an average of 40 per year. Cardiac surgeons can schedule a CABG anytime they wish. The small units have an operative mortality of 7% compared with 4% for the large unit. To control costs, the health planning council of CABGville closes the three less productive cardiac surgery units. Elective CABG surgeries now have a 1-month waiting list, and because of tight scheduling, surgeons are less likely to operate; the number of CABGs goes down from 420 to 340 per year; both the overall costs of CABG surgery and the unit cost per CABG operation drop, as does the mortality rate. Did CABGville achieve painful or painless cost control?

2. Pretend that total US health care expenditures have been capped and are controlled by a health services commission. Because of tight budgetary constraints, the commission must decide whether to fund an all-out program of mammography or to limit mammography and finance in its place high-cost chemotherapy regimens for patients with metastatic breast cancer, treatments whose effectiveness has not been proven, but which might help certain subgroups of women. Under the first option, several thousand cases of early-stage breast cancer could be treated with curative surgery each year, but women currently suffering from advanced-stage breast cancer would receive no benefit. Which is the more painful cost-control option from the point of view of women without breast cancer? From the perspective of women with metastatic breast cancer? From the perspective of society as a whole? Which of these two groups of women should have priority in this decision?

CHAPTER 9: MECHANISMS FOR CONTROLLING COSTS

▶ Discussion Topics

1. You are chair of the health planning council of CABGville, a town that continues to have a health care cost crisis. The town has 30 physicians, each seeing 30 patients a day at a cost of $30 per visit.

Total daily cost is $30 \times 30 \times 30 = \$27,000$. What methods are available to reduce the total cost of physician services? Would it work to reduce the fee per visit from \$30 to \$20? If an expenditure cap strategy (tying fees to volume) were used, how would it work?

2. The CABGville health planning council changes the mode of physician payment from fee-for-service to capitation: \$20 per patient per month to PCPs, with 20 PCPs each having 2,000 patients. (PCPs pay specialists from the \$20 capitation.) Total cost per month = \$800,000 (approximately \$27,000 per day). How could the health planning council reduce the monthly cost? Could physician costs still increase despite this method of cost control? Why or why not?

3. What are the arguments, pros and cons, of patient cost sharing as a cost-control strategy?

4. You are the President of the United States, and your first term ends in a year. The cost-control mechanism you instituted 2 years ago, based on patient cost sharing and managed competition, has not worked, and the American people are upset about persistent health care inflation. You are preparing for a major television address on health care costs. What will you propose? Can you convince the public that yours is a painless cost-control strategy?

CHAPTER 10: QUALITY OF HEALTH CARE

▶ Discussion Topics

1. Have you ever experienced or witnessed a medical care encounter of poor quality? What did you do about it? What should you have done?

2. In the vignette about Shelley Rush, who do you think was responsible for the error in giving insulin to the wrong patient?

3. In the vignette about Nina Brown, had the physician been working in a fee-for-service environment rather than a cost-conscious HMO, do you think he or she would have admitted Ms. Brown to the hospital?

4. Reread the example of the 23-year-old graduate student whose x-ray report was lost. If you were the administrator of the hospital, what would you do

to prevent such an error from taking place again? If you were the office manager of the internist's office that never received the x-ray report, what would you do to avoid a recurrence of this problem?

5. What is wrong with the malpractice system? What would you do to fix it?

CHAPTER 11: PREVENTION OF ILLNESS

1. Why did tuberculosis (TB) decline prior to the identification of the TB bacillus? Why did polio morbidity and mortality decline? Why did Hodgkin's disease mortality fall in the late 20th century?

2. What are the first and the second epidemiologic revolutions?

▶ Discussion Topics

1. Two people are campaigning for the consumer board of their group practice. The incumbent is running on a platform of charging tobacco users higher premiums than nonusers, because their use of tobacco costs the group practice more money. The opponent believes that society rather than the individual is responsible for tobacco addiction and that the group practice should become involved in social action against cigarette smoking. Conduct a debate between these two views.

2. What are the medical vs. public health models of prevention? Which is the better model for lowering cholesterol levels to reduce heart attacks?

3. You are named as head of the breast cancer prevention section of the US Centers for Disease Control and Prevention. What primary and secondary prevention programs would you favor to reduce the incidence of and mortality from breast cancer?

CHAPTER 12: LONG-TERM CARE

1. What are activities of daily living and instrumental activities of daily living?

2. What are the two largest funders of long-term care?

3. Which long-term care services are covered by Medicare and which are not?

Discussion Topics

1. You are president of LTC Insurance Company and are testifying before a Senate Committee on long-term care. You are asked two questions: Why do only a few million people carry private long-term care insurance? How do you answer the complaints that senior citizen advocacy groups make about the terms of private long-term care insurance policies? What do you say to the committee?

2. Your mother's Alzheimer's disease is getting worse; she wanders around the neighborhood, sometimes unable to find her way home; she sleeps during the day and stays up most of the night; and she has become incontinent. Your father died 2 years ago. You and your spouse both work, you have three school-aged children, and you have an extra room in your home. The hospital social worker calls and says that your mother needs 24-hour-a-day help. Your choices are:

   (a) hiring a homemaker to live with your mother at $16,000 per year;

   (b) placing your mother in a nursing home whose bill will be paid by Medicaid; and

   (c) taking your mother home with you. What do you decide?

   What reforms in the United States long-term care system might have benefited you in this situation? How should such reforms be financed?

CHAPTER 13: MEDICAL ETHICS AND RATIONING OF HEALTH CARE

Discussion Topics

1. Pretend that the Lakeberg family discussed in this chapter belongs to a vertically integrated, globally budgeted health system like Kaiser and, that you are the system's medical director. The Lakeberg parents want surgery to separate the Siamese twins at the cost of $1 million. The list of benefits covered in the Lakebergs' insurance policy neither affirms nor denies their right to the surgery, so the responsibility to approve or deny the surgery falls on you. What do you decide? If you approve the surgery, who will end up paying for it? Is an ethical dilemma involved or not?

2. You are Dr. Marco Intensivo, as described in the vignette in the section "What is Rationing?" What do you do?

3. In the case of Mr. Elder and Mr. Younger described in the organ transplant section, which patient should receive the donor heart?

4. You are the PCP for Rodolfo, a 58-year-old man who suffered a cerebral hemorrhage and has been in a persistent vegetative state for 18 months. He lives in a nursing home, requires tube feedings and round-the-clock nursing attention, and his care is paid for by Medicaid. He never discussed his health wishes with anyone. Rodolfo's daughter is a nurse in the intensive care unit of your hospital. Rodolfo's wife is deeply religious and has faith that Rodolfo will get better.

   Every 6 weeks, Rodolfo develops a urinary tract infection with septicemia and must be admitted to the hospital—often to the ICU—for treatment. Over the course of 2 years, Rodolfo's care has cost $460,000. The hospital ethics committee discussed the case and recommended that tube feedings be withdrawn, or that the next episode of septicemia not be treated, thereby allowing Rodolfo to die. When you discussed the ethics committee recommendations with the family, the daughter agreed but the wife demanded that everything possible be done to continue Rodolfo's life. As Rodolfo's physician, what do you do? Which ethical dilemmas are involved? Autonomy versus beneficence? Autonomy versus nonmaleficence? Autonomy versus distributive justice? Beneficence versus distributive justice? If Rodolfo's care were withdrawn, what would happen to the money saved?

5. Evidence from public opinion polls suggests that people in the United States want the right to health care but don't want to pay for it.

   At midnight, a new mother awakens to hear her 2-week-old infant scream. The mother and baby are Medicaid recipients. If she were experienced, the mother would know that the scream is normal, but she is frightened. She phones the emergency department and asks to bring the baby in to be seen. No amount of telephone advice seems to reassure her. Does the right to health care include society paying for her visit to the emergency department? Who is actually paying? Should the mother be advised to come into the emergency department if she is uninsured and wealthy? Uninsured and poor?

6. Should physicians be responsible to serve one master—their patient—or two masters—their patient and the broader needs of society? In your discussion, draw from the examples of the Lakebergs, Dr. Intensivo, and Rodolfo. How has the distribution system for organ transplantation tried to balance these two masters?

CHAPTER 14: HEALTH CARE IN FOUR NATIONS

1. You are a secretary in a large company in Germany (Canada, United Kingdom, or Japan). How is your health care paid for? You become sick and are forced to retire from your job. How is your health care paid for in Germany (Canada, United Kingdom, or Japan)?

2. If you developed a urinary tract infection, what would you do in Germany (Canada, United Kingdom, or Japan)? What if you needed cataract surgery? What if you had a sudden abdominal pain in the middle of the night? What if you developed leukemia and needed a bone marrow transplant? In each of these cases, which physician would care for you and where would you be cared for?

3. You are a general practitioner in Germany (Canada, United Kingdom, or Japan). How are you paid? You are a specialist in Germany (Canada, United Kingdom, or Japan). How are you paid? You are a hospital administrator in Germany (Canada, UK, or Japan). How is your hospital paid?

CHAPTER 15: HEALTH CARE REFORM AND NATIONAL HEALTH INSURANCE

1. Describe how a government-financed national health insurance plan, an employer mandate plan, and an individual mandate plan would work.

2. What is the difference between a social insurance and a public assistance approach to government-financed national health insurance? Use Medicare and Medicaid as examples.

3. What are the main features of the 2010 Affordable Care Act (ACA)?

▶ **Discussion Topics**

1. You are the speech writer for two candidates for the Democratic presidential nomination. One candidate favors a mixed employer and individual mandate and the other a single-payer approach. What points would you have each candidate make about the strengths of his or her position and the weaknesses of the other candidate's position?

2. Why do you think that there has been such a polarized debate over the ACA?

CHAPTER 16: CONFLICT AND CHANGE IN AMERICA'S HEALTH CARE SYSTEM

1. Describe how the payers of health care services increased their power between 1945 and 1995.

2. Describe changes in the relationships between physicians and insurance companies between 1945 and 1995.

3. Describe the 1995 to 2000 backlash against managed care.

4. Give examples of the recent merging of the purchaser, insurer, provider, and supplier actors in the health care system.

▶ **Discussion Topics**

1. Discuss potential conflicts between the profit motive and the principles of beneficence and nonmaleficence in the following situations:
   (a) a private surgeon receiving fee-for-service reimbursement;
   (b) a primary physician in a small group practice that receives capitation payments covering primary care, laboratory, x-ray, and specialty referrals;
   (c) a physician who is the utilization manager of a large for-profit HMO receiving requests from her employed physicians to authorize expensive MRI scans for their patients;
   (d) the administrator of a nonprofit hospital who has calculated that a new cardiac surgery unit will be profitable even if only one surgery is performed each week;

(e) the CEO of a group practice deciding whether to accept Medicaid patients, for whom the state government pays 30% less than payments for private patients.

(f) What changes in the organization of health care could be made that would minimize such conflicts?

2. Discuss how health care is organized in your community—who are the payers, insurers, and providers? To what degree has your local health care system moved from a dispersed set of institutions to a small number of horizontally, vertically, or virtually integrated health care conglomerates?

3. Where in the health care system of the 21st century would you like to be—as a provider and as a patient? What are your fears and hopes for the future?

Index

Page numbers followed by f refer to figures; page numbers followed by t refer to tables.